Kidney Biomarkers: Clinical Aspects

Kidney Biomarkers: Clinical Aspects

Editor: Kristina Camarillo

MURPHY & MOORE
www.murphy-moorepublishing.com

www.murphy-moorepublishing.com

MURPHY & MOORE

Cataloging-in-Publication Data

Kidney biomarkers : clinical aspects / edited by Kristina Camarillo.
p. cm.
Includes bibliographical references and index.
ISBN 978-1-63987-791-1
1. Kidneys--Diseases--Molecular diagnosis. 2. Kidneys--Diseases--Treatment.
3. Biochemical markers. I. Camarillo, Kristina.
RC904 .K53 2023
616.61--dc23

Murphy & Moore Publishing
1 Rockefeller Plaza,
New York City,
NY 10020, USA

ISBN 978-1-63987-791-1

Contents

Preface

Renal diseases or kidney diseases are a set of chronic diseases or conditions that affect the functioning of the kidneys. They are classified into two major categories, namely, inflammatory kidney diseases (nephritis) or non-inflammatory kidney diseases (nephrosis). A biomarker or biologic marker is a measurable indicator of a specific biological state, particularly one relevant to the risk for, presence of, or stage of a disease. Biomarkers of renal diseases are used to screen and diagnose the activity of renal diseases, and guide molecularly targeted therapy or therapeutic response. The most accurate and promising biomarkers for detecting chronic kidney disease (CKD) are neutrophil gelatinase-associated lipocalin (NGAL), cystatin C and FGF-23. The risk stratification for the progression and mortality of kidney diseases can be improved by using ratio calculated by glomerular filtration rate (eGFR) and albuminuria (UACR). This book describes the most important biomarkers researched and studied in the context of renal diseases. Those in search of information to further their knowledge will be greatly assisted by it.

This book is a result of research of several months to collate the most relevant data in the field.

When I was approached with the idea of this book and the proposal to edit it, I was overwhelmed. It gave me an opportunity to reach out to all those who share a common interest with me in this field. I had 3 main parameters for editing this text:

1. Accuracy - The data and information provided in this book should be up-to-date and valuable to the readers.

2. Structure - The data must be presented in a structured format for easy understanding and better grasping of the readers.

3. Universal Approach - This book not only targets students but also experts and innovators in the field, thus my aim was to present topics which are of use to all.

Thus, it took me a couple of months to finish the editing of this book.

I would like to make a special mention of my publisher who considered me worthy of this opportunity and also supported me throughout the editing process. I would also like to thank the editing team at the back-end who extended their help whenever required.

Editor

1

Urinary Extracellular Vesicles as Biomarkers of Kidney Disease: From Diagnostics to Therapeutics

In O. Sun [1,2] and Lilach O. Lerman [1,*]

1 Division of Nephrology and Hypertension, Mayo Clinic, Rochester, MN 55905, USA; inogood77@gmail.com
2 Division of Nephrology, Department of Internal Medicine, Presbyterian Medical Center, Jeonju 54987, Korea
* Correspondence: Lerman.Lilach@Mayo.Edu.

Abstract: Cell-derived extracellular vesicles (EVs) can be isolated from various body fluids, including urine. Urinary EVs have gained important recognition as potential diagnostic biomarkers in renal disease since their cargo includes nucleic acids, proteins, and other cellular components, which likely mirror the physiological and possibly pathophysiological state of cells along the nephron. Accumulating evidence highlights the feasibility of using EVs as biomarkers for diagnostic, prognostic, and therapeutic purposes in several forms of renal disease, such as acute kidney injury, glomerulonephritis, and renal transplantation. Additionally, exogenous delivery of EVs released in vitro by cells in culture may have salutary benefits for renal diseases. In this review, we introduce recent studies that attempt to identify urinary EVs as candidate biomarkers for human kidney diseases and consider their potential implication as a therapeutic option in key kidney diseases.

Keywords: urine; exosomes; biomarkers; kidney diseases

---

1. Introduction

Extracellular vesicles (EVs) are membrane-bound nanosized structures generated and released into the extracellular fluid by cells under stressful conditions. They serve the role of intercellular communication and transfer their cargo to alter the phenotype of the recipient cells [1]. EVs contain various molecules, including proteins, lipids, DNA, mRNA, and microRNA (miRNA), and are characterized by the common proteins that they carry, including tumor susceptibility gene-101, tetraspanins (CD9, CD63), heat shock proteins, annexins, and apoptosis-linked gene-2-interacting protein-X. Additionally, EVs can also display surface markers from their cell of origin, such as aquaporin-2 in the collecting duct, sodium/hydrogen exchanger-1 in the proximal tubule, and podocalyxin in podocytes. The main types of EVs are exosomes, microparticles, and apoptotic bodies, which are distinguishable by their cellular origin, size, and cargo [2,3].

EVs have been detected in blood and urine, as well as in other body fluids. Urine is a highly useful specimen for biomarker discovery that is used to diagnose and monitor kidney diseases because it can be collected repeatedly using non-invasive techniques. Proteomic analysis has shown that the majority of urinary EV cargo represents glomerular, tubular, prostate, and bladder cells, whereas circulating EVs presumably cannot cross the filtration barrier, at least under physiological conditions, supporting the notion that urinary EVs derive primarily from cells in the genitourinary tract facing the urinary space [4]. Therefore, analysis of urinary EVs may serve as a logical and novel diagnostic approach in kidney disease since changes in the number or characteristics of released EVs may be linked to the development of disease or response to therapy.

2. Urinary EV Isolation

The isolation of urinary EVs needs to take into account several practical considerations. For studies using urine EVs, it is important to maintain optimal storage conditions of urine samples to prevent proteolysis. Storage at −80 °C, rather than 4 °C or −20 °C, is preferable to prevent degradation, although the use of freshly processed urine is most optimal. Urine can be collected as a spot or timed sample, and the process of EV isolation begins with a low speed and/or a low centrifugal force (3000× *g*) centrifugation step for a short time (< 10 min) and at a low temperature (4 °C) [5]. Then, urine is carried forward through to the urinary EV isolation step. Several methods for isolating EVs have been described and frequently used. Traditionally, EVs are isolated and purified using differential centrifugation and ultracentrifugation. However, ultracentrifugation is not only labor-intensive and time-consuming but also requires expensive laboratory equipment, making it impractical for high throughput clinical applications. Ultrafiltration represents a faster and simpler method of isolating urinary EVs and usually involves the use of a polyethersulfone nanomembrane filter [5]. However, this method is inefficient in patients with nephrotic syndrome because of protein adherence to the nanomembrane and high protein retention. Precipitation followed by centrifugation has also been explored for rapid exosome isolation. Several commercial precipitation reagents have been introduced over the last few years. Kits such as ExoQuick-TC™ and Total EX isolation reagent from Invitrogen™ are based on aggregating agents followed by low-speed centrifugation [6]. Isolation of urinary EVs using a commercial kit is quicker than other methods because it does not require ultracentrifugation, yet may be more costly. The amounts of EVs collected may also vary between isolation methods and has been reported to be around (2–4) × 10^8 particles/mL of urine [7].

3. Urinary EVs as Diagnostic Biomarkers for Kidney Diseases

3.1. Acute Kidney Injury

Most cell types in the kidney produce and secrete EVs. Proteomic analysis of urinary EVs has confirmed that proteins within them may arise from all nephron segments, including podocytes, proximal tubules, the thick ascending limb of Henle's Loop, the distal tubule, and the collecting duct. Therefore, exosomal proteins may be leveraged as biomarkers for location-specific diseases [4]. The exosomal content may vary in response to various pathophysiological conditions such that exosomal proteins may be biomarkers for specific diseases. For example, the aquaporin-1 (AQP1) protein level in urinary exosomes has been identified as a potential biomarker for acute kidney injury (AKI). During renal ischemia/reperfusion in rats, urinary exosomal AQP1 decreased significantly [8]. Similarly, the Na^+/H^+ exchange type-3 and fetuin-A levels in urinary exosomes have been identified as potential biomarkers for AKI. Increased levels of Na^+/H^+ exchange type-3 in urinary exosomes were observed in acute tubular necrosis but not in prerenal azotemia or other causes of AKI, which may help differentiate those causes of AKI [9]. In a rat model of cisplantin-induced AKI, a marked increase in urine exosome fetuin-A was detected not only before an elevation in serum creatinine levels but also before any evidence of morphological injury. Zhou et al. suggested the diagnostic utility of this biomarker in a limited number of intensive care unit patients with AKI [10]. Additionally, urinary levels of the exosomal transcription factor ATF3 increased in AKI patients before the elevation of serum creatinine, indicating that ATF3 may be useful as a biomarker for the early diagnosis of AKI [11]. Subsequently, urine ATF3 was also shown to be a biomarker for sepsis-induced AKI [12]. Therefore, elevated urinary levels of a specific exosome might provide an early index of etiology-specific AKI.

3.2. Glomerular Disease

Urinary biomarkers may mitigate the need for an invasive kidney biopsy in glomerular disease. Podocytes, which are specialized epithelial cells forming the glomerular filtration barrier with the glomerular basement membrane, are the main cell-types affected in glomerular disease. Thus, podocyte-derived EVs may be a promising index of glomerular injury. In focal segmental glomerulosclerosis (FSGS), a disease with significant podocyte damage, Wilm's tumor-1 (WT-1), a transcriptional factor required for normal kidney development, was examined in urinary exosomes as a marker for podocyte damage. Increased expression of WT-1 in urinary exosomes preceded urinary albumin excretion by one week in a mouse model of collapsing glomerulopathy [13]. Additionally, in human subjects with FSGS, exosomal WT-1 levels were significantly higher in children with active nephrotic syndrome caused by FSGS compared with healthy controls or patients with steroid-sensitive nephrotic syndrome (SSNS). Furthermore, a significant fall in urinary exosomal WT-1 was also shown in patients in remission of SSNS following steroid treatment [13]. WT-1 expression in urinary EVs was also found to be elevated in patients with diabetes, in which podocyte injury is an early feature. Kalani et al. identified WT-1 in urinary exosomes of diabetic patients, which correlated with declining renal function, highlighting exosomal WT-1 as a biomarker of podocyte injury in diabetic nephropathy [14]. Notably, we recently identified elevated numbers of podocyte-derived exosomes in obese compared with lean human subjects and pigs [15], which might represent early markers of kidney disease.

Urinary EVs may also help to differentiate early IgA nephropathy from thin basement membrane nephropathy. Moon et al. used proteomic analysis to compare levels of exosomal proteins in these two diseases and found that levels of aminopeptidase-N and vasorin precursor were higher in the thin basemen-membrane nephropathy group, whereas α-1-antitrypsin and ceruloplasmin levels were elevated in IgA patients [16]. Moreover, urinary exosomal chemokine ligand-2 (CCL2) levels are upregulated in IgA nephropathy patients compared with healthy controls and correlate with renal function and histologic injury [17]. Hence, different forms of glomerular disease might show specific profiles of urinary EV protein expression.

3.3. *Tubular Disease*

Urinary EVs often contain solute transporters, such as Na-Cl cotransporter (NCC), which was found to be absent in patients with Gitelman's syndrome or Bartter syndrome type-1 [18], a genetic disorder caused by a mutation of the gene encoding for this cotransporter-2 [19]. Yet, while urinary EV phenotyping might be useful in the diagnosis of Gitelman's and Bartter syndromes [20], additional studies are needed to address whether these EVs can be used as a preliminary screening tool in patients suspected of having these genetic disorders.

Polycystic kidney disease (PKD) is the most common inherited kidney disease and is caused by a mutation in genes encoding for proteins involved in the function of primary cilia, including polycystin (PC)-1, PC-2, and fibrocystin. EVs may be important elements in cilia biology and biomarkers for PKD, as cystin and ADP ribosylation-factor-like-6 are abnormally expressed in urinary EVs of patients with PKD [21]. Recently, the presence of transmembrane protein-2 (TMEM2) in urinary exosomes was shown to be more than twofold higher in patients with PKD1 mutations compared with controls. The PC-to-TMEM ratio correlated inversely with kidney volume, suggesting that urine exosomal PC-1/TMEM2 or PC-2/TMEM2 may provide a novel technique to assess disease progression in patients with PKD. Recently, levels of plakins and complement in urinary EVs have also been implicated as disease-associated proteins in autosomal dominant PKD [22].

3.4. *Aging*

Aging is associated with a high prevalence of chronic degenerative diseases that impose an increasing burden of morbidities in a growing demographic of elderly people. Circulating plasma levels of EVs decrease with age, possibly due to increased internalization of vesicles into B-cells [23]. Aging also involves activation of both autonomous and non-autonomous cell mechanisms, a dominant among which is senescence. Cellular senescence is a form of cell-cycle arrest that changes cellular characteristics toward a pro-inflammatory phenotype. Regarding urinary EVs, six proteins (TSN1, PODXL, IDHC, PPAP, ACBP, and ANXA5) were found to express differently between subjects that were 25–50 and 50–70 years old [24]. Furthermore, the numbers of urinary exosomes, juxtaglomerular cells, and podocyte marker-positive EVs in human subjects decrease with increasing age, and several populations of EVs derived from glomerular and other nephron cells correlate with the development of nephron hypertrophy or nephrosclerosis [25]. Recently, we also found that mitochondrial dysfunction might be associated with cellular senescence in the early stage of atherosclerotic renal artery stenosis [26]. In short, aging impacts the renal cellular composition and its urinary representation.

3.5. Renovascular Disease

Renovascular disease (RVD) is the main cause of secondary hypertension, and prolonged renal ischemia may result in irreversible kidney damage [27]. Kwon et al. reported differential expression of miRNA in urinary EVs obtained from hypertensive patients [28]. The level of miRNA-21, -93, and -200b were lower in urinary EVs of patients with essential hypertension than in RVD, suggesting them as useful markers for discriminating different forms of renal damage in hypertension. Furthermore, urinary podocyte-derived EVs were also elevated in RVD patients and might be useful for monitoring glomerular damage in these patients [29]. Subsequently, we identified elevated urinary levels of exosomes derived from $p16^+$ tubular cells in hypertensive patients, suggesting increased tubular cellular senescence [30], and from peritubular capillaries, reflecting renal microcirculation injury [31].

3.6. Renal Transplantation

Renal transplantation is the best option for end-stage renal disease. The use of urinary EVs as biomarkers for kidney injury after renal transplantation was reported by Alvarez et al., who demonstrated the presence of neutrophil gelatinase-associated lipocalin (NGAL), a member of the lipocalin family that is largely expressed in tubular cells in response to inflammation, in cellular fraction and urinary exosomes from transplanted patients [32]. Despite no change in urinary free NGAL levels, its levels in urinary exosomes distinguished grafts harvested from deceased compared to living donors, and increased in patients with delayed graft function, suggesting that urinary exosomal NGAL could be a biomarker of injury or delayed graft function after kidney transplantation.

Decreased urinary $CD133^+$ EV levels are also associated with delayed graft function and vascular damage [33]. These $CD133^+$ EVs were detectable at high levels in urine from healthy donors but not in patients with end-stage renal disease, possibly indicating that these vesicles are only released by functioning renal tissue. In transplant patients, urinary $CD133^+$ EVs are present at low levels on the first day after transplantation and increase thereafter at day 7. Contrarily, in patients with severe pre-transplant vascular damage of the graft, $CD133^+$ EVs do not increase on day 7. Thus, $CD133^+$ EVs may reflect restored tubular function and the regenerative potential of the nephron after renal transplantation.

Intra-graft infiltration of T-cells is one of the hallmarks for the diagnosis of acute cellular rejection after kidney transplantation. A recent study showed that CD3-positive urinary exosomes in patients with acute cellular rejection could reflect T-cell infiltration in the allografts [34]. In the case of antibody-mediated rejection, mRNA transcript profiles, such as gp130, SH2D1B, TNFα, and CCL4, were increased in plasma exosomes of the patients [35].

4. EVs as a Therapeutic Approach in Kidney Disease

Mesenchymal stem cells (MSCs) are multipotent cells with robust self-renewal, regenerative, proliferative, and multi-lineage differentiation potential. Harvesting and delivery of MSC-derived EVs emerged as a novel non-cellular alternative to cell-based therapy. A potential therapeutic role of EVs in AKI has been examined extensively in animal models. Several studies have shown that MSC-derived EVs confer renoprotective effects in kidney injury models. The first evidence of the beneficial effect of EVs shed by bone-marrow MSC was reported by Bruno et al. in 2009, in a model of AKI induced by glycerol injection in immune-deficient mice [36]. They reported that MSC-derived EVs improved tubular injury and renal function by inducing tubular cell proliferation and that this may occur via horizontal transfer of mRNAs by the EVs. Recently, our group tested intrarenal delivery of autologous MSC-derived EVs in a porcine model of metabolic syndrome and renal artery stenosis.

We found that intrarenal injection of MSC-derived EVs in these pigs ameliorated renal inflammation, increased the number of reparative macrophages, and upregulated expression of IL-10, suggesting that the protective effects of EVs on the stenotic kidney are due to anti-inflammatory properties [37]. Furthermore, intra-renal delivery of MSC-derived EVs bearing pro-angiogenic properties restored renal microcirculation, hemodynamics, and function in an experimental animal model [38]. Interestingly, we subsequently found that intrarenal injection of MSC-derived EVs was helpful to mitigate the myocardial injury in experimental RVD likely via improvement of kidney function [39]. Furthermore, a recent study revealed that the delivery of exosomes secreted by urine-derived stem cells was useful in alleviating stress urinary incontinence and kidney complications from type-I diabetes in rats [40]. Additional studies are needed to determine whether the delivery of other types of exosomes isolated from the urine can serve as therapeutic tools in human subjects as well [41].

5. Urinary EVs as Monitors of Drug Therapy

Recently, circulating EVs, especially tumor-derived exosomes, have been evoking interest as surrogates of response to anti-cancer therapy, as well as diagnostic biomarkers. For example, circulating microvesicles allow for real-time monitoring of cancer's response to chemotherapy [42,43]. However, few studies have assessed the role of urinary EVs in monitoring the effects of drug therapy. In essential hypertensive patients, hydrochlorothiazide-induced reduction of blood pressure is correlated with NCC abundance in urinary exosomes [44]. The increase in NCC abundance in urinary exosomes was detected in responders but not in non-responders, implying that characteristics of urinary EVs may help direct therapy. More studies are needed to investigate the role of urinary EVs as a monitoring tool in drug therapy.

6. Urinary EVs as Vehicles for Drug Delivery

Recently, EVs have gained prominence as drug delivery vehicles thanks to their ability to deliver proteins, lipids, and nucleic acids to recipient cells [45]. Exosomes provide important advantages compared to other nanoparticle drug delivery systems, such as liposomes and polymeric nanoparticles [46]. Different cell sources for EVs have been investigated because the parental cell has been shown to influence their biological activity and subsequent therapeutic effect [47]. These include model cell lines, such as various tumor cell lines, dendritic cells from bone marrow, and mesenchymal stem/stromal cells.

The process of loading EVs with specific cargos can be attained by manipulating their parental cells (endogenous loading), or the isolated EVs (exogenous loading) themselves when endogenous loading is infeasible. Indeed, these versatile approaches may expand the applications of EVs of a wider variety of sources. Zhuang et al. reported that exosomes effectively delivered curcumin to the brain to treat neuroinflammation-related diseases, without adverse effects [48]. Endogenous loading techniques leverage the biological cellular apparatus to sort and pack molecules into EVs during their biogenesis. For example, incubating parental cells with chemotherapeutic paclitaxel and doxorubicin led to their incorporation [49,50] such that EV-encapsulated drugs could be isolated from the culture-conditioned media. Furthermore, to boost their delivery and biodistribution, EVs can be engineered to recognize specific cell surface receptors [51]. Thus, EVs can be loaded with therapeutic substances for delivery to target cells, exciting developments that may be used in future clinical trials. Whether these would apply to EVs isolated from urine remains to be tested.

7. Summary

Investigation of various types of EVs is currently among the most stimulating areas in cell biology. In the field of kidney biology and disease, studies have particularly centered on the potential of EVs as biomarkers, focusing primarily on EVs detected in urine (Figure 1).

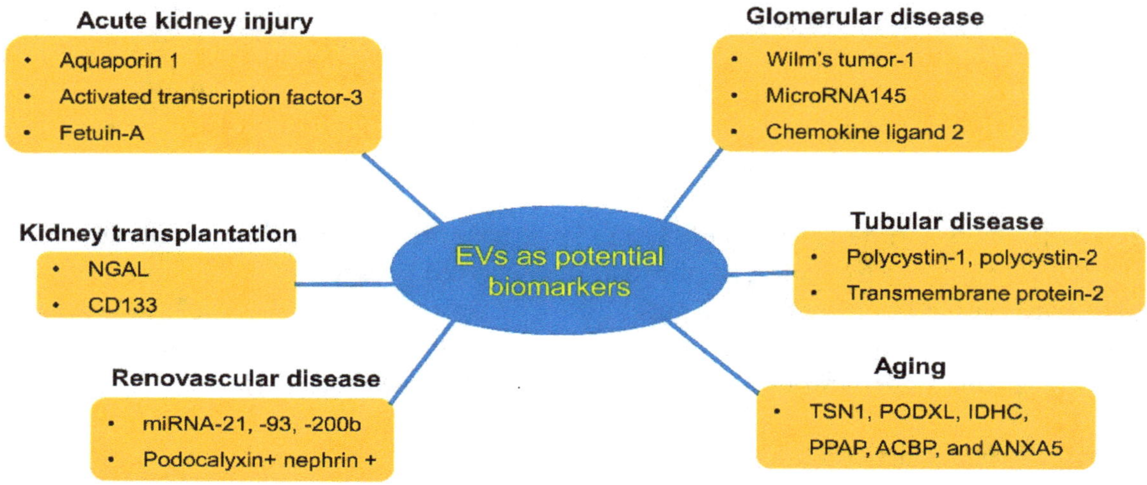

Figure 1. Potential biomarkers of urinary extracellular vesicles (EVs) in kidney diseases. Urinary EVs may augment the ability to diagnose and monitor renal conditions. Their most useful application may be predicting the clinical outcome of patients with kidney disease and guiding treatment decisions.

Such urinary EVs are appropriate and useful for diagnosis given the ease of collection and ability to serve as a "liquid biopsy" to provide information on the pathophysiological state of kidneys. The availability of a reliable and quick urinary assay of EV biomarkers might support a non-invasive diagnosis and facilitate adequate individualized management approaches. Additionally, further studies showing the relationship between the number of EVs and renal diseases are needed. The use of EVs as indices of the response to therapy is underutilized and needs further validation. Rigorous studies to detect and portray EVs will also extend our understanding of their diverse roles in health and disease, and provide new insight into the origins, diagnosis, and treatment options for renal disease.

Author Contributions: I.O.S. performed the initial literature search and wrote the manuscript. L.O.L. supervised, reviewed, obtained funding, corrected the manuscript, and provided final approval of publication for this manuscript. All authors have read and agreed to the published version of the manuscript.

Abbreviations

AKI	acute kidney injury
AQP1	aquaporin-1
CCL2	chemokine ligand-2
EV	extracellular vesicle
FSGS	focal segmental glomerulosclerosis
MiRNA	microRNA
MSC	mesenchymal stem cell
NCC	Na-Cl cotransporter
NGAL	neutrophil gelatinase-associated lipocalin
PC	polycystin
PKD	polycystic kidney disease
RVD	renovascular disease
SSNS	steroid-sensitive nephrotic syndrome
TMEM2	transmembrane protein-2
WT-1	Wilm's tumor-1

References

1. Hessvik, N.P.; Llorente, A. Current knowledge on exosome biogenesis and release. *Cell. Mol. Life Sci.* **2018**, *75*, 193–208. [CrossRef]
2. van der Pol, E.; Boing, A.N.; Harrison, P.; Sturk, A.; Nieuwland, R. Classification, functions, and clinical relevance of extracellular vesicles. *Pharmacol. Rev.* **2012**, *64*, 676–705. [CrossRef]
3. Zaborowski, M.P.; Balaj, L.; Breakefield, X.O.; Lai, C.P. Extracellular vesicles: Composition, biological relevance, and methods of study. *Bioscience* **2015**, *65*, 783–797. [CrossRef] [PubMed]
4. Pisitkun, T.; Shen, R.F.; Knepper, M.A. Identification and proteomic profiling of exosomes in human urine. *Proc. Natl. Acad. Sci. USA* **2004**, *101*, 13368–13373. [CrossRef] [PubMed]
5. Merchant, M.L.; Rood, I.M.; Deegens, J.K.J.; Klein, J.B. Isolation and characterization of urinary vesicles: Implications for biomarker discovery. *Nat. Rev. Nephrol.* **2017**, *13*, 731–749. [CrossRef] [PubMed]
6. Alvarez, M.L.; Khosroheidari, M.; Kanchi, R.R.; DiStefano, J.K. Comparison of protein, microRNA, and mRNA yields using different methods of urinary exosomes isolation for the discovery of kidney disease biomarkers. *Kidney Int.* **2012**, *82*, 1024–1032. [CrossRef] [PubMed]
7. Musante, L.; Bontha, S.V.; La Salvia, S.; Fernandez-Piñeros, A.; Lannigan, J.; Le, T.H.; Erdbrügger, U. Rigorous characterization of urinary extracellular vesicles (uEVs) in the low centrifugation pellet—A neglected source for uEVs. *Sci. Rep.* **2020**, *28*, 3701. [CrossRef] [PubMed]
8. Sonoda, H.; Yokota-Ikeda, N.; Oshikawa, S.; Kanno, Y.; Yoshinaga, K.; Uchida, K.; Ueda, Y.; Kimiya, K.; Uezono, S.; Ueda, A.; et al. Decreased abundance of urinary exosomal aquaporin-1 in renal ischemic-reperfusion injury. *Am. J. Physiol. Renal Physiol.* **2009**, *297*, F1006–F1016. [CrossRef] [PubMed]
9. dU Cheyron, D.; Daubin, C.; Poggioli, J.; Ramakers, M.; Houillier, P.; Charbonneau, P.; Paillard, M. Urinary measurement of Na+/H+ exchanger isoform 3 (NHE3) protein as new marker of tubule injury in critically ill patients with ARF. *Am. J. Kidney Dis.* **2003**, *42*, 497–506. [CrossRef]
10. Zhou, H.; Pisitkun, T.; Aponte, A.; Yuen, P.S.; Hoffert, J.D.; Yasuda, H.; Hu, X.; Chawla, L.; Shen, R.F.; Knepper, M.A.; et al. Exosomal Fetuin-A identified by proteomics: A novel urinary biomarker for detecting acute kidney injury. *Kidney Int.* **2006**, *70*, 1847–1857. [CrossRef]
11. Zhou, H.; Cheruvanky, A.; Hu, X.; Matsumoto, T.; Hiramatsu, N.; Cho, M.E.; Berger, A.; Leelahavanichkul, A.; Doi, K.; Chawla, L.S.; et al. Urinary exosomal transcription factors, a new class of biomarkers for renal disease. *Kidney Int.* **2008**, *74*, 613–621. [CrossRef] [PubMed]
12. Panich, T.; Chancharoenthana, W.; Somparn, P.; Issara-Amphorn, J.; Hirankarn, N.; Leelahavanichkul, A. Urinary exosomal activating transcriptional factor 3 as the early diagnostic biomarker for sepsis induced acute kidney injury. *BMC Nephrol.* **2017**, *18*, 10. [CrossRef] [PubMed]
13. Zhou, H.; Kajiyama, H.; Tsuji, T.; Hu, X.; Leelahavanichkul, A.; Vento, S.; Frank, R.; Kopp, J.B.; Trachtman, H.; Star, R.A.; et al. Urinary exosomal Wilms' tumor-1 as a potential biomarker for podocyte injury. *Am. J. Physiol. Renal Physiol.* **2013**, *305*, F553–F559. [CrossRef] [PubMed]
14. Kalani, A.; Mohan, A.; Godbole, M.M.; Bhatia, E.; Gupta, A.; Sharma, R.K.; Tiwari, S. Wilm's tumor-1 protein levels in urinary exosomes from diabetic patients with or without proteinuria. *PLoS ONE* **2013**, *8*, e60177. [CrossRef] [PubMed]
15. Zhang, L.H.; Zhu, X.Y.; Eirin, A.; Nargesi, A.A.; Woollard, J.R.; Santelli, A.; Sun, I.O.; Textor, S.C.; Lerman, L.O. Early podocyte injury and elevated levels of urinary podocyte-derived extracellular vesicles in swin with metabolic syndrome: Role of podocyte mitochondria. *Am. J. Physiol. Renal Physiol.* **2019**, *317*, F12–F22. [CrossRef]
16. Moon, P.G.; Lee, J.E.; You, S.; Kim, T.K.; Cho, J.H.; Kim, I.S.; Kwon, T.H.; Kim, C.D.; Park, S.H.; Hwang, D.; et al. Proteomic analysis of urinary exosomes from patients of early IgA nephropathy and thin basement membrane nephropathy. *Proteomics* **2011**, *11*, 2459–2475. [CrossRef]
17. Feng, Y.; Lv, L.L.; Wu, W.J.; Li, Z.L.; Chen, J.; Ni, H.F.; Zhou, L.T.; Tang, T.T.; Wang, F.M.; Wang, B.; et al. Urinary exosomes and exosomal CCL2 mRNA as biomarkers of active histologic injury in IgA nephropathy. *Am. J. Pathol.* **2018**, *188*, 2542–2552. [CrossRef]
18. Gonzales, P.A.; Pisitkun, T.; Hoffert, J.D.; Tchapyjnikov, D.; Kleta, R.; Wang, N.S.; Knepper, M.A. Large-scale proteomics and phosphoproteomics of urinary exosomes. *J. Am. Soc. Nephrol.* **2009**, *20*, 363–379. [CrossRef]

19. Joo, K.W.; Lee, J.W.; Jang, H.R.; Heo, N.J.; Jeon, U.S.; Oh, Y.K.; Lim, C.S.; Na, K.Y.; Kim, J.; Cheong, H.I.; et al. Reduced urinary excretion of thiazie-sensitive Na-Cl cotransporter in Gitelman syndrome: Preliminary data. *Am. J. Kidney Dis.* **2007**, *50*, 765–773. [CrossRef]
20. Corbetta, S.; Raimondo, F.; Tedeschi, S.; Syren, M.L.; Rebora, P.; Savoia, A.; Baldi, L.; Bettinelli, A.; Pitto, M. Urinary exosomes in the diagnosis of Gitelman and Bartter syndromes. *Nephrol. Dial. Transplant.* **2015**, *30*, 621–630. [CrossRef]
21. Hogan, M.C.; Manganelli, L.; Wollard, J.R.; Masyuk, A.I.; Masyuk, T.V.; Tammachote, R.; Huang, B.Q.; Leontovich, A.A.; Beito, T.G.; Madden, B.J.; et al. Characterization of PKD protein-positive exosome-like vesicles. *J. Am. Soc. Nephrol.* **2009**, *20*, 278–288. [CrossRef] [PubMed]
22. Salih, M.; Demmers, J.A.; Bezstarosti, K.; Leonhard, W.N.; Losekoot, M.; van Kooten, C.; Gansevoort, R.T.; Peters, D.J.; Zietse, R.; Hoorn, E.J.; et al. Proteomics of urinary vesicles links plakins and complement to polycystic kidney disease. *J. Am. Soc. Nephrol.* **2016**, *27*, 3079–3092. [CrossRef] [PubMed]
23. Eitan, E.; Green, J.; Bodogai, M.; Mode, N.A.; Bæk, R.; Jørgensen, M.M.; Freeman, D.W.; Witwer, K.W.; Zonderman, A.B.; Biragyn, A.; et al. Age-related changes in plasma extracellular vesicle characteristics and internalization by leukocytes. *Sci. Rep.* **2017**, *7*, 1342. [CrossRef] [PubMed]
24. Raj, D.A.; Fiume, I.; Capasso, G.; Pocsfalvi, G. A multiplex quantitative proteomics strategy for protein biomarker studies in urinary exosomes. *Kidney Int.* **2012**, *81*, 1263–1272. [CrossRef]
25. Turco, A.E.; Lam, W.; Rule, A.D.; Denic, A.; Lieske, J.C.; Miller, V.M.; Larson, J.J.; Kremers, W.K.; Jayachandran, M. Specific renal parenchymal-derived urinary extracellular vesciles identify age-associated structural changes in living donor kidneys. *J. Extracell. Vesicles* **2016**, *5*, 29642. [CrossRef]
26. Kim, S.R.; Eirin, A.; Zhang, X.; Lerman, A.; Lerman, L.O. Mitochondria protection partly mitigates kidney cellular senescence in swine atherosclerotic renal artery stenosis. *Cell. Physiol. Biochem.* **2019**, *52*, 617–632.
27. Hansen, K.J.; Edwards, M.S.; Craven, T.E.; Cherr, G.S.; Jackson, S.A.; Appel, R.G.; Burke, G.L.; Dean, R.H. Prevalence of renovascular disease in the elderly: A population-based study. *J. Vasc. Surg.* **2002**, *36*, 443–451. [CrossRef]
28. Kwon, S.H.; Tang, H.; Saad, A.; Woollard, J.R.; Lerman, A.; Textor, S.C.; Lerman, L.O. Differential expression of microRNAs in urinary extracellular vesicles obtained from hypertensive patients. *Am. J. Kidney Dis.* **2016**, *68*, 331–332. [CrossRef]
29. Kwon, S.H.; Woollard, J.R.; Saad, A.; Garovic, V.D.; Zand, L.; Jordan, K.L.; Textor, S.C.; Lerman, L.O. Elevated urinary podocyte-derived extracellular microvesicles in renovascular hypertensive patients. *Nephrol. Dial. Transplant.* **2017**, *32*, 800–807. [CrossRef]
30. Santelli, A.; Sun, I.O.; Eirin, A.; Abumoawad, A.M.; Woollard, J.R.; Lerman, A.; Textor, S.C.; Puranik, A.S.; Lerman, L.O. Senescent kidney cells in hypertensive patients release urinary extracellular vesicles. *J. Am. Heart Assoc.* **2019**, *8*, e012584. [CrossRef]
31. Sun, I.O.; Santelli, A.; Abumoawad, A.; Eirin, A.; Ferguson, C.M.; Woollard, J.R.; Lerman, A.; Textor, S.C.; Puranik, A.S.; Lerman, L.O. Loss of renal peritubular capillaries in hypertensive patients is detectable by urinary endothelial microparticle levels. *Hypertension* **2018**, *72*, 1180–1188. [CrossRef] [PubMed]
32. Alvarz, S.; Suazo, C.; Boltansky, A.; Ursu, M.; Carvajal, D.; Innocenti, G.; Vukusich, A.; Hurtado, M.; Villanueva, S.; Carreno, J.E.; et al. Urinary exosomes as a source of kidney dysfunction biomarker in renal transplantation. *Transplant. Proc.* **2013**, *45*, 3719–3723. [CrossRef] [PubMed]
33. Dimuccio, V.; Ranghino, A.; Pratico Barbato, L.; Fop, F.; Biancone, L.; Camussi, G.; Bussolati, B. Urinary CD133+ extracellular vesicles are decreased in kidney transplanted patients with slow graft function and vascular damage. *PLoS ONE* **2014**, *9*, e104490. [CrossRef]
34. Park, J.; Lin, H.Y.; Assaker, J.P.; Jeong, S.; Huang, C.H.; Kurdi, T.; Lee, K.; Fraser, K.; Min, C.; Eskandari, S.; et al. Integrated kidney exosome analysis for the detection of kidney transplant rejection. *ACS Nano* **2017**, *11*, 11041–11046. [CrossRef] [PubMed]
35. Zhang, H.; Huang, E.; Kahwaji, J.; Nast, C.C.; Li, P.; Mirocha, J.; Thomas, D.L.; Ge, S.; Vo, A.A.; Jordan, S.C.; et al. Plasma exosomes from HLA-sensitized kidney transplant recipients contain mRNA transcripts which predict development of antibody-mediated rejection. *Transplantation* **2017**, *101*, 2419–2428. [CrossRef] [PubMed]
36. Bruno, S.; Grange, C.; Deregibus, M.C.; Calogero, R.A.; Saviozzi, S.; Collino, F.; Morando, L.; Busca, A.; Falda, M.; Bussolati, B.; et al. Mesenchymal stem cell-derived microvesicles protect against acute tubular injury. *J. Am. Soc. Nephrol.* **2009**, *20*, 1053–1067. [CrossRef] [PubMed]

37. Eirin, A.; Zhu, X.Y.; Puranik, A.S.; Tang, H.; McGurren, K.A.; van Wijnen, A.J.; Lerman, A.; Lerman, L.O. Mesenchymal stem cell-derived extracellular vesicles attenuate kidney inflammation. *Kidney Int.* **2017**, *92*, 114–124. [CrossRef]
38. Eirin, A.; Zhu, X.Y.; Jonnada, S.; Lerman, A.; van Wijnen, A.J.; Lerman, L.O. Mesenchymal stem cell-derived extracellular vesicles improve the renal microvasculature in metabolic renovascular disease in swine. *Cell Transplant.* **2018**, *27*, 1080–1095. [CrossRef]
39. Zhang, L.; Zhu, X.Y.; Zhao, Y.; Eirin, A.; Liu, L.; Ferguson, C.M.; Tang, H.; Lerman, A.; Lerman, L.O. Selective intrarenal delivery of mesenchymal stem cell-derived extracellular vesicles attenuates myocardial injury in experimental metabolic renovascular disease. *Basic Res. Cardiol.* **2020**, *115*, 16. [CrossRef]
40. Wu, R.; Huang, C.; Wu, Q.; Jia, X.; Liu, M.; Xue, Z.; Qiu, Z.; Niu, X.; Wang, Y. Exosomes secreted by urine-derived stem cells improve stress urinary incontience by promoting repair of pubococcygeus muscle injury in rats. *Stem Cell Res. Ther.* **2019**, *10*, 80. [CrossRef]
41. Jiang, Z.Z.; Liu, Y.M.; Niu, X.; Yin, J.Y.; Hu, B.; Guo, S.C.; Fan, Y.; Wang, Y.; Wang, N.S. Exosomes secreted by human urine-derived stem cells could prevent kidney complications from type I diabetes in rats. *Stem Cell Res. Ther.* **2016**, *7*, 24. [CrossRef] [PubMed]
42. Shao, H.; Chung, J.; Balaj, L.; Charest, A.; Bigner, D.D.; Carter, B.S.; Hochberg, F.H.; Breakefield, X.O.; Weissleder, R.; Lee, H. Protein typing of circulating microvesicles allows real-time monitoring of gliblastoma therapy. *Nat. Med.* **2012**, *18*, 1835–1840. [CrossRef] [PubMed]
43. Aubertin, K.; Silva, A.K.; Luciani, N.; Espinosa, A.; Djmat, A.; Charue, D.; Gallet, F.; Blanc-Brude, O.; Wilhelm, C. Massive release of extracellular vesicles from cancer cells after photodynamic treatment or chemotherapy. *Sci. Rep.* **2016**, *6*, 35376.
44. Pathare, G.; Tutakhel, O.A.Z.; van der Wel, M.C.; Shelton, L.M.; Deinum, J.; Lenders, J.W.M.; Hoenderop, J.G.J.; Bindels, R.J.M. Hydrochlorothiazide treatment increases the abundance of the NaCl cotransporter in urinary extracellular vesicles of essential hypertensive patients. *Am. J. Physiol. Renal Physiol.* **2017**, *312*, F1063–F1072. [CrossRef]
45. Turturici, G.; Tinnirello, R.; Sconzo, G.; Geraci, F. Extracellular membrane vesicles as a mechanism of cell-to-cell communication: Advantages and disadvantages. *Am. J. Physiol. Cell Physiol.* **2014**, *306*, C621–C633. [CrossRef]
46. Ha, D.; Yang, N.; Nadithe, V. Exosomes as therapetic drug carriers and delivery vehicles across biological membrane: Current perspectives and future challenges. *Acta Pharm. Sin. B* **2016**, *6*, 287–296. [CrossRef]
47. Villa, F.; Quarto, R.; Tasso, R. Extracellular vesicles as natural, safe and efficient drug delivery systems. *Pharmaceutics* **2019**, *11*, 557. [CrossRef]
48. Zhuang, X.; Xiang, X.; Grizzle, W.; Sun, D.; Zhang, S.; Axtell, R.C.; Ju, S.; Mu, J.; Zhang, L.; Steinman, L.; et al. Treatment of brain inflammatory diseases by delivering exosome encapsulated anti-inflammatory drugs from the nasal region to the brain. *Mol. Ther.* **2011**, *19*, 1769–1779. [CrossRef]
49. Melzer, C.; Rehn, V.; Yang, Y.; Bahre, H.; von der Ohe, J.; Hass, R. Taxol-loaded MSC-derived exosomes provide a therapeutic vehicle to target metastatic breast cancer and other carcinoma cells. *Cancers* **2019**, *11*, 798. [CrossRef]
50. Goh, W.J.; Lee, C.K.; Zou, S.; Woon, E.C.; Czarny, B.; Pastorin, G. Doxorubicin-loaded cell-derived nanovesicles: An alternative targeted approach for anti-tumor therapy. *Int. Nanomed.* **2017**, *12*, 2759–2767. [CrossRef]
51. Antes, T.J.; Middleton, R.C.; Luther, K.M.; Ijichi, T.; Peck, K.A.; Liu, W.J.; Valle, J.; Echavez, A.K.; Marban, E. Targeting extracellular vesicles to injuired tissue using membrane cloaking and surface display. *J. Nanobiotechnol.* **2018**, *16*, 1–15. [CrossRef] [PubMed]

2

The Utility of Novel Renal Biomarkers in Assessment of Chronic Kidney Disease of Unknown Etiology (CKDu)

T.D.K.S.C. Gunasekara [1], P. Mangala C.S. De Silva [1,2,*], Chula Herath [3], Sisira Siribaddana [4], Nipuna Siribaddana [5], Channa Jayasumana [6], Sudheera Jayasinghe [7], Maria Cardenas-Gonzalez [2,8] and Nishad Jayasundara [9,10]

1 Department of Zoology, Faculty of Science, University of Ruhuna, Matara 81000, Sri Lanka; gunasekara.sc166@fgs.ruh.ac.lk
2 Renal Division, Brigham and Women's Hospital, Harvard Medical School, Boston, MA 02115, USA; mariana.cardenas@conacyt.mx
3 Department of Nephrology, Sri Jayawardenapura General Hospital, Sri Jayawardenepura Kotte 10100, Sri Lanka; chulaherath@gmail.com
4 Department of Medicine, Faculty of Medicine and Allied Sciences, Rajarata University of Sri Lanka, Mihintale 50300, Sri Lanka; sisira.siribaddana@gmail.com
5 Department of Parasitology, Faculty of Medicine and Allied Sciences, Rajarata University of Sri Lanka, Mihintale 50300, Sri Lanka; nipunas@gmail.com
6 Department of Pharmacology, Faculty of Medicine and Allied Sciences, Rajarata University of Sri Lanka, Mihintale 50300, Sri Lanka; channajayasumana@gmail.com
7 Department of Pharmacology, Faculty of Medicine, University of Ruhuna, Matara 81000, Sri Lanka; sudheerasj@med.ruh.ac.lk
8 Mexican Council of Science and Technology, Consejo Nacional de Ciencia y Tecnología, Mexico City 03940, Mexico
9 The Nicholas School of the Environment, Duke University, Durham, NC 27708, USA; nishad.jayasundara@duke.edu
10 The School of Marine Sciences, University of Maine, Orono, ME 04469, USA
* Correspondence: chathura@zoo.ruh.ac.lk

Abstract: Chronic Kidney Disease (CKD) is a globally prevalent non-communicable disease with significant mortality and morbidity. It is typically associated with diabetes and hypertension; however, over the last two decades, an emergence of CKD of unknown etiology (CKDu) has claimed thousands of lives in several tropical agricultural communities. CKDu is associated with gradual loss of renal function without initial symptoms until reaching complete kidney failure and eventually death. The most impacted are young adult males of lower socio-economic strata. Since the disease progression can be successfully attenuated through early detection, the development of superior screening and management measures is of utmost importance. In contrast to the conventional biomarkers, novel biomarkers with improved sensitivity and specificity are being discussed as promising tools for early diagnosis of the disease. This review summarizes emerging novel biomarkers used in assessing CKD and discusses the current utility and diagnostic potential of such biomarkers for CKDu screening in clinical settings of different communities impacted by CKDu. Our goal is to provide a framework for practitioners in CKDu impacted regions to consider the use of these novel biomarkers through this synthesis. The increased use of these biomarkers will not only help to validate their diagnostic power further and establish potential prognostic value but may also provide critical insights into sites and mechanisms of renal damage.

Keywords: CKD; CKDu; novel biomarkers; renal function; rural farmers; Sri Lanka

1. Background

Chronic Kidney Disease (CKD) is a non-communicable disease that carries a high morbidity and mortality and affects more than~10% of the global population. CKD is defined as "abnormalities of kidney structure or function, present for more than three months" [1]. Clinically, reduction of Glomerular Filtration Rate (GFR) to less than 60 mL/min/1.73 m^2 or increase in albumin to creatinine ratio (ACR $\geq$ 30 mg/g (3 mg/mmol)) is the main criteria for the diagnosis. The leading etiologies of the disease worldwide are type 2 diabetes mellitus, hypertension and chronic glomerulonephritis [2,3]. The estimated number of disability-adjusted life years (DALYS), a measurement of health and wellness lost, attributable to CKD has increased by 26% globally from 1990 to 2013 [4].

In contrast to CKD associated with typical risk factors, a new form of renal disease has emerged in several parts of the world, including in tropical farming communities in Central American and South Asian countries [5] (Figure 1). Both CKD and chronic kidney disease of unknown etiology (CKDu) are characterized by a progressive decline in renal function. However, the exact causes of this disease are highly debated, and given this ambiguity, it is commonly referred to as chronic kidney disease of unknown etiology (CKDu) or, in some instances, as chronic interstitial nephritis in agricultural communities (CINAC) [6]. Among other factors, epidemiological studies suggest a role for environmental contaminant exposures, heat stress, and dehydration associated with farming, infections, and mycotoxins. Recent studies posit that synergistic effects of multiple environmental factors coupled with genetic predisposing may contribute to the initiation, continuous renal injury, and kidney dysfunction progression.

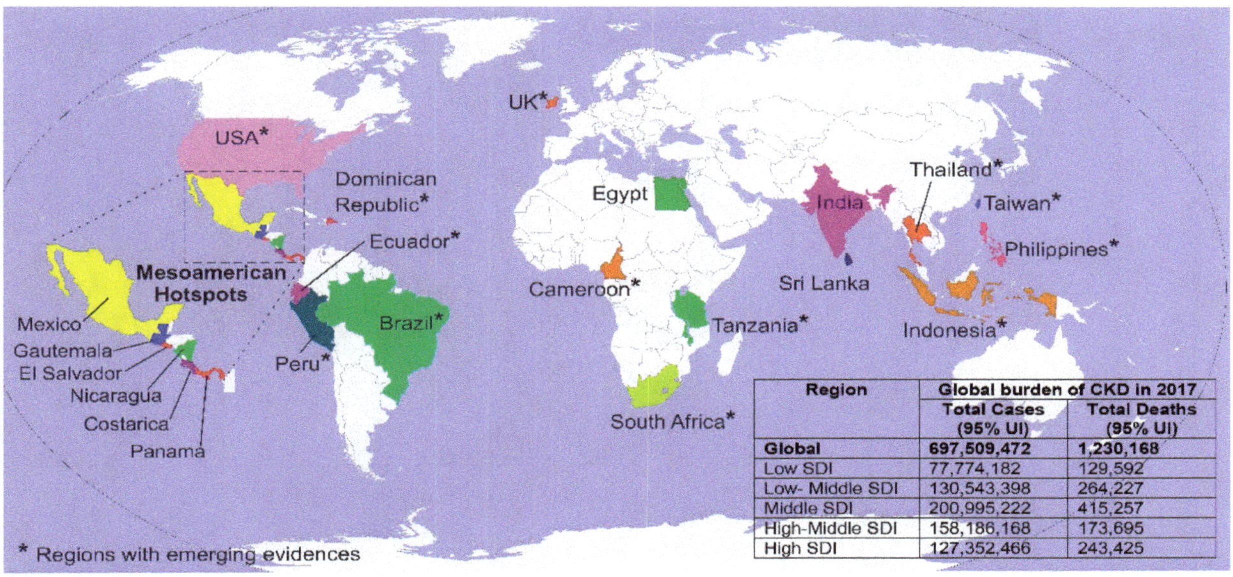

Region	Global burden of CKD in 2017	
	Total Cases (95% UI)	Total Deaths (95% UI)
Global	**697,509,472**	**1,230,168**
Low SDI	77,774,182	129,592
Low- Middle SDI	130,543,398	264,227
Middle SDI	200,995,222	415,257
High-Middle SDI	158,186,168	173,695
High SDI	127,352,466	243,425

Figure 1. Endemic chronic kidney disease of unknown etiology (CKDu) hotspots and regions with emerging evidence of CKDu and chronic kidney disease (CKD) of nontraditional causes (CKDnT) around the world. Global burden is illustrated as all forms of CKD, including CKDu in countries of low to high socio-demographic index (SDI)-based economic strata.

A major challenge in mitigating CKDu is the lack of early diagnostic assays, and the potential to use renal injury markers as early indicators of CKDu manifestation is beginning to be explored. In CKDu patients, the main clinical manifestations such as elevated serum creatinine, protein excretion and urinary albumin to creatinine ratio (ACR), become apparent only after a significant damage to the renal tissues. However, renal tissues express a variety of molecules such as KIM-1, NGAL, and NAG in response to renal injury (Figure 2). These may have the potential to reflect renal damage earlier than conventional markers with a high degree of specificity. They are indeed emerging as potential early predictors of renal damage in CKD and may contribute to the early diagnosis of CKDu. However, convenient assessment strategies and precise reference standards have not been established yet; hence the transformation of these novel biomarkers into clinical screening tools in CKDu requires further studies, and their prognostic power remains to be validated. The objective of this review is to highlight the current use and limitations of novel biomarkers in CKDu studies to provide an initial framework for practitioners in CKDu affected communities when considering the use of these novel biomarkers.

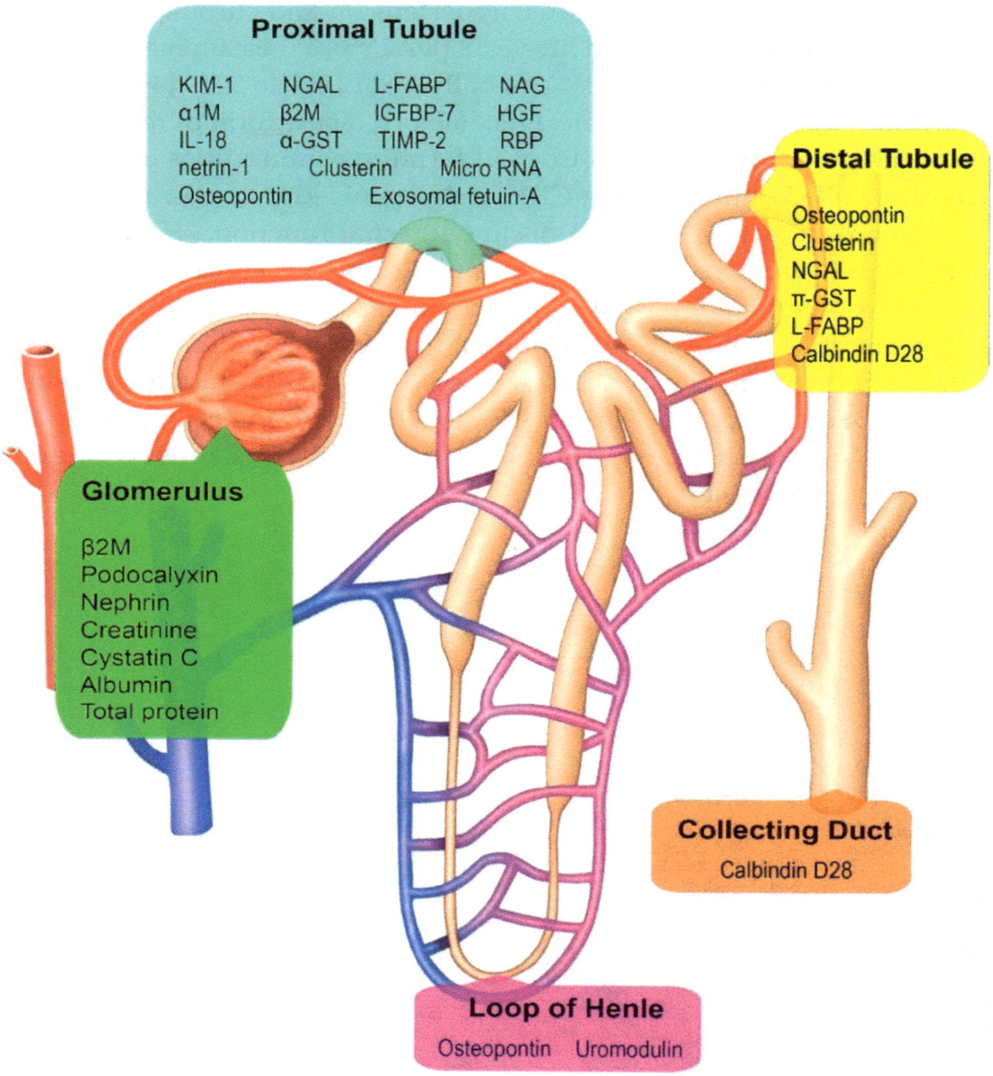

Figure 2. Macromolecules that may serve as biomarkers and their sites of expression. (KIM-1: Kidney Injury Molecule-1; NGAL: Neutrophil Gelatinase-Associated Lipocalin; TIMP-2: Tissue Inhibitor Metalloproteinase-2; IGFBP-7: Insulin- like Growth Factor Binding Protein-7; Pi-GST: Glutathione S-Transferase; NAG: N-acetyl-beta-D-glucosaminidase; IL-18: Interleukin-18; RBP: Retinol Binding Protein; L-FABP: Liver type Fatty Acid Binding Protein; α1M: α1- Microglobulin; β2M: β2-Microglobulin; HGF: Hepatocyte Growth Factor.).

2. Chronic Kidney Disease of Unknown Etiology (CKDu)

Similar to most other forms of CKD, CKDu is also asymptomatic until later stages. It is initially relatively non-proteinuric (less than 1 g/24 h), and early identification has been challenging. Histopathology of patients from later stages shows a chronic tubulo-interstitial disease with secondary glomerulosclerosis [7].

CKDu incidences first emerged in several Mesoamerican countries, including El Salvador, Nicaragua, Guatemala, Mexico, Panama, and Costa Rica [8], Andhra Pradesh in India, the El-Minia

Governorate in Egypt, and several provinces of Sri Lanka [9]. Current evidence presented in various studies suggests incidences in several other South East Asian countries, including Thailand [10], Indonesia [11], the Philippines, and Taiwan; in Tanzania, South Africa, Cameroon, Brazil, Peru, Ecuador, and Dominican Republic [12]; in parts of the United States of America [11] and Belfast in the United Kingdom [13]. Clinical, histological, biochemical, environmental, and socio-economic factors associated with CKDu are comparable across its geographical distribution and are considered a rapidly growing public health concern worldwide [14,15]. CKDu is predominant in rural agricultural communities, disproportionately affecting young to middle-aged male farmers [16,17].

The disease is characterized by prominent histopathological features that tend to be consistent over the global CKDu hotspots. In a study with Indian CKDu patients, glomerular sclerosis, interstitial infiltration with lymphocytic infiltration, interstitial fibrosis, and tubular atrophy were noted prominently. Importantly, significant histological changes have been noted in early-stage CKDu patients [18]. In a study with 64 renal biopsies from CKDu patients in Sri Lanka, interstitial fibrosis and tubular atrophy with or without nonspecific interstitial mononuclear cell infiltration were the dominant histopathological manifestations. In addition, glomerular sclerosis, glomerular collapse, and features of vascular pathology such as fibrous intimal thickening and arteriolar hyalinosis were also noted commonly [19]. The same histopathological and biochemical profiles have been observed in Mesoamerica [15,20].

Since its emergence, CKDu has claimed thousands of lives in Central America and South Asia [21,22], devastating impacted rural communities. Most affected communities are predominantly rural and rarely undergo regular medical checkups due to socio-economic limitations as well as the absence of other risk factors (e.g., type 2 diabetes and hypertension). The disease predominantly affects males, and lack of optimal disease management strategies has led to end-stage renal failure and death in most cases [23]. As illustrated in Figure 1, CKDu prevalence has increased across the globe and several CKDu hotspots have emerged, making it a global public health concern [24].

CKDu hotspots are defined based on the high prevalence of CKD attributed to unexplained causes. However, characterizing precise CKDu prevalence has been difficult due to several factors, including the ambiguity in defining geographical boundaries of impacted and non-impacted regions. In most community studies, declined renal function in the absence of diabetes mellitus, hypertension, and glomerular diseases is treated as CKDu or CKD of nontraditional causes. These clinical manifestations associated with CKDu were confirmed in a recent study with CKDu patients in Sri Lanka [25]. Nonetheless, several community studies conducted in 2019 in CKDu affected regions indicate the gravity of this epidemic. In one such study conducted in the disease endemic North Central Province in Sri Lanka, CKDu prevalence among adults was reported as 6.0% [17], while it was estimated as 13.3% among adults in the Uddanam region in India [26]. Similar cross-sectional studies of CKDu in other farming communities such as among the west Javanese rice farmers in Indonesia (18.6%) [11], residents of León in Nicaragua (7.4–8.4%) [27], suggest a high prevalence of this disease, although these statistics vary depending on the study. Another key limitation is the lack of a standardized disease diagnosis approach as well as the lack of intensive data collection from population surveys. An important step towards facilitating better health policies and intervention strategies is developing early detection markers of CKDu.

3. Etiology of CKDu

Although the exact etiology is yet to be determined, several environmental, socio-economic, and occupational factors are strongly associated with CKDu. Studies have suggested a role for a multitude of contributing factors such as chronic low dose exposure to multiple heavy metals and agrochemicals [28,29], heat stress and recurrent dehydration [30,31], nephrotoxic pharmaceuticals [32], high fluoride levels and water hardness [33], hyperuricemia and hyperuricosuria [34], leptospirosis [35], and genetic predisposition [36]. Heat stress, coupled with dehydration, are considered key driving factors in Mesoamerican CKDu patients [12,37]. However, a recent meta-analysis suggested that pesticide exposure, heat stress, and pharmaceutical use were not associated with CKDu in Mero-America [8]. In South Asia, environmental contaminants are believed to play a significant role in disease initiation and progression [29,38]. Notably, a recent review of studies focused on the etiologies of CKDu has shown that many exposures are heterogeneous and vary by region [39]. Accordingly, a combination of factors are likely contributors to this disease at different stages [9], and below, we summarize the three most prominently discussed drivers of CKDu.

3.1. Heat Stress and CKDu

According to the heat stress/dehydration hypothesis, recurrent mild acute kidney injury caused by recurrent work-associated dehydration episodes leads to CKD [40]. Dehydration causes hyperosmolarity, which activates the aldose reductase enzyme in the proximal tubule of the nephron. This enzyme is involved in the polyol pathway of glucose metabolism that converts glucose to fructose. Metabolism of fructose by fructokinase results in oxidative stress leading to tubular injury. In addition, this hyperosmolarity increases vasopressin, affecting kidney tubules. The predominant distribution of global CKDu hotspots in warmer climates favors this hypothesis. Indeed, CKDu is commonly observed in individuals working strenuously in agricultural fields under extreme heat and are dehydrated [12]. While some studies have argued that there is no clear association between ambient temperature and CKDu [41], this theory's more detailed rebuttal has been published recently [42]. Thus, the hypothesis warrants further validation in different communities through in-depth studies.

3.2. Environmental Contaminants, Water Quality, and CKDu

Several classes of naturally occurring and anthropogenic chemical compounds have been discussed to play a significant role in CKDu. This hypothesis was further supported by a recent study that examined 34 renal biopsies of patients with CKD stage 2–3 (who were diagnosed as CKDu patients) from Sri Lanka, India, El Salvador, and France. Lysosomal proximal tubulopathy with abnormal enlarged dysmorphic lysosomes containing dispersed dark electron-dense aggregates, under light and electron microscopy, indicating a toxin-induced proximal tubular nephropathy in CKDu patients [6,43]. Indeed, varying levels of heavy metals such as mercury, cadmium and lead, arsenic, vanadium, and other agrochemical constituents as well as other nephrotoxic compounds have been found in soil, drinking water, and food in CKDu endemic regions [29,44,45]. In contrast, in a recent study in CKDu prevalent areas in Sri Lanka, analysis of urine, hair, and renal tissue samples did not provide evidence to support cadmium or arsenic toxicity in CKDu patients. Further, Cd and as levels in water and rice samples were within the recommended levels [46]. Animal model studies demonstrated that chemical mixtures found in the environment might induce renal damage and alter kidney development [29]. Additionally, the same substances have been found in urine, blood, hair, and nail samples collected from affected populations [14,47,48], providing strong evidence for an association with environmental toxins with renal diseases, including CKDu. Further, studies from multiple geographic regions suggest clear associations of groundwater fluoride and water hardness with the onset of renal diseases, including interstitial tubule damage [49] coupled with experimental validation through animal studies [33]. Certain nephrotoxic mycotoxins (e.g., aflatoxins, ochratoxins, fumonisins) and phytotoxins such as aristolochic acid, are other environmental factors known to cause chronic tubule-interstitial disease. Among the nephrotoxic agents, a role for aristolochic acid is well documented. Aristolochic acid nephropathy (AAN), formerly known as "Chinese herbal nephropathy" has accounted for a number of cases of chronic renal failure in countries where traditional herbal medicines are widely used [50,51]. Balkan endemic nephropathy (BEN), a severe kidney disease reported in the Balkan Peninsula, is also attributed to AAN. Histology studies show that AAN results in an interstitial fibrosis with a typical corticomedullary gradient and tubular atrophy [52], which has been validated in several animal studies [53,54]. However, there is a lack of clear evidence linking them to CKDu in South Asia and Mesoamerica. Further research is warranted to examine mechanisms of toxicity, underlying initiation and propagation of renal damage by toxic substances.

3.3. *Infectious Origin*

Two studies have shown a possible link between CKDu and an infectious etiology. One study demonstrated elevated levels of Hantavirus IgG antibodies in CKDu patients in Sri Lanka [55], and the other indicated leptospirosis as a risk factor for CKDu in several farming communities [35]. Although these data may provide an association between CKDu and an infectious etiology, further research is required to substantiate a causal link.

4. Renal Biomarkers

The National Institutes of Health (NIH), USA defines a biomarker as "a characteristic that is objectively measured and evaluated as an indicator of normal biological processes, pathogenic processes, or pharmacologic responses to a therapeutic intervention" [56]. In a clinical context, biomarkers can be applied as tools for screening, diagnosing, and monitoring diseases as well as assessing the response of therapeutic interventions [57].

The progression of renal diseases can be successfully alleviated if diagnosed at the potentially treatable and reversible earlier phases. Thus, early detection is of utmost importance, especially for CKDu patients. Biomarkers play a distinct role in aiding the prediction of disease progression and monitoring therapeutic outcomes, and developing more potent biomarkers has become essential in kidney disease management strategies [58].

Cellular stress responses in various renal structures produce several macromolecules at different locations that can serve as markers of kidney dysfunction or damage (Figure 2). For example, a wide spectrum of molecules including urinary and blood-borne proteins and recently discovered micro RNAs might serve as biomarkers in kidney disease screening. However, the sensitivity, specificity, and predictive value of these biomarkers are diverse.

At present, the CKDu epidemic in predominantly agricultural communities has been characterized using conventional renal biomarkers such as serum creatinine (SCr), cystatin C, blood urea nitrogen (BUN), estimated GFR (eGFR), and albumin to creatinine ratio (ACR). These markers have deficiencies in sensitivity and/or specificity to detect kidney injury (or response to injury), especially prior to significant renal function loss. For example, CKDu is a relatively non-proteinuric condition and will often not show a significant elevation of ACR. Furthermore, the elevation of SCr occurs only when significant renal damage has occurred. Hence, the utility of more specific and sensitive biomarkers and better-designed population studies are important, especially for an early diagnosis.

In contrast to conventional renal damage markers, emerging novel biomarkers can serve as early predictors of renal diseases and help locate the site of injury [59,60]. Despite the emerging use of a wide range of novel biomarkers in acute kidney injury and CKD, such approaches are just beginning to be applied in monitoring CKDu. Kidney injury molecule -1 (KIM-1), neutrophil gelatinase-associated lipocalin (NGAL), α1-microglobulin (A1M), β2- macroglobulin (B2M), N-acetyl-beta-D-glucosaminidase (NAG), clusterin (CLU), osteopontin (OPN), and cystatin-C (CysC) are promising examples of new biomarkers. In 2018, the Food and Drug Administration (FDA) approved the qualification of KIM-1, NGAL, NAG, CLU, CysC, and OPN as biomarkers to facilitate the detection of renal tubular injury in phase 1 trials in healthy individuals [61]. A summary of these novel kidney injury biomarkers' characteristics and clinical significance and their utilization in CKDu contexts across the world are given in Table 1 and the site of release is illustrated in Figure 2. These can potentially help to (i) predict and monitor CKDu outcomes in preclinical and clinical settings and (ii) gain critical insights into renal damage sites at the early stages of the disease.

Table 1. Examples of novel kidney injury biomarkers used in CKDu around the globe with their characteristics and clinical significance. (Abbreviations: KIM-1—kidney injury molecule -1; NGAL—neutrophil gelatinase-associated lipocalin; A1M—α1-microglobulin; B2M—macroglobulin; NAG—N-acetyl-beta-D-glucosaminidase; CLU—clusterin; OPN—osteopontin; CysC—cystatin-C; IL-18—Interleukin 18; MCP-1—monocyte chemoattractant protein).

Bio-Marker	Biochemical Significance	Site of Release in the Kidney	Clinical Significance
CLU	Referred to as apolipoprotein J (Apo J). 75–80 kDa glycoprotein.	Proximal tubule Dedifferentiated tubular cells Distal tubule	Elevated urinary expression observed in rat models of tubular proteinuria, but not in glomerular proteinuria.
CysC	Low molecular weight protein (13 kDa). Freely filtered at the glomerulus, subjected to reabsorption and catabolism, but not to tubular secretion.	Glomerulus Proximal tubule	Sensitive serum marker of GFR Prognostic marker of adverse outcomes such as renal replacement therapy. A predictive biomarker of cardiovascular events in patients with kidney diseases.
KIM-1	A Highly conserved phosphatidylserine receptor of 38.7 kDa with a mucin-rich extracellular region.	Proximal tubule Dedifferentiated tubular cells	Proximal tubular injury marker A sensitive and early diagnostic marker of renal injury. Associated with tubule-interstitial fibrosis, tubular damage, and inflammation.
NAG	A proximal tubule lysosomal enzyme.	Proximal tubule	A sensitive and robust indicator of AKI Increased in impaired glucose tolerance, rheumatoid arthritis, and hyperthyroidism.
NGAL	25 kDa lipocalin superfamily protein. A glycoprotein bound to matrix MMP-9 in human neutrophils.	Proximal tubule Distal tubule	A sensitive and early diagnostic marker of renal injury and AKI. Marked upregulation in proximal tubules within 3 h of ischemia/reperfusion injury. Also expressed in salivary glands, uterus, prostate, trachea, lung, stomach in addition to the kidney.
OPN	44 kDa extracellular matrix glycol-phosphoprotein. Produced in high levels in bone tissue and epithelial cells.	Proximal tubule Loop of Henle Distal tubule	Marker of nephrotoxicity. Expressed with inflammation and tubulo-interstitial fibrosis in progressive idiopathic membranous nephropathy, crescentic glomerulonephritis, IgA nephritis, and diffuse proliferative lupus nephritis. Involved in remodeling and calcification of bones, cell adhesion, migration, and survival, immune responses and tumorigenesis.
A1M	27 -30 kDa glycoprotein primarily synthesized by the liver. Detectable in human urine, serum and cerebrospinal fluid. Freely filtered at the glomerulus, subjected to complete reabsorption and catabolized by proximal tubular cells.	Proximal tubule	Elevated levels in urine reflects proximal tubular injury or dysfunction. Urinary levels increase with age. Plasma level varies with age, gender, liver diseases, ulcerative colitis, HIV infection, and mood disorders.
B2M	13.7 kDa light chain MHC-I protein Expressed on all nucleated cells, serum, urine, and synovial fluid. Filtered at the glomerulus and almost entirely reabsorbed and catabolized by the proximal tubular cells.	Proximal tubule	Tubular injury marker in AKI and CKD. Increase in serum reflects the decrease in glomerular function in CKD. Elevated in cadmium toxicity, following cardiac surgery, liver and renal transplantation and idiopathic membranous nephropathy.
IL-18	18 kDa proinflammatory cytokine, activated via cleavage by caspase-1. Induced and cleaved mainly in the proximal tubules in human kidney and released into the urine.	Proximal tubule	Elevated urinary IL-18 levels are apparent in patients with kidney injury.
MCP-1	8.7 kDa protein of Chemotactic cytokine (chemokine) family. Produced in renal cells in response to proinflammatory cytokines.	Glomerular mesangial cells Podocytes Tubular epithelial cells	Expressed by renal cells following renal injury. Urinary MCP-1 is upregulated in inflammatory renal disease and diabetic nephropathy.

5. Current Use of Novel Biomarkers in CKDu Hotspots and Their Diagnostic Potential

5.1. Mesoamerica

Mesoamerican countries with CKDu include Mexico, Belize, Guatemala, El Salvador, Honduras, Nicaragua, Peru, and the northern part of Costa Rica. The first published study on Mesoamerican CKDu appeared in 2002, describing 205 newly dialyzed patients from 1999–2000 in El Salvador. As it is commonly observed today, the patients were predominantly men (87%), working in the sugarcane industry (63%), with an average age of 51 years. A majority of them (73%) had been exposed to agrochemicals. The cause of kidney failure was unknown, and it was proposed to be of toxic origin [62]. Subsequently, similar patients were recorded from several Mesoamerican countries. Among diverse Mesoamerican farming communities, impaired renal function has been characterized in terms of conventional renal biomarkers, including eGFR, SCr (serum creatinine), and ACR [63,64]. However, novel biomarkers are beginning to be used in Mesoamerica, and here we describe some of these studies, emphasizing their use and diagnostic potential (Figure 3).

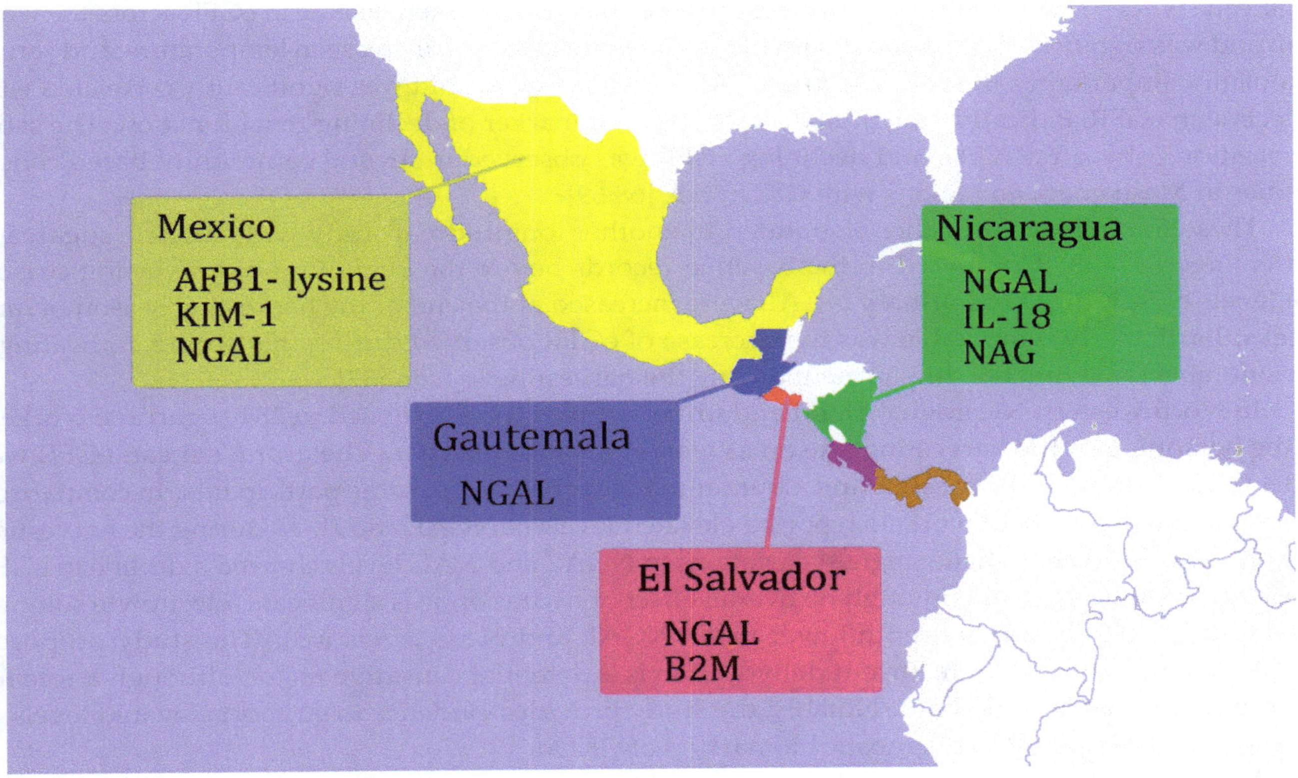

Figure 3. Overview of commonly used renal biomarkers for screening CKDu affected communities in the Mesoamerican region.

A recent study in a CKDu impacted community established renal dysfunction based on eGFR and urinary NGAL [65]. The population composed of 350 apparently healthy young adults in the age range 18–30 from affected areas in northwest Nicaragua, of whom 74% of participants were males working outdoors. Serum and urine creatinine, urinary albumin, urinary NGAL (uNGAL), serum cystatin C, and eGFR were monitored as diagnostic measures during the follow-up of two years. Based on the baseline eGFR values, participants were divided into three groups, group 1 (established renal dysfunction), group 2 (rapidly declining renal function), and group 3 (control). Group 1 individuals showed higher baseline uNGAL levels in comparison to other groups. Furthermore, 16% of group 1 and 4.7% of group 3 participants showed urinary ACR $\geq$ 30 mg/g. A model based only on a single eGFR measurement was predictive of renal dysfunction in group 1 compared to group 3, and the addition of uNGAL showed no improvement in predictive value. While looking for an effective model for predicting the decline in renal function, using eGFR at baseline, 6 months, and 12 months showed the best outcomes, and incorporation of uNGAL in the model showed the same predictive capacity. The findings indicate that a minimum follow-up period of one year with measurements starting from baseline and then at six-month intervals is necessary to differentiate between the progressive loss of eGFR and stable kidney function [66]. However, this study does not provide strong evidence for any added value of uNGAL in CKDu screening.

Similar findings were evident in a cross-sectional study with 189 sugar cane cutters (18–49 years old) in El Salvador. Elevated SCr and uric acid levels were commonly observed in both males and females. Reduced eGFR was observed in slightly older individuals. Elevated BUN levels, SCr, and uNGAL were observed in participants with proteinuria compared to the non-proteinuric. Serum creatinine, urea nitrogen, and uric acid showed significant cross-shift (during the work shift) increases. The participants' working hours were in the range 1.4 to 11 h and the day temperature ranged between 34 to 42 °C. Thus, recurrent dehydration from strenuous work under high heat exposure might be a factor for observed cross shift renal stress [30]. However, uNGAL decreased over their work shift. Similarly, Sorensen et al. (2019) [67] reported a significant decrease in uNGAL across Guatemalan sugarcane workers' work shift. This decrease was coupled to a marked decline in eGFR across the work shift and was significantly associated with BUN, increased uric acid, increase in temperature, and serum osmolality. Importantly, this increase in uNGAL across the work shift was significantly correlated with a decline in eGFR, indicating the utility of uNGAL as a marker of declining renal function. The same association between uNGAL and declining eGFR was observed in several community-based cohort studies in Mesoamerican regions with CKDu risk [68,69].

These findings were further elaborated in another longitudinal study with 29 male sugarcane cutters aged 17–38. Compared to the baseline records before the beginning of harvesting season, the levels of SCr, BUN and urinary NGAL were increased at the end of the harvesting season of nine weeks. Particularly remarkable was the decrease of eGFR observed during this period, indicating a considerable renal function impairment during the harvesting season [37].

In Northwestern Nicaragua, blood and urine samples were analyzed in 284 sugarcane workers at the beginning of the harvesting season as well as six months later. The group's mean eGFR was 113 mL/min/1.73 m^2 at the baseline and albuminuria was observed in some participants. In comparison to non-field workers, field workers reported elevated levels of NGAL and IL-18 during the harvesting season. Also, workers with the highest elevations in NGAL and NAG levels showed a decline in eGFR during harvesting season. Although no overall effect of hydration was significant, electrolyte solution consumption was associated with lower mean NGAL and NAG levels [69]. The study proposed that exposure to heat with recurrent dehydration is a potential causative factor, although a role for nephrotoxins was not ruled out. Notably, the study provides evidence to support elevated levels of NGAL, NAG, and IL-18 as diagnostic biomarkers of CKDu.

Novel and conventional biomarkers were used in another small descriptive study with 10 females diagnosed as CKDu stage 2 and 3 in El Salvador's agricultural communities. Their kidney biopsies showed renal damage restricted mostly to the tubulo-interstitium, and increased urinary excretion of B2M and NGAL was observed [70].

To investigate kidney disease initiation early in childhood, kidney injury biomarkers were assessed in 200 young school students aged 12–18 from different CKDu affected regions of Nicaragua. Comparisons were made with some schools located in CKDu risk areas. The presence of urinary glucose and protein, hemoglobinuria, and leucocyte esterase were rarely observed, while dysuria was common. A higher incidence of increased urine concentration was observed in girls compared to boys. Generally, NGAL, NAG, and IL-18 levels were significantly higher in boys than girls. However, higher NGAL levels were observed in leukocyte esterase positive girls and mean IL-18 levels were also higher in girls with hematuria [71]. Another recent study with 210 primary and secondary school students (7–17 years of age) from regions with a high prevalence of CKDu along the pacific coast of Nicaragua, reported consistent findings. Urinary KIM-1, NGAL, and IL-18 levels of the students were higher than those reported from healthy children in the USA and Poland. Although urinary monocyte chemoattractant protein 1 (MCP-1), and chitinase-3-like protein 1 (YKL-40) were assessed, researchers could not establish a clear association with renal function. However, girls reported significantly higher levels of these five biomarkers in urine than the boys [72], which notably contrasts the male predominance among CKDU patient cohorts [71,72]. However, this sex effect on renal injury and related biomarker expression, has not been adequately studied. Particularly elevated NGAL, NAG, KIM-1 and IL-18 levels in urine were observed in the students from regions with higher CKDu and adult mortality rates. This indicates the potential early onset of kidney disease in CKDu endemic areas and the potential to use these markers as early diagnostic tools. A similar risk of impaired renal function was observed in a study with 1058 boys and 1057 girls (age < 18 years) from CKDu regions in El Salvador using conventional markers [73]. These findings are also consistent with data on Sri Lankan children in CKDu endemic areas, where they are at a higher risk of kidney impairment [74]. These data strongly support a role for nephrotoxins potentially initiating the disease early on and further illustrate the critical need for markers predictive of early-stage renal damage and/or dysfunction.

While few studies have examined links between toxic insults and CKDu in Mesoamerica, novel biomarkers have rarely been used in this context. However, a recent pilot study in indigenous Mexican women measured their exposure to aflatoxin-B1 (AFB1) and was assessed using AFB1-lysine as a biomarker. AFB1-Lys was found in the majority of the study population, indicating a serious toxic exposure. There was also a strong significant correlation of AFB1-lysine with KIM-1 and Cystatin C expression, but not with NGAL [75].

In Mesoamerica, leptospirosis was also proposed as a possible causative factor underlying CKDu. In a study involving 282 sugarcane workers, 47 endemic controls, and 160 workers from other industries, Leptospira sero-positive individuals were higher among sugarcane cutters than other groups. These sero-positive individuals had higher NGAL expression than the sero-negative candidates, suggesting an association between leptospirosis and Mesoamerican nephropathy [76].

In summary, the use of novel biomarkers in Mesoamerica mainly focused on agricultural workers and other established conventional renal markers. Urinary NGAL was the most frequently used novel biomarker combined with other markers such as NAG and AFB1-lysine. While these biomarkers, with a few exceptions, generally followed tends demonstrated by conventional markers indicating their diagnostic potential, further studies are needed to confirm their prognostic value. Future studies may consider including one or more of the biomarkers discussed in this review to establish their use as early markers of CKDu risk potentially.

5.2. *Sri Lanka*

CKDu in Sri Lanka was first identified in the early 1990s among the farming communities in the Anuradhapura district. The disease was predominantly observed among the middle-aged male farmers [77]. Since its recognition, the disease has emerged as a significant threat to inhabitants in the agricultural communities in 11 districts [78] (Figure 4) in the country's dry zone. The disease is primarily characterized by conventional markers such as ACR, eGFR, and proteinuria [74,79], although recent studies have utilized novel biomarkers. Rathnayake et al. (2017) found Cystatin C as the best functional marker over creatinine and ACR in detecting CKDu in endemic regions in their attempt to select the best marker for community screening. However, the comparatively high analytical cost associated with Cystatin C (Supplementary Materials Table S1) tends to hinder its application in community screening [79]. Thus, identifying cost-effective novel biomarkers will be more economical for community screening, particularly with increasing disease prevalence.

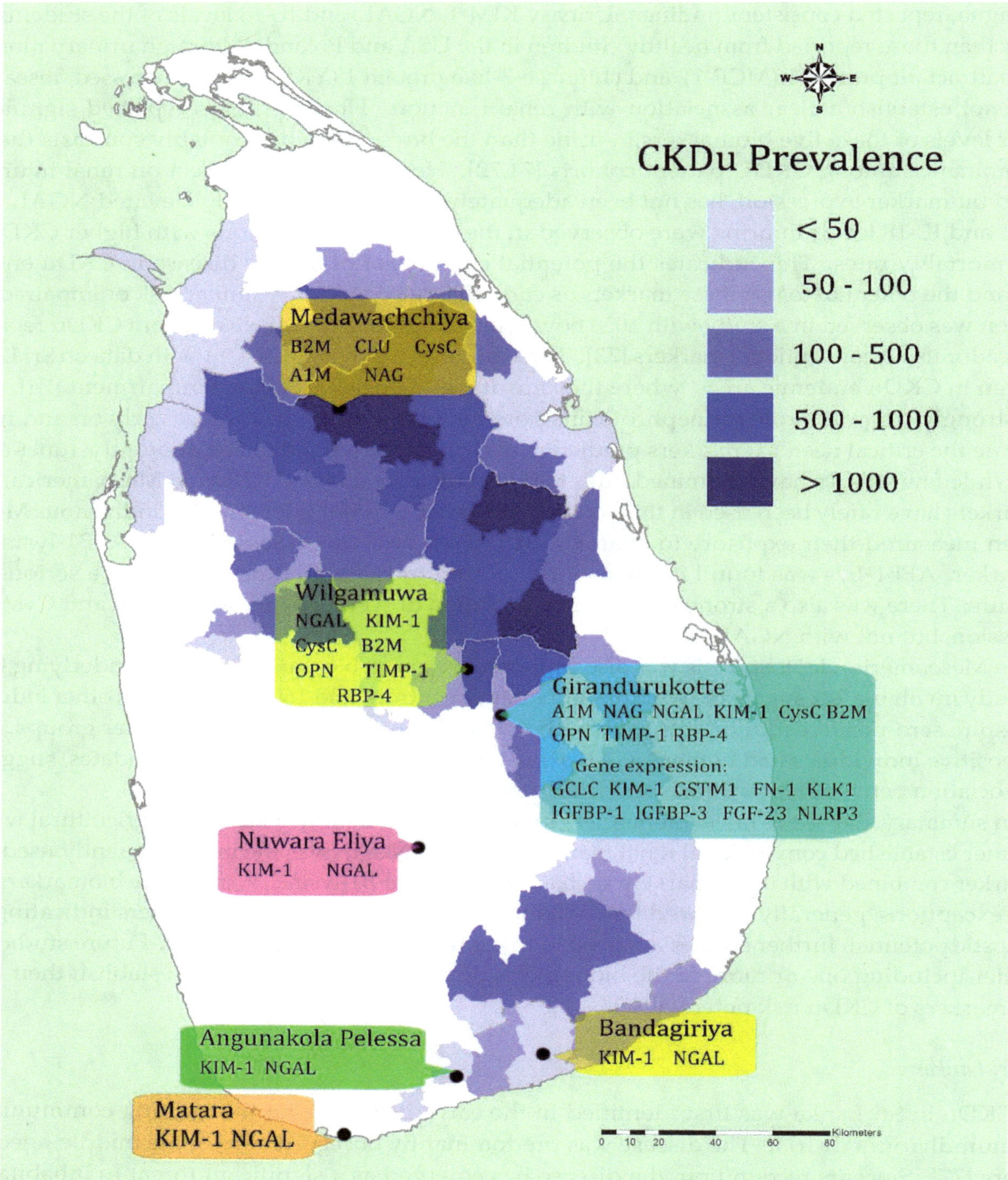

Figure 4. Regional distribution of CKDu in Sri Lanka and currently assessed biomarkers in different communities. Prevalence is illustrated in terms of the number of reported cases in the level of Divisional Secretariat Divisions.

The potential applicability of novel biomarkers KIM-1 and NGAL in CKDu characterization in Sri Lankan farming communities was first illustrated by De Silva et al. (2016) [80]. This study showed that NGAL and KIM-1 expression in urine is significantly correlated with high urinary ACR levels in the participants from CKDu endemic and emerging locations in comparison to healthy controls. Importantly, NGAL and KIM-1 levels were elevated in apparently healthy farmers with normal urinary ACR, indicating the potential early prognostic capacity of these markers in the CKDu context [77].

Elevated KIM-1 and NGAL were also found in CKDu non-endemic locations indicating early renal damage among rural farming communities.

Chung et al. (2017) [81] adopted a novel technique called micro-urine nanoparticle detection (μUNPD) and assessed urine samples of 42 candidates, including three acute kidney injury

(AKI) patients, 18 CKD patients from Western Province, and healthy participants from North Central Province in Sri Lanka. AKI patients showed an increase in urinary KIM-1 levels, and both KIM-1 and cystatin were elevated in CKD patients, suggesting that these biomarkers can be used for disease diagnosis.

In another study, a group of patients with CKD and CKDu from Girandurukotte (a CKDu endemic area) and healthy controls were examined for genetic biomarker-based differentiation of CKDu and CKD. Significant differences in expression of genes coding for insulin-like growth factor binding protein 1 (IGFBP1), KIM1, Glutathione-S-transferase mu 1 (GSTM1), glutamate-cysteine ligase catalytic subunit (GCLC) was observed in CKD and CKDu patients in varying degrees compared to healthy controls. In addition, significant correlations of differentially expressed genes with serum creatinine and, in turn, with eGFR were observed. The overall analysis suggested that a combined panel of IGFBP1, KIM1, GCLC, and GSTM1 genes could be used for early screening of CKDu and these genes in addition to fibronectin 1 (FN1), IGFBP3, and kallikrein 1 (KLK1) could be used for monitoring CKDu progression. However, further validation may be required prior to clinical use [82]. A similar study was conducted to assess gene expression changes associated with oxidative stress in CKD and CKDu patients in comparison to healthy controls from CKDu endemic and non-endemic areas. Compared to the controls from non-endemic areas, genes coding for glutamate-cysteine ligase catalytic subunit (GCLC), glutathioneS-transferasemu1 (GSTM1), fibroblast growth factor-23 (FGF23), and NLR family pyrin domain containing 3 (NLRP3) were upregulated in CKD and CKDu patients in varying degrees [83]. These studies indicate that redox imbalance may play a mechanistic role in initiation or progression of this disease, and oxidative stress markers may serve as early biomarkers of renal cellular dysfunction. However, oxidative stress markers are associated with many disease etiologies and may need significant validation prior to clinical use.

Several renal biomarkers' predictive performance was assessed in a recent cross-sectional study incorporating CKDu patients and CKD patients along with healthy controls from endemic and non-endemic areas. Compared to healthy controls, CKDu and CKD patients showed elevated median levels of several biomarkers including α1-microglobulin, β2-microglobulin, cystatin C, and retinol binding protein 4 (RBP4) and NGAL in varying degrees. Further, in terms of specificity and sensitivity, A1M, KIM1, and RBP4 were found to be the best minimum marker combination for differentiation of CKD and CKDu from healthy controls. OPN, KIM1, and RBP4 combination showed a high diagnostic value for CKDu and CKD patients [84].

A comparative cross-sectional study with 37 CKDu patients and control groups from CKDu endemic and non-endemic areas also showed significantly elevated levels of several urinary biomarkers, including fibrinogen, CLU, CysC, and B2M in CKDu patients. Fibrinogen and B2M were the most significant markers in distinguishing CKDu patients from healthy controls. Urinary fibrinogen and B2M also showed positive correlations with arsenic and urinary mercury levels, respectively. In workers with lead exposure, urinary KIM1 showed a better correlation with lead levels in blood [85].

Urinary levels of B2M were assessed in a study with 30 CKDu patients and 30 controls, who were matched for age and sex from Medawachchiya, a CKDu endemic area in Sri Lanka. Urinary B2M was significantly higher in CKDu patients, and the mean urinary B2M level of CKDu patients showed a gradual increase with the progression of the disease as indicated by the deterioration of renal function. The study aimed to evaluate the effect of staple foods such as rice on kidney dysfunction as defined by urinary B2M levels, but no link was detected [86]. Levels of urinary biomarkers and cadmium exposure were investigated with a group of 106 CKDu affected patients in North Central Province. A control group of non-affected blood relatives of the selected CKDu patients and non-affected individuals from Japan served as controls. When compared to controls, urinary A1M was observed at a significantly higher level in CKDu stage 1 and a steady increase was observed through CKDu stage 1 to 3 (defined as eGFR stratification). Urinary NAG levels showed a significant difference only in CKDu stage 5 patients, suggesting A1M may be a useful early stage renal disease marker. In comparison to Japanese controls, Sri Lankan participants reported remarkably low urinary cadmium levels, and no significant correlation was observed between the studied biomarkers and cadmium urine excretion. Familial clustering analysis with patients and their relatives strongly suggested a potential genetic predisposition to this disease [47].

In summary, the use of novel biomarkers in identifying CKDu in Sri Lanka is very promising. Several biomarkers have been utilized and a few of them (e.g., KIM-1, NGAL, A1M) can be used in a broad clinical set up. However, the sensitivity and specificity of the biomarkers warrant further studies. Additionally, most studies were focused on CKDu endemic locations, and the levels of biomarkers in healthy adult populations and children among the rural farming communities remain unclear. The use of novel markers in Sri Lanka may largely depend on future longitudinal cohort studies, where the markers' prognostic value could be further evaluated.

5.3. *India*

Characteristics of CKDu India share some similarities with that of CKDu patients in Sri Lanka and Mesoamerica. For example, a recent study with 2210 participants above 18 years of age reported a high prevalence of 18.23% of CKD in rural Indian communities in the Uddanam region. Importantly, 73% of the diagnosed CKD patients did not have diabetes, long-standing hypertension, or significant proteinuria (>1), indicating a higher prevalence of CKDu [26]. Most were farmers, and 55.7% of them were women. A creatinine level above 1.2 mg/dL was seen in 13%, and 59% were males. Low eGFR (<60) was seen in 13.9% of the population. Urinary protein creatinine ratio (more than 0.2) was seen in 9.04% and when eGFR and proteinuria were both taken together, 18.2% of the population was deemed to have CKD. However, none of India's published clinical studies on CKDu appeared to have utilized any of the novel biomarkers described in the current review.

5.4. *Egypt*

CKD has been identified in Egyptian communities via several studies. In a cohort of 587 children, CKD patients with stage one to five were detected. Obstructive uropathy, primary glomerulonephritis, reflux/urinary tract infection, aplasia/ hypoplasia, and familial/metabolic diseases were associated with renal dysfunction, while 20.6% of participants had no identified etiology, classifying them in CKDu [87]. In another study with 1004 known CKD patients in the El-Sharkia Governorate in Egypt, hypertension and diabetes were the main causes found, while 17.7% of participants were classified as CKDu [88]. However, no novel biomarker-based studies on CKDu in Egyptian communities are available in the literature.

5.5. *Indonesia*

A recent cross-sectional study with male rice farmers in Karawang and Bogor Regency, in West Java Province in Indonesia, evidenced the presence of CKDu. Out of the 354 healthy male farmers, the total CKD prevalence was 24.9%, and CKDu prevalence was 18.6% [11]. The determination was based on conventional markers, and no novel biomarker-based studies were reported from Indonesia.

6. Conclusions

CKDu has been clinically characterized using both novel and conventional biomarkers in many of the impacted regions. Within the spectrum of clinical findings, a variety of factors, including heavy metals, heat stress, agrochemicals, nephrotoxins, infections, geography, and socio-economic factors appear to be contributing to CKDu. The significance of each factor may vary depending on the patient population, and the continuous use of conventional and novel biomarkers will contribute to an improved understanding of this disease.

To date, SCr, eGFR, Cys-C, and ACR have been used extensively for screening. Considering studies on different communities with CKDu, a decline in eGFR was observed along with elevated SCr and BUN levels. Although these markers appear valid when distinguishing prospective patients, they are suboptimal when evaluating kidney health in cross-sectional studies. To this end, longitudinal studies will identify and validate biomarkers that may predict renal outcomes. For example, in some Mesoamerican studies, a decline in renal function is characterized by reduced eGFR, increased SCr, BUN, and novel biomarkers. However, these studies did not examine chronicity or progressive decline in renal function over a considerable period. It is possible that participants of some of the Mesoamerican studies could have had reduced renal function with normal serum creatinine at the entry to the study, and the elevation of serum creatinine in response to dehydration may have been an epiphenomenon of underlying CKD rather than the cause of CKDu. Therefore, more longitudinal studies with longer follow-up using multiple renal biomarkers will help unravel such confounding factors and provide more insights into the validity of the marker and potential causative factors.

In addition to early predictive markers, it is critical to have markers with higher sensitivity and specificity to define CKDu pathology. The most common traditional markers such as SCr, proteinuria, ACR, and eGFR are quite useful in determining renal impairment and renal function variation over time. However, these are generic markers that indicate renal impairment and are not informative on the damage's nature. The novel biomarkers discussed in this review have begun to gain importance in the clinical setting for their rapid and site-specific expression. For example, biomarkers such as KIM-1 and NGAL become detectable in renal damage earlier than detectable changes in creatinine and eGFR. NGAL is especially becoming recognized as a biomarker for monitoring CKD progression. However, each biomarker has different pathologies, and therefore a panel of defined biomarkers would be more revealing in clinical screening for CKD or CKDu. Validation and establishment of reference levels for novel biomarkers such as CysC, NGAL, and KIM-1, some of which are potentially important in the diagnosis of prerenal dysfunction [89], and other lesser-known biomarkers such as insulin-like growth factor binding protein (IGFBP) that could possibly predict renal recovery [90], would be useful in demonstrating the AKI-CKD continuum in agricultural workers.

While it is clear that the use of strategic batteries of biomarkers with diagnostic, monitoring, predictive, prognostic and/or susceptibility/risk characteristics is needed to detect better, monitor, and risk screening CKDu endemic regions, costs of these may become prohibitive. Many of the novel biomarkers discussed here remain inaccessible in low resource settings (Supplementary Materials Table S1), primarily due to lack of equipment and high costs per sample. In fact, to date, no novel biomarker has been incorporated beyond the research level into clinical laboratories for public access at affordable rates. The currently available analytical techniques, most commonly Enzyme Linked Immunosorbent Assays (ELISA), are expensive and time-consuming compared to conventional markers. Therefore, although a large spectrum of potential novel biomarkers has emerged in recent years, their value in clinical application is yet to be established, especially in the context of CKDu. This indicates that, in addition to advancements in high throughput technologies (e.g., proteomics), sample conditioning, and analytical trajectories in search of superior biomarkers for renal diseases, efforts to reduce the cost of analysis of existing novel biomarkers are also critical. For example, with the emergence of CKDu cases in Sri Lanka, governmental and non-governmental efforts helped implement clinical laboratory facilities in rural settings to assess conventional markers such as creatinine and microalbumin. Upon recognizing the potential value of novel biomarkers, local authorities and practitioners can play an important role in soliciting equipment and resources to be added to these locations enabling other biomarker assays.

Finally, as CKDu is largely non-proteinuric with normal creatinine levels in the earlier phases, conventional tests are likely missing opportunities to diagnose this disease early. Although CKDu is commonly diagnosed in adults, children in CKDu prevalent communities are also at risk, as shown in

Nicaragua [71,72] and Sri Lanka [74]. This critical situation highlights the paramount importance of detailed and intensive studies for characterizing the early development of CKDu. Longitudinal studies involving children cohorts may provide ideal follow-up studies to identify biomarkers with improved predictability and may complement ongoing efforts to validate the prognostic power of novel renal biomarkers before translation into broad clinical practices. Nonetheless, we emphasize that the use of these markers in CKDu impacted communities warrants greater attention, since they may be the key to mitigating this complex disease.

Author Contributions: T.D.K.S.C.G. and P.M.C.S.D.S. collated all the information, developed the figures, and developed the initial draft. N.J. provided extensive edits and reviewed the manuscript. C.H., S.S., N.S., C.J., S.J. and M.C.-G. contributed equally to reviewing existing biomarkers associated with kidney disease and edited and revised the manuscript over multiple iterations. All authors have read and agreed to the published version of the manuscript.

Acknowledgments: We thank all our laboratory members for their continuous support and helpful feedback.

Abbreviations

A1M	α1-microglobulin.
ACR	albumin–creatinine ratio
AFB1	aflatoxin-B1
AKI	acute kidney injury
B2M	β2- macroglobulin
BUN	blood urea nitrogen
CKD	chronic kidney disease
CKDu	chronic kidney disease of unknown etiology
CLU	clusterin
CysC	cystatin-C
DALYS	disability-adjusted life years
eGFR	estimated glomerular filtration rate
FDA	food and drug administration
FN1	fibronectin- 1
GCLC	glutamate-cysteine ligase catalytic
GFR	glomerular filtration rate
GSTM1	glutathione-S-transferase mu 1
HGF	hepatocyte growth factor
HIV	human immune virus
IGFBP	insulin-like growth factor binding protein
IL-18	interleukin-18
KDIGO	Kidney disease: improving global outcomes
KIM-1	kidney injury molecule -1
L-FABP	liver type fatty acid binding protein
KLK1	kallikrein-1
NAG	N-acetyl-beta-D-glucosaminidase
NGAL	neutrophil gelatinase-associated lipocalin
NIH	National Institutes of Health
NLR	nod-like receptor
NLRP3	NLR family pyrin domain containing 3

Abbreviations

OPN	osteopontin
Pi-GST	glutathione S-transferase

RBP	retinol binding protein
RRT	renal replacement therapy
SCR	serum creatinine
TIMP-2	tissue inhibitor metalloproteinase-2
uNGAL	urinary neutrophil gelatinase-associated lipocalin
μUNPD	micro-urine nano particle detection

References

1. Inker, L.A.; Astor, B.C.; Fox, C.H.; Isakova, T.; Lash, J.P.; Peralta, C.A.; Kurella Tamura, M.; Feldman, H.I. KDOQI US Commentary on the 2012 KDIGO Clinical Practice Guideline for the Evaluation and Management of CKD. *Am. J. Kidney Dis.* **2014**, *63*, 713–735. [CrossRef] [PubMed]
2. Barsoum, R.S. Chronic Kidney Disease in the Developing World. *N. Engl. J. Med.* **2006**, *354*, 997–999. [CrossRef] [PubMed]
3. Jha, V.; Garcia-Garcia, G.; Iseki, K.; Li, Z.; Naicker, S.; Plattner, B.; Saran, R.; Wang, A.Y.-M.; Yang, C.-W. Chronic Kidney Disease: Global Dimension and Perspectives. *Lancet Lond. Engl.* **2013**, *382*, 260–272. [CrossRef]
4. Murray, C.J.L.; Barber, R.M.; Foreman, K.J.; Lopez, A.D.; Vos, T.; GBD 2013 DALYs and HALE Collaborators. Global, Regional, and National Disability-Adjusted Life Years (DALYs) for 306 Diseases and Injuries and Healthy Life Expectancy (HALE) for 188 Countries, 1990–2013: Quantifying the Epidemiological Transition. *Lancet Lond. Engl.* **2015**, *386*, 2145–2191. [CrossRef]
5. Mendley, S.R.; Levin, A.; Correa-Rotter, R.; Joubert, B.R.; Whelan, E.A.; Curwin, B.; Koritzinsky, E.H.; Gaughan, D.M.; Kimmel, P.L.; Anand, S.; et al. Chronic Kidney Diseases in Agricultural Communities: Report from a Workshop. *Kidney Int.* **2019**, *96*, 1071–1076. [CrossRef]
6. Vervaet, B.A.; Nast, C.C.; Jayasumana, C.; Schreurs, G.; Roels, F.; Herath, C.; Kojc, N.; Samaee, V.; Rodrigo, S.; Gowrishankar, S.; et al. Chronic Interstitial Nephritis in Agricultural Communities is a Toxin-Induced Proximal Tubular Nephropathy. *Kidney Int.* **2020**, *97*, 350–369. [CrossRef]
7. Athuraliya, N.T.C.; Abeysekera, T.D.J.; Amerasinghe, P.H.; Kumarasiri, R.; Bandara, P.; Karunaratne, U.; Milton, A.H.; Jones, A.L. Uncertain Etiologies of Proteinuric-Chronic Kidney Disease in Rural Sri Lanka. *Kidney Int.* **2011**, *80*, 1212–1221. [CrossRef]
8. González-Quiroz, M.; Pearce, N.; Caplin, B.; Nitsch, D. What Do Epidemiological Studies Tell Us about Chronic Kidney Disease of Undetermined Cause in Meso-America? A Systematic Review and Meta-Analysis. *Clin. Kidney J.* **2018**, *11*, 496–506. [CrossRef]
9. Gifford, F.J.; Gifford, R.M.; Eddleston, M.; Dhaun, N. Endemic Nephropathy Around the World. *Kidney Int. Rep.* **2017**, *2*, 282–292. [CrossRef]
10. Jha, V.; Ur-Rashid, H.; Agarwal, S.K.; Akhtar, S.F.; Kafle, R.K.; Sheriff, R. ISN South Asia Regional Board. The State of Nephrology in South Asia. *Kidney Int.* **2019**, *95*, 31–37. [CrossRef]
11. Fitria, L.; Prihartono, N.A.; Ramdhan, D.H.; Wahyono, T.Y.M.; Kongtip, P.; Woskie, S. Environmental and Occupational Risk Factors Associated with Chronic Kidney Disease of Unknown Etiology in West Javanese Rice Farmers, Indonesia. *Int. J. Environ. Res. Public. Health* **2020**, *17*, 4521. [CrossRef]
12. Glaser, J.; Lemery, J.; Rajagopalan, B.; Diaz, H.F.; García-Trabanino, R.; Taduri, G.; Madero, M.; Amarasinghe, M.; Abraham, G.; Anutrakulchai, S.; et al. Climate Change and the Emergent Epidemic of CKD from Heat Stress in Rural Communities: The Case for Heat Stress Nephropathy. *Clin. J. Am. Soc. Nephrol.* **2016**, *11*, 1472–1483. [CrossRef] [PubMed]
13. McKinley, J.M.; Mueller, U.; Atkinson, P.M.; Ofterdinger, U.; Cox, S.F.; Doherty, R.; Fogarty, D.; Egozcue, J.J.; Pawlowsky-Glahn, V. Chronic Kidney Disease of Unknown Origin Is Associated with Environmental Urbanisation in Belfast, UK. *Environ. Geochem. Health* **2020**. [CrossRef] [PubMed]
14. Jayasumana, C.; Orantes, C.; Herrera, R.; Almaguer, M.; Lopez, L.; Silva, L.C.; Ordunez, P.; Siribaddana, S.; Gunatilake, S.; De Broe, M.E. Chronic Interstitial Nephritis in Agricultural Communities: A Worldwide Epidemic with Social, Occupational and Environmental Determinants. *Nephrol. Dial. Transpl.* **2017**, *32*, 234–241. [CrossRef]
15. Wijkström, J.; Jayasumana, C.; Dassanayake, R.; Priyawardane, N.; Godakanda, N.; Siribaddana, S.; Ring, A.;

Hultenby, K.; Söderberg, M.; Elinder, C.-G.; et al. Morphological and Clinical Findings in Sri Lankan Patients with Chronic Kidney Disease of Unknown Cause (CKDu): Similarities and Differences with Mesoamerican Nephropathy. *PLoS ONE* **2018**, *13*, e0193056. [CrossRef]

16. Ranasinghe, A.V.; Kumara, G.W.G.P.; Karunarathna, R.H.; De Silva, A.P.; Sachintani, K.G.D.; Gunawardena, J.M.C.N.; Kumari, S.K.C.R.; Sarjana, M.S.F.; Chandraguptha, J.S.; De Silva, M.V.C. The Incidence, Prevalence and Trends of Chronic Kidney Disease and Chronic Kidney Disease of Uncertain Aetiology (CKDu) in the North Central Province of Sri Lanka: An Analysis of 30,566 Patients. *BMC Nephrol.* **2019**, *20*, 338. [CrossRef]
17. Ruwanpathirana, T.; Senanayake, S.; Gunawardana, N.; Munasinghe, A.; Ginige, S.; Gamage, D.; Amarasekara, J.; Lokuketagoda, B.; Chulasiri, P.; Amunugama, S.; et al. Prevalence and Risk Factors for Impaired Kidney Function in the District of Anuradhapura, Sri Lanka: A Cross-Sectional Population-Representative Survey in Those at Risk of Chronic Kidney Disease of Unknown Aetiology. *BMC Public Health* **2019**, *19*, 763. [CrossRef]
18. Selvarajah, M.; Weeratunga, P.; Sivayoganthan, S.; Rathnatunga, N.; Rajapakse, S. Clinicopathological Correlates of Chronic Kidney Disease of Unknown Etiology in Sri Lanka. *Indian J. Nephrol.* **2016**, *26*, 357–363. [CrossRef]
19. Nanayakkara, S.; Komiya, T.; Ratnatunga, N.; Senevirathna, S.T.M.L.D.; Harada, K.H.; Hitomi, T.; Gobe, G.; Muso, E.; Abeysekera, T.; Koizumi, A. Tubulointerstitial Damage as the Major Pathological Lesion in Endemic Chronic Kidney Disease among Farmers in North Central Province of Sri Lanka. *Environ. Health Prev. Med.* **2012**, *17*, 213–221. [CrossRef]
20. López-Marín, L.; Chávez, Y.; García, X.A.; Flores, W.M.; García, Y.M.; Herrera, R.; Almaguer, M.; Orantes, C.M.; Calero, D.; Bayarre, H.D.; et al. Histopathology of Chronic Kidney Disease of Unknown Etiology in Salvadoran Agricultural Communities. *Med. Rev.* **2014**, *16*, 49–54.
21. Cohen, J. Mesoamerica's Mystery Killer. *Science* **2014**, *344*, 143–147. [CrossRef] [PubMed]
22. Wanigasuriya, K. Update on Uncertain Etiology of Chronic Kidney Disease in Sri Lanka's North-Central Dry Zone. *Med. Rev.* **2014**, *16*, 61–65.
23. Murray, C.J.L.; Lopez, A.D. Measuring the Global Burden of Disease. *N. Engl. J. Med.* **2013**, *369*, 448–457. [CrossRef] [PubMed]
24. GBD Chronic Kidney Disease Collaboration. Global, Regional, and National Burden of Chronic Kidney Disease, 1990-2017: A Systematic Analysis for the Global Burden of Disease Study 2017. *Lancet Lond. Engl.* **2020**, *395*, 709–733. [CrossRef]
25. Fernando, B.N.T.W.; Sudeshika, T.S.H.; Hettiarachchi, T.W.; Badurdeen, Z.; Abeysekara, T.D.J.; Abeysundara, H.T.K.; Jayasinghe, S.; Ranasighe, S.; Nanayakkara, N. Evaluation of Biochemical Profile of Chronic Kidney Disease of Uncertain Etiology in Sri Lanka. *PLoS ONE* **2020**, *15*, e0232522. [CrossRef]
26. Tatapudi, R.R.; Rentala, S.; Gullipalli, P.; Komarraju, A.L.; Singh, A.K.; Tatapudi, V.S.; Goru, K.B.; Bhimarasetty, D.M.; Narni, H. High Prevalence of CKD of Unknown Etiology in Uddanam, India. *Kidney Int. Rep.* **2019**, *4*, 380–389. [CrossRef]
27. Lebov, J.F.; Valladares, E.; Peña, R.; Peña, E.M.; Sanoff, S.L.; Cisneros, E.C.; Colindres, R.E.; Morgan, D.R.; Hogan, S.L. A Population-Based Study of Prevalence and Risk Factors of Chronic Kidney Disease in León, Nicaragua. *Can. J. Kidney Health Dis.* **2015**, *2*, 6. [CrossRef]
28. Jayasumana, C.; Paranagama, P.; Agampodi, S.; Wijewardane, C.; Gunatilake, S.; Siribaddana, S. Drinking Well Water and Occupational Exposure to Herbicides Is Associated with Chronic Kidney Disease, in Padavi-Sripura, Sri Lanka. *Environ. Health Glob. Access Sci. Source* **2015**, *14*, 6. [CrossRef]
29. Babich, R.; Ulrich, J.C.; Ekanayake, E.M.D.V.; Massarsky, A.; De Silva, P.M.C.S.; Manage, P.M.; Jackson, B.P.; Ferguson, P.L.; Di Giulio, R.T.; Drummond, I.A.; et al. Kidney Developmental Effects of Metal-Herbicide Mixtures: Implications for Chronic Kidney Disease of Unknown Etiology. *Environ. Int.* **2020**, *144*, 106019. [CrossRef]
30. García-Trabanino, R.; Jarquín, E.; Wesseling, C.; Johnson, R.J.; González-Quiroz, M.; Weiss, I.; Glaser, J.; José Vindell, J.; Stockfelt, L.; Roncal, C.; et al. Heat Stress, Dehydration, and Kidney Function in Sugarcane Cutters in El Salvador—A Cross-Shift Study of Workers at Risk of Mesoamerican Nephropathy. *Environ. Res.* **2015**, *142*, 746–755. [CrossRef]
31. Roncal-Jimenez, C.; Lanaspa, M.A.; Jensen, T.; Sanchez-Lozada, L.G.; Johnson, R.J. Mechanisms by Which

Dehydration May Lead to Chronic Kidney Disease. *Ann. Nutr. Metab.* **2015**, *66* (Suppl. 3), 10–13. [CrossRef] [PubMed]

32. Xing, W.M.; Yuan, T.J.; Xu, J.D.; Gu, L.L.; Liang, P.; Lu, H. Proteomic Identification of Mitochondrial Targets Involved in Andrographolide Sodium Bisulfite-Induced Nephrotoxicity in a Rat Model. *Environ. Toxicol. Pharm.* **2015**, *40*, 592–599. [CrossRef] [PubMed]
33. Perera, T.; Ranasinghe, S.; Alles, N.; Waduge, R. Experimental Rat Model for Acute Tubular Injury Induced by High Water Hardness and High Water Fluoride: Efficacy of Primary Preventive Intervention by Distilled Water Administration. *BMC Nephrol.* **2020**, *21*, 103. [CrossRef] [PubMed]
34. Roncal-Jimenez, C.; García-Trabanino, R.; Barregard, L.; Lanaspa, M.A.; Wesseling, C.; Harra, T.; Aragón, A.; Grases, F.; Jarquin, E.R.; González, M.A.; et al. Heat Stress Nephropathy from Exercise-Induced Uric Acid Crystalluria: A Perspective on Mesoamerican Nephropathy. *Am. J. Kidney Dis.* **2016**, *67*, 20–30. [CrossRef] [PubMed]
35. Yang, C.-W. Leptospirosis Renal Disease: Emerging Culprit of Chronic Kidney Disease Unknown Etiology. *Nephron* **2018**, *138*, 129–136. [CrossRef] [PubMed]
36. Nanayakkara, S.; Senevirathna, S.T.M.L.D.; Parahitiyawa, N.B.; Abeysekera, T.; Chandrajith, R.; Ratnatunga, N.; Hitomi, T.; Kobayashi, H.; Harada, K.H.; Koizumi, A. Whole-Exome Sequencing Reveals Genetic Variants Associated with Chronic Kidney Disease Characterized by Tubulointerstitial Damages in North Central Region, Sri Lanka. *Environ. Health Prev. Med.* **2015**, *20*, 354–359. [CrossRef] [PubMed]
37. Wesseling, C.; Aragón, A.; González, M.; Weiss, I.; Glaser, J.; Bobadilla, N.A.; Roncal-Jiménez, C.; Correa-Rotter, R.; Johnson, R.J.; Barregard, L. Kidney Function in Sugarcane Cutters in Nicaragua—A Longitudinal Study of Workers at Risk of Mesoamerican Nephropathy. *Environ. Res.* **2016**, *147*, 125–132. [CrossRef] [PubMed]
38. Correa-Rotter, R.; Wesseling, C.; Johnson, R.J. CKD of Unknown Origin in Central America: The Case for a Mesoamerican Nephropathy. *Am. J. Kidney Dis.* **2014**, *63*, 506–520. [CrossRef] [PubMed]
39. Lunyera, J.; Mohottige, D.; Von Isenburg, M.; Jeuland, M.; Patel, U.D.; Stanifer, J.W. CKD of Uncertain Etiology: A Systematic Review. *Clin. J. Am. Soc. Nephrol.* **2016**, *11*, 379–385. [CrossRef] [PubMed]
40. Wesseling, C.; Aragón, A.; González, M.; Weiss, I.; Glaser, J.; Rivard, C.J.; Roncal-Jiménez, C.; Correa-Rotter, R.; Johnson, R.J. Heat Stress, Hydration and Uric Acid: A Cross-Sectional Study in Workers of Three Occupations in a Hotspot of Mesoamerican Nephropathy in Nicaragua. *BMJ Open* **2016**, *6*, e011034. [CrossRef]
41. VanDervort, D.R.; López, D.L.; Orantes, C.M.; Rodríguez, D.S. Spatial Distribution of Unspecified Chronic Kidney Disease in El Salvador by Crop Area Cultivated and Ambient Temperature. *Med. Rev.* **2014**, *16*, 31–38.
42. Herath, C.; Jayasumana, C.; De Silva, P.M.C.S.; De Silva, P.H.C.; Siribaddana, S.; De Broe, M.E. Kidney Diseases in Agricultural Communities: A Case Against Heat-Stress Nephropathy. *Kidney Int. Rep.* **2018**, *3*, 271–280. [CrossRef]
43. Weaver, V.M.; Fadrowski, J.J.; Jaar, B.G. Global Dimensions of Chronic Kidney Disease of Unknown Etiology (CKDu): A Modern Era Environmental and/or Occupational Nephropathy? *BMC Nephrol.* **2015**, *16*, 145. [CrossRef] [PubMed]
44. Petejova, N.; Martinek, A.; Zadrazil, J.; Teplan, V. Acute Toxic Kidney Injury. *Ren. Fail.* **2019**, *41*, 576–594. [CrossRef] [PubMed]
45. Orr, S.E.; Bridges, C.C. Chronic Kidney Disease and Exposure to Nephrotoxic Metals. *Int. J. Mol. Sci.* **2017**, 18. [CrossRef]
46. Nanayakkara, S.; Senevirathna, S.T.M.L.D.; Harada, K.H.; Chandrajith, R.; Hitomi, T.; Abeysekera, T.; Muso, E.; Watanabe, T.; Koizumi, A. Systematic Evaluation of Exposure to Trace Elements and Minerals in Patients with Chronic Kidney Disease of Uncertain Etiology (CKDu) in Sri Lanka. *J. Trace Elem. Med. Biol.* **2019**, *54*, 206–213. [CrossRef] [PubMed]
47. Nanayakkara, S.; Senevirathna, S.T.M.L.D.; Karunaratne, U.; Chandrajith, R.; Harada, K.H.; Hitomi, T.; Watanabe, T.; Abeysekera, T.; Aturaliya, T.N.C.; Koizumi, A. Evidence of Tubular Damage in the Very Early Stage of Chronic Kidney Disease of Uncertain Etiology in the North Central Province of Sri Lanka: A Cross-Sectional Study. *Environ. Health Prev. Med.* **2012**, *17*, 109–117. [CrossRef]
48. Kim, N.H.; Hyun, Y.Y.; Lee, K.-B.; Chang, Y.; Ryu, S.; Rhu, S.; Oh, K.-H.; Ahn, C. Environmental Heavy Metal Exposure and Chronic Kidney Disease in the General Population. *J. Korean Med. Sci.* **2015**, *30*, 272–277. [CrossRef]

49. Chandrajith, R.; Dissanayake, C.B.; Ariyarathna, T.; Herath, H.M.J.M.K.; Padmasiri, J.P. Dose-Dependent Na and Ca in Fluoride-Rich Drinking Water–Another Major Cause of Chronic Renal Failure in Tropical Arid Regions. *Sci. Total Environ.* **2011**, *409*, 671–675. [CrossRef]
50. Vanherweghem, J.L.; Depierreux, M.; Tielemans, C.; Abramowicz, D.; Dratwa, M.; Jadoul, M.; Richard, C.; Vandervelde, D.; Verbeelen, D.; Vanhaelen-Fastre, R. Rapidly Progressive Interstitial Renal Fibrosis in Young Women: Association with Slimming Regimen Including Chinese Herbs. *Lancet Lond. Engl.* **1993**, *341*, 387–391. [CrossRef]
51. Debelle, F.D.; Vanherweghem, J.-L.; Nortier, J.L. Aristolochic Acid Nephropathy: A Worldwide Problem. *Kidney Int.* **2008**, *74*, 158–169. [CrossRef] [PubMed]
52. Depierreux, M.; Van Damme, B.; Vanden Houte, K.; Vanherweghem, J.L. Pathologic Aspects of a Newly Described Nephropathy Related to the Prolonged Use of Chinese Herbs. *Am. J. Kidney Dis.* **1994**, *24*, 172–180. [CrossRef]
53. Cosyns, J.P.; Dehoux, J.P.; Guiot, Y.; Goebbels, R.M.; Robert, A.; Bernard, A.M.; van Ypersele de Strihou, C. Chronic Aristolochic Acid Toxicity in Rabbits: A Model of Chinese Herbs Nephropathy? *Kidney Int.* **2001**, *59*, 2164–2173. [CrossRef]
54. Sato, N.; Takahashi, D.; Chen, S.-M.; Tsuchiya, R.; Mukoyama, T.; Yamagata, S.; Ogawa, M.; Yoshida, M.; Kondo, S.; Satoh, N.; et al. Acute Nephrotoxicity of Aristolochic Acids in Mice. *J. Pharm. Pharmacol.* **2004**, *56*, 221–229. [CrossRef] [PubMed]
55. Gamage, C.D.; Yoshimatsu, K.; Sarathkumara, Y.D.; Kulendiran, T.; Nanayakkara, N.; Arikawa, J. Serological Evidence of Hantavirus Infection in Girandurukotte, an Area Endemic for Chronic Kidney Disease of Unknown Aetiology (CKDu) in Sri Lanka. *Int. J. Infect. Dis.* **2017**, *57*, 77–78. [CrossRef]
56. FDA-NIH Biomarker Working Group. *BEST (Biomarkers, EndpointS, and Other Tools) Resource*; Food and Drug Administration (US): Silver Spring, MD, USA; National Institutes of Health (US): Bethesda, MD, USA, 2020.
57. Etzioni, R.; Urban, N.; Ramsey, S.; McIntosh, M.; Schwartz, S.; Reid, B.; Radich, J.; Anderson, G.; Hartwell, L. The Case for Early Detection. *Nat. Rev. Cancer* **2003**, *3*, 243–252. [CrossRef]
58. Yu, A.; Chertow, G.; Luyckx, V.; Marsden, P.; Skorecki, K.; Taal, M. *Brenner & Rector's the Kidney*, 11th ed.; Elsevier Inc: Philadelphia, PA, USA, 2019.
59. Ostermann, M.; Philips, B.J.; Forni, L.G. Clinical Review: Biomarkers of Acute Kidney Injury: Where Are We Now? *Crit. Care Lond. Engl.* **2012**, *16*, 233. [CrossRef]
60. Murray, P.T.; Mehta, R.L.; Shaw, A.; Ronco, C.; Endre, Z.; Kellum, J.A.; Chawla, L.S.; Cruz, D.; Ince, C.; Okusa, M.D.; et al. Potential Use of Biomarkers in Acute Kidney Injury: Report and Summary of Recommendations from the 10th Acute Dialysis Quality Initiative Consensus Conference. *Kidney Int.* **2014**, *85*, 513–521. [CrossRef]
61. Food and Drug Administration US (FDA). *List of Qualified Biomarkers*; FDA: Silver Spring, MD, USA, 2020.
62. Trabanino, R.G.; Aguilar, R.; Silva, C.R.; Mercado, M.O.; Merino, R.L. End-stage renal disease among patients in a referral hospital in El Salvador. *Rev. Panam. Salud Publica* **2002**, *12*, 202–206. [CrossRef]
63. Torres, C.; Aragón, A.; González, M.; López, I.; Jakobsson, K.; Elinder, C.-G.; Lundberg, I.; Wesseling, C. Decreased Kidney Function of Unknown Cause in Nicaragua: A Community-Based Survey. *Am. J. Kidney Dis.* **2010**, *55*, 485–496. [CrossRef]
64. Sanoff, S.L.; Callejas, L.; Alonso, C.D.; Hu, Y.; Colindres, R.E.; Chin, H.; Morgan, D.R.; Hogan, S.L. Positive Association of Renal Insufficiency with Agriculture Employment and Unregulated Alcohol Consumption in Nicaragua. *Ren. Fail.* **2010**, *32*, 766–777. [CrossRef]
65. González-Quiroz, M.; Camacho, A.; Faber, D.; Aragón, A.; Wesseling, C.; Glaser, J.; Le Blond, J.; Smeeth, L.; Nitsch, D.; Pearce, N.; et al. Rationale, Description and Baseline Findings of a Community-Based Prospective Cohort Study of Kidney Function amongst the Young Rural Population of Northwest Nicaragua. *BMC Nephrol.* **2017**, *18*, 16. [CrossRef]
66. Gonzalez-Quiroz, M.; Smpokou, E.-T.; Pearce, N.; Caplin, B.; Nitsch, D. Identification of Young Adults at Risk of an Accelerated Loss of Kidney Function in an Area Affected by Mesoamerican Nephropathy. *BMC Nephrol.* **2019**, *20*, 21. [CrossRef] [PubMed]
67. Sorensen, C.J.; Butler-Dawson, J.; Dally, M.; Krisher, L.; Griffin, B.R.; Johnson, R.J.; Lemery, J.; Asensio, C.; Tenney, L.; Newman, L.S. Risk Factors and Mechanisms Underlying Cross-Shift Decline in Kidney Function in Guatemalan Sugarcane Workers. *J. Occup. Environ. Med.* **2019**, *61*, 239–250. [CrossRef]

68. Gonzalez-Quiroz, M.; Smpokou, E.-T.; Silverwood, R.J.; Camacho, A.; Faber, D.; Garcia, B.L.R.; Oomatia, A.; Hill, M.; Glaser, J.; Le Blond, J.; et al. Decline in Kidney Function among Apparently Healthy Young Adults at Risk of Mesoamerican Nephropathy. *J. Am. Soc. Nephrol.* **2018**, *29*, 2200–2212. [CrossRef] [PubMed]
69. Laws, R.L.; Brooks, D.R.; Amador, J.J.; Weiner, D.E.; Kaufman, J.S.; Ramírez-Rubio, O.; Riefkohl, A.; Scammell, M.K.; López-Pilarte, D.; Sánchez, J.M.; et al. Biomarkers of Kidney Injury Among Nicaraguan Sugarcane Workers. *Am. J. Kidney Dis.* **2016**, *67*, 209–217. [CrossRef] [PubMed]
70. Herrera Valdés, R.; Orantes, C.M.; Almaguer López, M.; López Marín, L.; Arévalo, P.A.; Smith González, M.J.; Morales, F.E.; Bacallao, R.; Bayarre, H.D.; Vela Parada, X.F. Clinical Characteristics of Chronic Kidney Disease of Non-Traditional Causes in Women of Agricultural Communities in El Salvador. *Clin. Nephrol.* **2015**, *83* (Suppl. 1), 56–63. [CrossRef]
71. Ramírez-Rubio, O.; Amador, J.J.; Kaufman, J.S.; Weiner, D.E.; Parikh, C.R.; Khan, U.; McClean, M.D.; Laws, R.L.; López-Pilarte, D.; Friedman, D.J.; et al. Urine Biomarkers of Kidney Injury among Adolescents in Nicaragua, a Region Affected by an Epidemic of Chronic Kidney Disease of Unknown Aetiology. *Nephrol. Dial. Transpl.* **2016**, *31*, 424–432. [CrossRef] [PubMed]
72. Leibler, J.H.; Ramirez-Rubio, O.; Velázquez, J.J.A.; Pilarte, D.L.; Obeid, W.; Parikh, C.R.; Gadupudi, S.; Scammell, M.K.; Friedman, D.J.; Brooks, D.R. Biomarkers of Kidney Injury among Children in a High-Risk Region for Chronic Kidney Disease of Uncertain Etiology. *Pediatr. Nephrol. Berl. Ger.* **2020**. [CrossRef] [PubMed]
73. Orantes Navarro, C.; Herrera-Valdés, R.; Almaguer-López, M.; Brizuela-Díaz, E.; Alvarado-Ascencio, N.; Morales, E.; Bayarre, H.; Calero-Brizuela, D.; Vela Parada, X.; Zelaya-Quezada, S. Chronic Kidney Disease in Children and Adolescents in Salvadoran Farming Communities: NefroSalva Pediatric Study (2009–2011). *Med. Rev.* **2016**, *18*, 15–21. [CrossRef]
74. Agampodi, S.B.; Amarasinghe, G.S.; Naotunna, P.G.C.R.; Jayasumana, C.S.; Siribaddana, S.H. Early Renal Damage among Children Living in the Region of Highest Burden of Chronic Kidney Disease of Unknown Etiology (CKDu) in Sri Lanka. *BMC Nephrol.* **2018**, *19*, 115. [CrossRef] [PubMed]
75. Díaz de León-Martínez, L.; Díaz-Barriga, F.; Barbier, O.; Ortíz, D.L.G.; Ortega-Romero, M.; Pérez-Vázquez, F.; Flores-Ramírez, R. Evaluation of Emerging Biomarkers of Renal Damage and Exposure to Aflatoxin-B1 in Mexican Indigenous Women: A Pilot Study. *Environ. Sci. Pollut. Res. Int.* **2019**, *26*, 12205–12216. [CrossRef] [PubMed]
76. Riefkohl, A.; Ramírez-Rubio, O.; Laws, R.L.; McClean, M.D.; Weiner, D.E.; Kaufman, J.S.; Galloway, R.L.; Shadomy, S.V.; Guerra, M.; Amador, J.J.; et al. Leptospira Seropositivity as a Risk Factor for Mesoamerican Nephropathy. *Int. J. Occup. Environ. Health* **2017**, *23*, 1–10. [CrossRef] [PubMed]
77. Jayasumana, C.; Gajanayake, R.; Siribaddana, S. Importance of Arsenic and Pesticides in Epidemic Chronic Kidney Disease in Sri Lanka. *BMC Nephrol.* **2014**, *15*, 124. [CrossRef] [PubMed]
78. Kafle, K.; Balasubramanya, S.; Horbulyk, T. Prevalence of Chronic Kidney Disease in Sri Lanka: A Profile of Affected Districts Reliant on Groundwater. *Sci. Total Environ.* **2019**, *694*, 133767. [CrossRef]
79. Ratnayake, S.; Badurdeen, Z.; Nanayakkara, N.; Abeysekara, T.; Ratnatunga, N.; Kumarasiri, R. Screening for Chronic Kidney Disease of Uncertain Aetiology in Sri Lanka: Usability of Surrogate Biomarkers over Dipstick Proteinuria. *BMC Nephrol.* **2017**, *18*, 199. [CrossRef] [PubMed]
80. De Silva, P.M.C.S.; Mohammed Abdul, K.S.; Eakanayake, E.M.D.V.; Jayasinghe, S.S.; Jayasumana, C.; Asanthi, H.B.; Perera, H.S.D.; Chaminda, G.G.T.; Chandana, E.P.S.; Siribaddana, S.H. Urinary Biomarkers KIM-1 and NGAL for Detection of Chronic Kidney Disease of Uncertain Etiology (CKDu) among Agricultural Communities in Sri Lanka. *PLoS Negl. Trop. Dis.* **2016**, *10*, e0004979. [CrossRef] [PubMed]
81. Chung, H.J.; Pellegrini, K.L.; Chung, J.; Wanigasuriya, K.; Jayawardene, I.; Lee, K.; Lee, H.; Vaidya, V.S.; Weissleder, R. Nanoparticle Detection of Urinary Markers for Point-of-Care Diagnosis of Kidney Injury. *PLoS ONE* **2015**, *10*, e0133417. [CrossRef]
82. Sayanthooran, S.; Magana-Arachchi, D.N.; Gunerathne, L.; Abeysekera, T. Potential Diagnostic Biomarkers for Chronic Kidney Disease of Unknown Etiology (CKDu) in Sri Lanka: A Pilot Study. *BMC Nephrol.* **2017**, *18*, 31. [CrossRef]
83. Sayanthooran, S.; Magana-Arachchi, D.N.; Gunerathne, L.; Abeysekera, T.D.J.; Sooriyapathirana, S.S. Upregulation of Oxidative Stress Related Genes in a Chronic Kidney Disease Attributed to Specific Geographical Locations of Sri Lanka. *Biomed. Res. Int.* **2016**, *2016*, 7546265. [CrossRef]

84. Fernando, B.N.T.W.; Alli-Shaik, A.; Hemage, R.K.D.; Badurdeen, Z.; Hettiarachchi, T.W.; Abeysundara, H.T.K.; Abeysekara, T.D.J.; Wazil, A.; Rathnayake, S.; Gunaratne, J.; et al. Pilot Study of Renal Urinary Biomarkers for Diagnosis of CKD of Uncertain Etiology. *Kidney Int. Rep.* **2019**, *4*, 1401–1411. [CrossRef] [PubMed]
85. Wanigasuriya, K.; Jayawardene, I.; Amarasiriwardena, C.; Wickremasinghe, R. Novel Urinary Biomarkers and Their Association with Urinary Heavy Metals in Chronic Kidney Disease of Unknown Aetiology in Sri Lanka: A Pilot Study. *Ceylon Med. J.* **2017**, *62*, 210–217. [CrossRef] [PubMed]
86. Siriwardhana, E.A.R.I.E.; Perera, P.A.J.; Sivakanesan, R.; Abeysekara, T.; Nugegoda, D.B.; Weerakoon, K.G.A.D. Is the Staple Diet Eaten in Medawachchiya, Sri Lanka, a Predisposing Factor in the Development of Chronic Kidney Disease of Unknown Etiology?—A Comparison Based on Urinary B2-Microglobulin Measurements. *BMC Nephrol.* **2014**, *15*, 103. [CrossRef] [PubMed]
87. Safouh, H.; Fadel, F.; Essam, R.; Salah, A.; Bekhet, A. Causes of Chronic Kidney Disease in Egyptian Children. *Saudi J. Kidney Dis. Transpl.* **2015**, *26*, 806–809. [CrossRef]
88. Ghonemy, T.A.; Farag, S.E.; Soliman, S.A.; El-okely, A.; El-hendy, Y. Epidemiology and Risk Factors of Chronic Kidney Disease in the El-Sharkia Governorate, Egypt. *Saudi J. Kidney Dis. Transpl.* **2016**, *27*, 111–117. [CrossRef]
89. Nejat, M.; Pickering, J.W.; Devarajan, P.; Bonventre, J.V.; Edelstein, C.L.; Walker, R.J.; Endre, Z.H. Some Biomarkers of Acute Kidney Injury Are Increased in Pre-Renal Acute Injury. *Kidney Int.* **2012**, *81*, 1254–1262. [CrossRef]
90. Endre, Z.H. Recovery from Acute Kidney Injury: The Role of Biomarkers. *Nephron Clin. Pract.* **2014**, *127*, 101–105. [CrossRef]

3

Toll-Like Receptor as a Potential Biomarker in Renal Diseases

Sebastian Mertowski [1,*], Paulina Lipa [2], Izabela Morawska [1], Paulina Niedźwiedzka-Rystwej [3,*], Dominika Bębnowska [3], Rafał Hrynkiewicz [3], Ewelina Grywalska [1,*], Jacek Roliński [1] and Wojciech Załuska [4]

1 Department of Clinical Immunology and Immunotherapy, Medical University of Lublin, 20-093 Lublin, Poland; izabelamorawska19@gmail.com (I.M.); jacek.rolinski@gmail.com (J.R.)
2 Department of Genetics and Microbiology, Institute of Microbiology and Biotechnology, Faculty of Biology and Biotechnology, Maria Curie-Skłodowska University, Akademicka 19 St., 20-033 Lublin, Poland; paulina.lipa56@gmail.com
3 Institute of Biology, University of Szczecin, Felczaka 3c, 71-412 Szczecin, Poland; bebnowska.d@wp.pl (D.B.); rafal.hrynkiewicz@gmail.com (R.H.)
4 Department of Nephrology, Medical University of Lublin, 20-954 Lublin, Poland; wojciech.zaluska@umlub.pl
* Correspondence: mertowskisebastian@gmail.com (S.M.); paulina.niedzwiedzka-rystwej@usz.edu.pl (P.N.-R.); ewelina.grywalska@gmail.com (E.G.)

Abstract: One of the major challenges faced by modern nephrology is the identification of biomarkers associated with histopathological patterns or defined pathogenic mechanisms that may assist in the non-invasive diagnosis of kidney disease, particularly glomerulopathy. The identification of such molecules may allow prognostic subgroups to be established based on the type of disease, thereby predicting response to treatment or disease relapse. Advances in understanding the pathogenesis of diseases, such as membranous nephropathy, minimal change disease, focal segmental glomerulosclerosis, IgA (immunoglobulin A) nephropathy, and diabetic nephropathy, along with the progressive development and standardization of plasma and urine proteomics techniques, have facilitated the identification of an increasing number of molecules that may be useful for these purposes. The growing number of studies on the role of TLR (toll-like receptor) receptors in the pathogenesis of kidney disease forces contemporary researchers to reflect on these molecules, which may soon join the group of renal biomarkers and become a helpful tool in the diagnosis of glomerulopathy. In this article, we conducted a thorough review of the literature on the role of TLRs in the pathogenesis of glomerulopathy. The role of TLR receptors as potential marker molecules for the development of neoplastic diseases is emphasized more and more often, as prognostic factors in diseases on several epidemiological backgrounds.

Keywords: acute kidney injury; biomarker; diabetic nephropathy; focal segmental glomerulosclerosis; innate immunity; membranous nephropathy; minimal change diseases; TLR

1. Introduction

The term "biological marker" in the literature refers to the objective health status of the patient, which can be observed from the outside, i.e., in a way that can be measured in an extremely accurate and, most importantly, repeatable manner. Various medical symptoms can often contrast with each other, or, on the contrary, correlations between them are observed, which may contribute to a better and faster diagnosis of the disease or the effectiveness of the treatment process. A joint project of the World Health Organization together with the United Nations under the name of the International Program on Chemical Safety has attempted to standardize the term biomarker used in the literature.

Currently, a biomarker is defined as "any substance, structure or process that can be measured in the body or its products and that can influence or predict the occurrence of an outcome or disease" [1], which means that the modern definition of biomarkers covers every response of the body, whether functional, physiological, or biochemical, to the occurrence of a potential threat (physical, chemical, or biological) that may modify the body's reactions at the cellular or molecular level. Usually, biomarker is used with two meanings: (1) A biomarker is a component (analyte) of a human biological system (i.e., plasma, urine, etc.); or (2) a biomarker is a biological property (i.e., mass concentration of X in plasma) [2]. Currently, examples of biomarkers can be both simple parameters of heart rate and blood pressure, as well as the determination of complex constituent molecules present in our blood or tissues, which are indicative of health. Types and applications of biomarkers are constantly changing as it evaluates our knowledge about them. Thus, it has recently been shown that counts of urinary T-cell, renal tubular epithelial cells, and podocalyxin-positive cells provide an excellent biomarker for the detection of renal transplant rejection in routine clinical trials [3]. Currently, the role of TLR receptors as potential marker molecules for the development of neoplastic diseases is emphasized more and more often, e.g., TLR5 as a prognostic marker for gastric cancer [4]. It was also shown that the activity of TLR receptor is correlated with the state of injury of post-surgical patients who have a disorder of the immune response related to the interaction of TLR receptors with DAMP (damage-associated molecular pattern). Moreover, the analyses led to conclusions regarding the role of TLR receptors in predicting pathological conditions, including tissue damage, in these patients [5]. One of the increasing threats in today's world is chronic kidney disease, the cause of which may be both primary processes related to the kidneys, and secondary processes observed in the course of rheumatic, cardiological, or diabetic diseases. As indicated in the literature, one of the largest causes of the development of chronic kidney disease in highly developed countries as well as in developing countries is hypertension and type 2 diabetes, currently classified as diseases of civilization [6]. As far as type 2 diabetes and renal disorders are concerned, it was shown that polypharmacy has a great impact on the occurrence, course, and treatment of the disease [7].

Genetic, epigenetic, or environmental factors that play a more or less important role in different regions of the world may lead to diseases associated with kidney glomerular damage, which leads to their chronic hypofunction and subsequent renal failure. Research conducted by O'Shaughnessy et al. [6], aimed to analyze the data from centers dealing with chronic kidney diseases, where several types of nephropathy were considered. Analysis shows that there is a difference in the incidence of individual nephropathy depending on the region. It turned out that focal segmental glomerulosclerosis (FSGS) and diabetic nephropathy are the most numerous in the USA because it occurred in 19% of diagnosed patients; the second type that dominated was IgA nephropathy (12%), another was membranous nephropathy (12%) and lupus nephritis (10%). Furthermore, FSGS was also common in Latin America (16%), although lupus nephritis strongly dominated the region (38%), while diabetic nephropathy (DN) (4%) and IgA nephropathy (IgAN) (6%) were relatively rare. A reverse dependence than in the USA has been observed in Europe and Asia. In Europe, IgA nephropathy dominated the diagnosis, and the second most common diagnosis was FSGS (15%), while in Asia, IgA glomerulopathy included 40% of diagnoses and the second most common diagnosis was lupus nephritis (17%) [8].

All of these diseases are the subject of intensive research by many scientists around the world. The following review of the literature focuses on the problems of diseases associated with glomerular dysfunction, in which there are answers to questions about the participation in the pathogenesis of diseases on TLR, which may become a potential marker molecule.

2. Classification of Biomarkers

There are many different ways to classify biological molecules as biomarkers in the literature. One of the basic methods is division according to the type of marker molecule. These are DNA, mitochondrial DNA, RNA, or mRNA molecules that belong to the genomic biomarker category, but also proteins, peptides, or antibodies that are classified as proteomic biomarkers. The third group is metabolic markers (metabolomics), which includes lipids, carbohydrates, enzymes, and products of metabolism (metabolites). Our attention was drawn to a slightly different classification of these unusual molecules, i.e., classification based on genetics and molecular biology, due to the usefulness of biomarkers in diagnostic processes and due to their application (Figure 1). The first group includes three types of biomarkers. Type 0 are biomarkers that correlate over time with known clinical indications and show the natural course and history of the disease. Type I relates to biomarkers of drug activity, which can be divided into biomarkers of efficacy (taking into account the therapeutic effect of a given drug), mechanism (providing information about the drug's mechanism of action), and toxicity (including the toxic effect of a given drug). Type II is known as surrogate biomarkers to help evaluate and predict the effect of therapy [9].

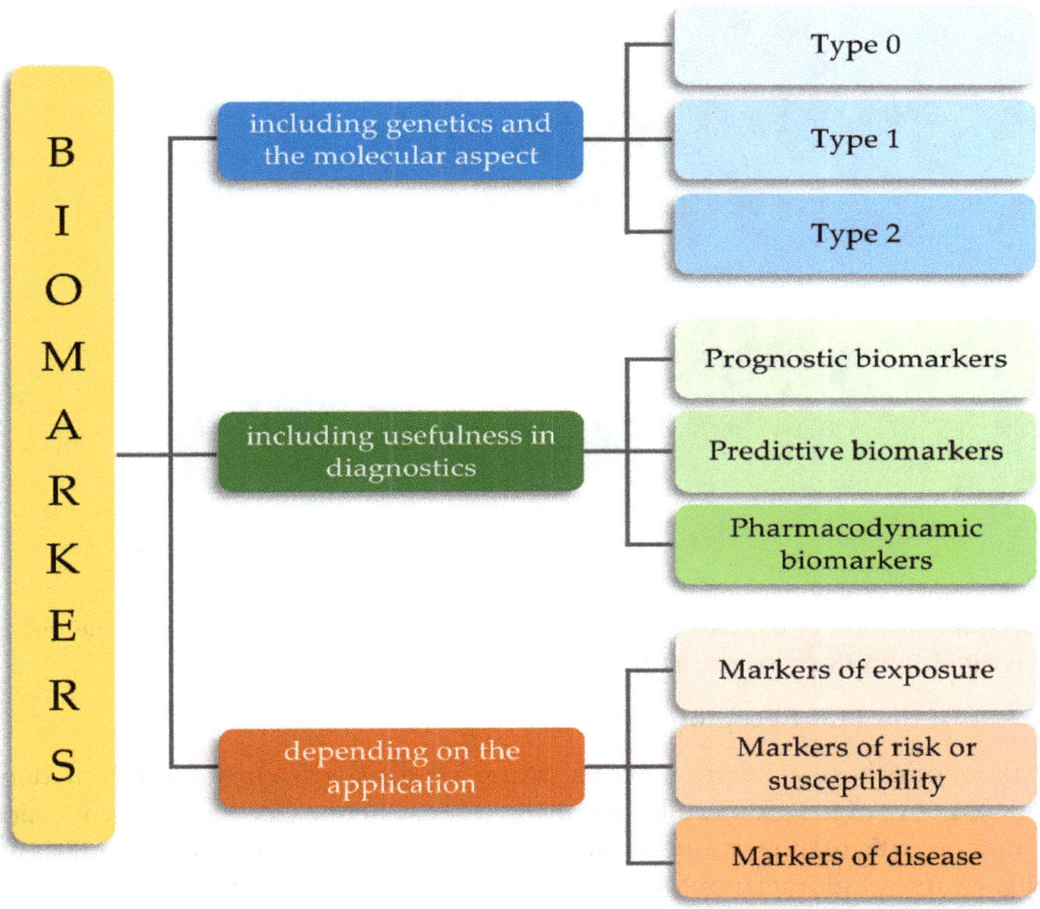

Figure 1. Classification of biomarkers due to the genetic and molecular aspect, the usefulness of biomarkers in diagnostic processes, and application.

Due to the usefulness of biomarkers in diagnostics, we can distinguish prognostic biomarkers; in other words, those that suggest the probable outcome of the disease in an untreated individual, and predictive biomarkers, the purpose of which is to identify patients for whom a specific therapy is most effective. Lastly, we can distinguish pharmacodynamic biomarkers that determine the pharmacological action of a given drug [10]. Another classification is based on the use of biomarkers. We distinguish here exposure markers and doses that are used to reconstruct and predict past accidental or occupational exposures. Risk or vulnerability markers, which relate to the identification of vulnerable individuals (or future patients) at increased risk of developing a disease, and disease markers represent the initial cellular or molecular changes that occur during the development of a particular disease entity. It is the latter group that includes TLR receptors [11,12]. However, what characteristics does an ideal biomarker need to meet? Is there an "ideal biomarker"? What features should a biomarker have to be close to the ideal? Well, according to the FDA, an ideal biomarker must meet the following six characteristics (Figure 2). First, it must be specific in the course of a particular disease entity and easy to differentiate between different physiological conditions of the patient. Secondly, such a biomarker must above all be easy to measure and safe. Then, the speed of its detection is also important, as it enables a quick diagnosis as well as the repeatability and accuracy of the results obtained. Attention is also paid to the cost of detecting such biomarkers, which must be relatively cheap. The advantage of such a biomarker is also the consistency between ethnic groups and genders of patients [13].

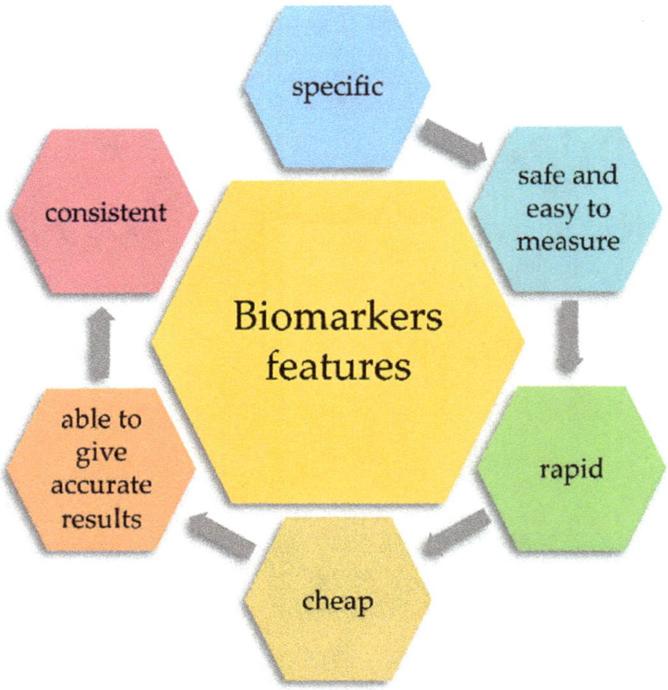

Figure 2. Classification of biomarkers due to the genetic and molecular aspect, the usefulness of biomarkers in diagnostic processes, and application.

3. Characteristic of the TLR Receptors

Glomerulonephritis is a heterogeneous group of diseases whose common denominator is inflammation, ongoing in the glomerulus, resulting from systemic (secondary glomerulonephritis) or only glomerulonephritis (primary glomerulonephritis) [14–19]. The etiopathogenesis and the cause of the variable course of glomerulopathy is the subject of numerous studies but remains unknown. Although the pathogenesis is not unequivocally elucidated, the literature data clearly indicate the involvement of various immune mechanisms in the etiopathogenesis of glomerulopathy. Researchers indicate the role of the immune system in the development of chronic kidney disease on the basis of primary and secondary disorders of the glomerular functions, and AKI (acute kidney injury) resulting from the above-mentioned entities and other disease states, e.g., sepsis [20]. The main elements involved in promoting kidney damage are dendritic cells, NK (natural killer) cells, macrophages, and proinflammatory cytokines. A critical role is played by the complement system, which can both protect and promote damage to the glomeruli [21].

Literature data suggest the contribution of innate immunity to TLRs in these processes. These receptors are a classic example of pattern recognition receptors (PRRs). Signals received by these receptors by recruiting specific molecules lead to activation of the transcription factors NF-κB (nuclear factor kappa-light-chain-enhancer of activated B cells) and IRF (interferon regulatory factor) and affect various elements of the host's innate immune response [22]. TLR mechanisms are based on the ability to recognize twofold signals. The first one is based on the detection of pathogen-associated molecular patterns (PAMPs), while the second reads molecules related to damage to the body's own cells (DAMPs; danger-associated molecular patterns) [23]. However, the origin of the signal, in the case of PAMP, is compounds of exogenous origin, while DAMP receives endogenous information. The result of receiving signals from both pathways is the effector reaction in which the production of costimulatory molecules and cytokines takes place. The location of TLRs is the cell surface or intracellular compartments, including ER (endoplasmic reticulum), lysosomes, and endosomes. It is pointed out that intracellular localization is important not only for ligand recognition but also for avoiding TLR contact with self-nucleic acids, which could cause autoimmunity. A high number of TLR receptors on cells of the immune system, such as monocytes, macrophages, dendritic cells, or lymphocytes, enables the thesis that they constitute a network allowing rapid cooperation of leukocytes and cells present at the site of infection or in the immediate vicinity of damaged host cells [23,24]. TLR synthesis begins in the rough endoplasmic reticulum, from where it goes to the Golgi apparatus and then to its destinations, in other words to the cell surface or to the intercellular compartments [22].

At present, there are 10 types of TLR receptors in humans and three additional types in mice, whereas others species may have more of these receptors (Table 1). Based on the amino acid sequence homology, TLRs occurring in vertebrates were divided into six subfamilies: TLR 1/2/6/10, TLR3, TLR4, TLR5, followed by TLR 7/8/9, and TLR 11 to the last 12/13 (Table 2). However, not all vertebrates have all types of receptors. PRRs have a specific structure in the form of transmembrane proteins, being an integral component of the cell membrane, in which the N-terminal part is responsible for ligand binding, whereas the C-terminal end is equipped with a signaling domain for IL-1 (TIR; toll IL-1 receptor), being part of the signal induction cascade for the production of anti-inflammatory mediators [23]. The transmembrane domain of TLRs contains about 20, mostly hydrophobic, amino acid residues. The N-terminal end (ECDs (extracellular domain) N-terminal ectodomains) is a glycoprotein of 500–800 amino acid residues. In their structure, we distinguish the presence of leucine-rich tandem repeats (LRRs), the number of which depends on the receptor type and ranges from 20–29 repeats (Table 1).

Table 1. Characteristics of individual TLRs (toll-like receptors).

Name	Location of Coding Genes	Location in the Cell	The Number of Amino Acids	Molecular Weight (kDa)	Number of LLR	Reference
TLR1	Chromosome 4	Golgi apparatus, Phagosome, Cell membrane	786aa	90.31	19	[25–27]
TLR2	Chromosome 4	Phagosome	784aa	89.83	19	[25,28,29]
TLR3	Chromosome 4	Early endosome, ER	904aa	103.82	23	[25,30,31]
TLR4	Chromosome 9	Cell membrane, Early endosome	839aa	95.68	21	[25,32,33]
TLR5	Chromosome 1	No data	858aa	97.83	20	[25,34,35]
TLR6	Chromosome 4	Golgi apparatus, Cell membrane, Phagosome	796aa	91.88	19	[25,36,37]
TLR7	Chromosome X	Endosomes, Lysosomes, ER, Phagosome	1049aa	120.92	25	[25,38]
TLR8	Chromosome X	No data	1041aa	119.82	25	[25,39,40]
TLR9	Chromosome 3	Endosomes, Lysosomes, ER, Phagosome	1032aa	115.86	25	[25,41]
TLR10	Chromosome 4	No data	811aa	94.56	19	[25,42,43]

Table 1. *Cont.*

Name	Location of Coding Genes	Location in the Cell	The Number of Amino Acids	Molecular Weight (kDa)	Number of LLR	Reference
TLR11	Expression in mice	No data	926aa	105.83	10	[44]
TLR12	Expression in mice	No data	906aa	99.94	17	[45]
TLR13	Expression in mice	Endosomes	991aa	114.44	25	[46]

TLRs also differ in the cell site. TLR 1/2/4/5/6/10/11/12 receptors are located on the outer membrane of cells, while 3/7/8/9 receptors are located inside of them. Several literature reports have identified specific PAMP and DAMP ligands, which are bound by particular TLRs (Table 2).

Table 2. Location and ligands bound by TLR.

Name	Occurrence	Ligand PAMP	The Origin of PAMP	Ligand DAMP	Reference
		Extracellular			
TLR1	Macrophages Neutrophils B lymphocytes Dendritic cells	Lipopeptides Soluble factors (lipoproteins)	Bacteria	No data	[47,48]
TLR2	Macrophages Neutrophils B lymphocytes Dendritic cells NK cells	Bacterial lipopeptides Teichoic acids, LAM Moduline, Glycolipids of bacteria, Porins, LPS,	Bacteria	Apolipoprotein CIII, Heparin sulphate, Hyaluronic acid, Hsp60, Hsp70, Peroxiredoxin	[47–50]
		Glycosinositolphospholipids	Protozoa, e.g., Trypanosoma cruzi		
		Zymosan	Fungi		
		Hemagglutinin	Measles virus		
		Protein	Herpesvirus		
		Hsp70 proteins	Host organism		
TLR4	Macrophages Neutrophils B lymphocytes Dendritic cells NK cells Treg cells	LPS	Bacteria	C-reactive protein, Fibronectin, Fibrinogen, Heparin sulphate, Neutrophil, Elastase, Angiotensin II, Hsp60	[48–51]
		Fusion proteins, Proteins present in the coating	Viruses, e.g., RSV virus		
		Taxol	Plants		
		Hsp60 protein Hsp70 protein A fragment of the A domain of fibronectin Hyaluronic acid oligosaccharide Fibrinogen Heparan sulphate	Host organism		
TLR5	Macrophages B lymphocytes Dendritic cells Treg cells	Flagellin	Bacteria (Gram-negative)	No data	[48,52]
TLR6	Macrophages Neutrophils Dendritic cells	Diacyl lipopeptides Lipoteichoic acids Zymosan	Bacteria Fungi	Versican	[47–50,53]
TLR10	Dendritic cells	No data	No data	No data	[54]
TLR11	Macrophages Dendritic cells	Flagellin Profilin	Bacteria Protozoa, e.g., Toxoplasma gondii	No data	[55,56]
TLR12	Dendritic cells	Profilin	Protozoa, e.g., Toxoplasma gondii	No data	[55]

Table 2. *Cont.*

Name	Occurrence	Ligand PAMP	The Origin of PAMP	Ligand DAMP	Reference
		Intracellular			
TLR3	Macrophages Neutrophils B lymphocytes Dendritic cells	Double-stranded RNA	Viruses	Own double-stranded RNA	[57,58]
TLR7	Macrophages Neutrophils Dendritic cells Treg cells	Single-stranded RNA Antiviral and anticancer compounds	Viruses Synthetic	Own single-stranded RNA	[48,59]
TLR8	Dendritic cells Treg cells	Single-stranded RNA Antiviral compounds	Viruses Synthetic	Own single-stranded RNA	[48,60]
TLR9	Macrophages Neutrophils Dendritic cells	Double-stranded DNA (containing unmethylated CpG sequences)	Bacteria, viruses and synthetic	HMGB1 Mitochondrial DNA	[48–50,61]

4. The Role of TLRs in Glomerulonephritis

Tissue damage glomerulonephritis predisposes many factors and individual characteristics. Most often, the first reveals hereditary predispositions in response to emerging environmental factors that can lead to a nephrogenic immune response. Then, there is a direct exposure to infectious etiological factors occurring in the environment (PAMP and DAMP), which may be subject to specific modification due to many epigenetic factors (such as physical exercise, microbes, environmental toxins, lifestyle, etc.) [62]. As a consequence of these changes, the innate immune system is activated as a result of interaction with TLRs present on circulating inflammatory cells (neutrophils, macrophages, basophils, and NK cells), as well as on resident glomerular cells and the complement system, which triggers a cascade of antigen-specific non-specific reactions [63]. These receptors are displayed on cells found inside the glomerulus (mesangial cells, monocytes, or dendritic cells) as well as in the renal interstitium (tubular epithelial cells, monocytes), where they interfere with potential ligands [63]. Part of the ligands, such as peptides, structural elements, or genetic material of both bacteria and viruses can be transmitted through the bloodstream to the inside of the nephron, in particular to the glomerulus. In the case of interstitial cells, in addition to the ligands of infectious origin, the potential ligands may also be fibrinogen, fibronectin, defensin 2, or necrotic cells (Figure 3).

In order to prevent over-activity of the immune system, TLRs are downregulated by numerous molecules and various mechanisms. Existing negative regulators target specific key molecules in TLR signaling, such as SOCS1 (suppressor of cytokine signaling 1), SOCS3 (suppressor of cytokine signaling 3), SARM (sterile α-and armadillo-motif containing protein), TANK (TRAF family member associated NF-κB activator), A20, and others [64–69]. Additionally, there are molecules that directly influence the inhibition of NF-kB and IRF-3 [70]. In addition, numerous mi-RNAs were discovered that affect the stability of mRNA encoding signaling molecules and mRNA for cytokines [69,71].

Activation of TLR releases the NF-κB transcription factor, which results in the production of inflammatory mediators (such as IL-1, IL-2, IL-6, IL-12, TNF-α (tumor necrosis factor alpha)), [72,73], and can cause glomerular damage. The next step is the conversion of the innate immune response that begins the antigen-specific reaction cycle. The transformation of the immune response includes several possible mechanisms, such as regulation of natural autoimmunity, conformational changes of epitopes, molecular mimicry, or the autoantigen complementarity phenomenon. TLRs are also required to activate the adaptive immune system by antigen-presenting cells that promote CD4 helper cell differentiation, B cell activation, and antibody production. Antibodies lead to the trapping of the circulating complex or the formation of in situ immune complexes that can activate both TLRs and complement components of the innate immune system [74]. CD4 Th1 and Th2 cells cause damage to the glomerular tissues indirectly, mainly through macrophages and basophils, whereas Th17 cells may directly mediate damage to kidney structures in particular diseases (Figure 4).

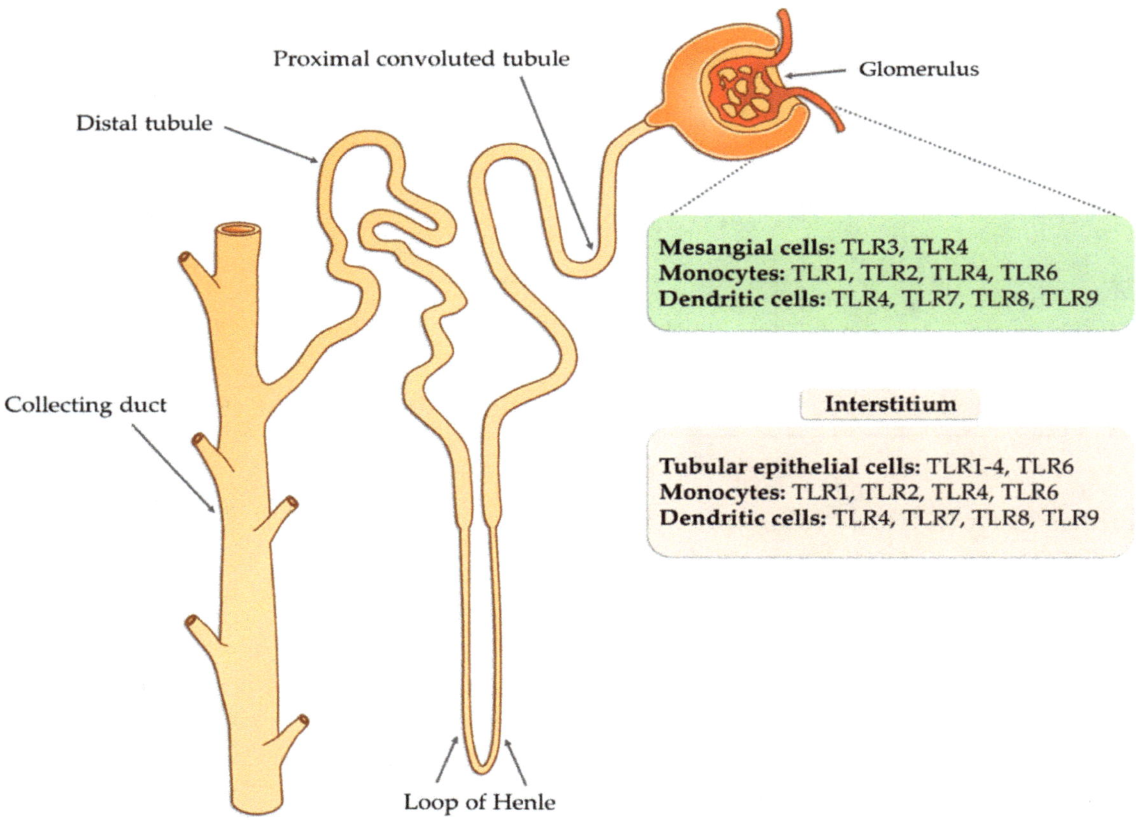

Figure 3. The potential occurrence of TLR receptors within the nephron (modified, based on [63]).

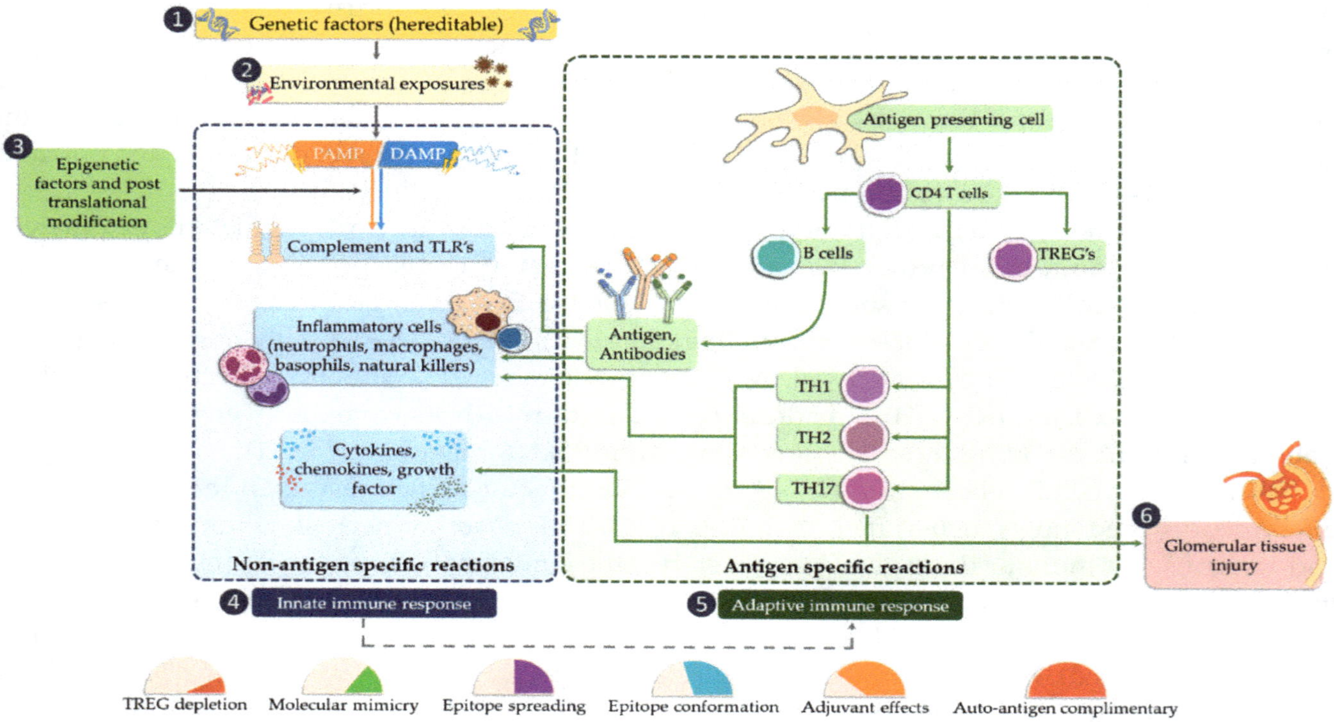

Figure 4. The potential occurrence of TLR receptors within the nephron (modified, based on [24]).

Various clinical situations affecting the kidneys, such as ischemic damage, toxic AKI, nephropathies secondary to diabetes mellitus, hypertension, or crystal deposition, are associated with aseptic inflammation caused, among others, by DAMP molecules [75,76]. These molecules can be released from dying parenchyma cells or during remodulation of the extracellular matrix. The presence of cells in the kidney capable of expressing TLR receptors makes it possible to initiate an immune response and inflammation [77,78]. In order to approximate the mode of action of these receptors in the disease state, their involvement in the most frequently diagnosed pathological conditions associated with glomerular dysfunction is presented in the further part of the material [8].

5. Biomarkers and Importance of the TLRs in Selected Glomerular Diseases

The literature classification divides the occurring nephropathies into two categories: Primary nephropathies, which are defined as those in which the systemic disease responsible for the condition cannot be established, and secondary nephropathies in which renal lesions appear as a result of other diseases accompanied by characteristic extrarenal symptoms. The first group includes diseases, such as: minimal change nephropathy (MCN), focal segmental glomerulosclerosis (FSGS), and membranous nephropathy (MN), which are also included in the nephrotic syndrome. The second group is primarily diabetic nephropathy and lupus nephropathy. In addition, the studies of our research group have resulted in the finding that the TLR-2 receptor may play an important role as a biomarker of primary non-proliferative nephropathies [79].

6. The Role of TLRs in Primary Non-Proliferative Nephropathies

6.1. Focal Segmental Glomerulosclerosis (FSGS)

FSGS is a diverse syndrome that arises after damage to podocytes for various reasons, some known and unknown. The sources of podocyte injury are diverse (circulating factors (primary FSGS), genetic abnormalities, viral infections, and medications) [80,81]. Most of the mutual interactions between these factors probably result in FSGS. There is a hypothesis about multistage pathogenic activation of autoimmunity in some forms of idiopathic FSGS [81]. Through the interaction of macrophages involved in kidney damage with many chemokines, the migration of monocytes to the site of damage occurs, which initiates the process of fibrosis. These macrophages also have the ability to self-spread and change into myofibroblasts that produce the extracellular matrix. Therefore, it can be assumed that excessive organ infiltration by monocytes and macrophages will cause an intensified fibrosis effect and, consequently, intensification of FSGS symptoms [82,83]. Currently, known biomarkers of FSGS are soluble urokinase-type plasminogen activator receptor (suPAR), soluble IL-2 receptor (sIL-2R), and ATP-binding cassette subfamily B member 1 glycoprotein-P (Figure 5). Damage to podocytes can release molecular patterns of proteins that are recognized by TLR as signals of danger. TLRs stimulate adapter proteins that activate a cascade of kinases, which amplify the signal and transmit it to the transcription factors regulating inflammatory genes. In the inflammatory microenvironment, the podocytes, acting as antigen-presenting cells, have a CD40 and CD80 receptor on their surface, thanks to which they capture antigens and present them to competent T-cells. However, in the case of abnormal expression of CD40 and CD80, they disorganize the cytoskeleton and filtration slit. In addition, CD40 can be identified as a foreign antigen, consequently leading to the production of anti-CD40 auto-antigen. Abnormal expression of CD40, CD80, and autoantibodies may lead to apoptosis of the podocytes, detachment of the podocytes from the glomerular basal membrane, proliferation of parietal epithelial cells, and attack on the glomeruli, and induction of segmental sclerosis [81]. In turn, other literature reports indicate the involvement of fibrinogen (Fg) in an inflammatory process mediated by the toll-like 4 receptor (TLR4) [84]. Fibrinogen is a protein that plays a proinflammatory role in vascular disorders, rheumatoid arthritis, glomerulonephritis, and certain cancers, e.g., myeloproliferative neoplasms [84,85]. Positive correlations have been noted between oxidative stress markers and, among others, fibrinogen, which may impact the course of several disorders [85]. Găman et al. [86] showed that obesity and diabetes are associated with increased levels of ROS (reactive oxygen species), accompanied by a simultaneous deficiency of antioxidants. The authors showed that the results of the free oxygen radical defense (FORT) and free oxygen radical defense (FORD) tests correlated with anthropometric/biochemical parameters in patients with obesity and diabetes. In studies carried out by Wang et al. [84], Fg has been shown to disrupt the actin cytoskeleton and induce apoptosis in podocytes via the TLR4-p38 MAPK-NF-κB p65 pathway in vitro and that co-expression of Fg and TLR4 is elevated in podocytes of Adriamycin-treated mice. It was also indicated that the level of fibrinogen in the urine may reflect the disease activity in patients with FSGS [84]. Literature data show that the use of synthetic small molecules lecinoxoids, which are inhibitors of TLR-2 and TLR-4, affects the activation and recruitment of monocytes in a rat model. The authors indicate [87] that the data demonstrate that targeting TLR-2-TLR-4 and/or monocyte migration directly affects the priming phase of fibrosis and may consequently perturb disease pathogenesis.

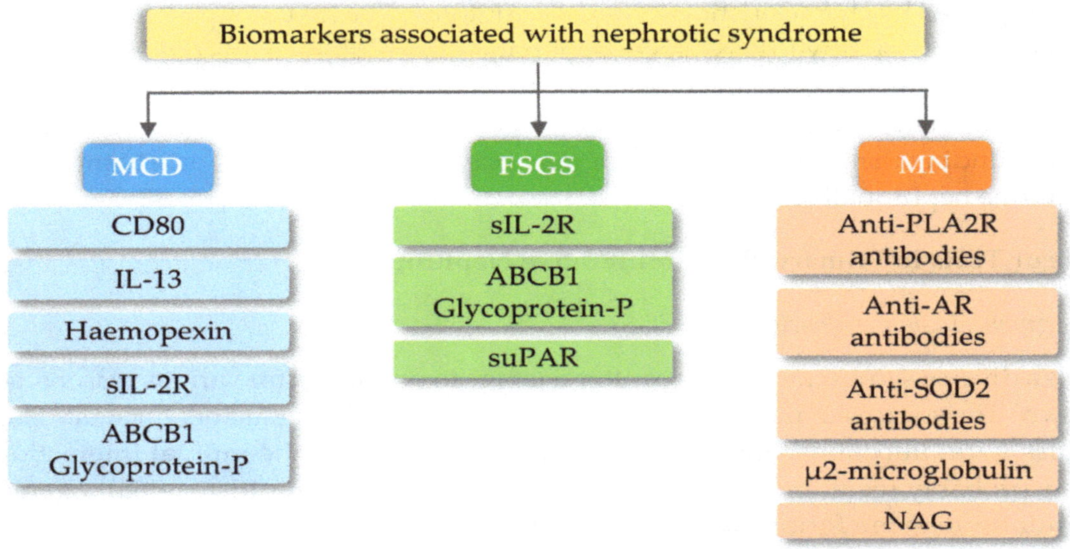

Figure 5. Biomarkers associated with nephrotic syndrome based on minimal change disease (MCD), focal segmental glomerulosclerosis (FSGS), and membranous nephropathy (MN) change based on [88]). CD80-Cluster of differentiation 80; IL-13-interleukin 13; sIL-2R-soluble IL-2 receptor; ABCB1 Glycoprotein-P-ATP-binding cassette subfamily B member 1 Glycoprotein-P; suPAR-soluble urokinase-type plasminogen activator receptor; PLA2R-M-type phospholipase A2 receptor; SOD2-manganese superoxide-dismutase 2; AR-Androgen Receptor; NAG-N-Acetyl-β-D Glucosaminidase.

6.2. Minimal Change Disease (MCD)

MCD is one of the most common glomerular kidney diseases in children and a common cause of nephrotic syndrome in adults. This disease entity is characterized by an outbreak of edema, selective proteinuria, and a clinical response to glucocorticoid therapy, as T-cell mechanisms are involved in the pathogenesis of the disease [89]. The pathogenesis is due to abnormalities in the functioning of podocytes, with the latest literature data suggesting the hypothesis that there are two initiating events. First, there are changes in the cytoskeleton of podocytes and, second, there are regulatory changes in T-cells that exacerbate abnormalities in podocytes [89,90]. Currently known biomarkers in MCD are urine levels and podocyte expression of CD80 (B7.1), interleukin 13, serum levels and protease activity of circulating hemopexin, serum levels of soluble interleukin 2 receptor, and ABCB1 and glycoprotein-P (Figure 5). The development of MCD may be significantly influenced by the body's innate immunity, in which TLRs are involved. Podocytes in the kidney glomeruli, due to their function and place of occurrence, are also equipped with the above receptors. In research conducted by Srivastava et al. [91], the presence of TLR receptors and their potential activity were checked on cell cultures stimulated with LPS (lipopolysaccharides) and the amino nucleoside puromycin (PAN). In the above studies, it was found that cultured human podocytes constitutively express TLR 1-6 and TLR-10 but not TLR 7–9.

Quantitative analysis using the RT-PCR method indicated that LPS at various concentrations and to varying degrees increased the expression of TLR (1–6) genes, the adapter molecule MyD88, and the transcription factor NF-κB within one hour. LPS also caused elevated levels of IL-6, IL-8, and MCP-1 (monocyte chemoattractant protein-1) without exerting any effect on TNF-α, IFN-α, or TGF-β1 after 24 h. It has also been shown that an increase in TLR 1 expression may attenuate the effect of TLR-4 activation, which is thought to be an indirect factor in LPS-induced podocyte damage [91]. Moreover, the increase in TLR-1 expression by LPS suggests that LPS damage to podocytes is associated with an increase in TLR-1 levels and its specific endogenous ligands (heat shock protein, heparin sulphate, and fibronectin). These results allow the conclusion that the main TLR4 ligand, which is LPS, can induce the expression of the genes of many TLR receptors, and thus may lead to changes being induced in podocytes, which may be related to the loss of receptor selectivity and stimulation of receptor interaction in podocytes [91]. An additional possibility indicating the involvement of TLRs in the development of MCD is the increase in the amount of the CD80 receptor in podocytes, after stimulation with ligands for TLR-and TLR-4 receptors. TLR ligands are usually microbial products and can be combined with a well-known association of viral infections as a causative agent of minimal lesion disease [92,93].

6.3. *Membranous Nephropathy (MN)*

MN is a common cause of nephrotic syndrome in adults. Patients with MN usually develop severe proteinuria, edema, hypoalbuminemia, and hyperlipidemia [94]. It is the most common cause of idiopathic nephrotic syndrome in non-diabetic white adults. About 80% of cases are restricted to the kidneys (primary MN, PMN, idiopathic membranous nephropathy) and 20% are related to other systemic diseases or exposure (secondary MN) [95]. MN is associated with a pathological alteration of the glomerular basement membrane. This change is due to the build-up of immune complexes that appear as granular immunoglobulin (Ig)G deposits after immunofluorescence imaging and as electron-dense deposits of high electron density. Deposits of these immune complexes between podocytes and the basement membrane have a complex that attacks the complement membrane (C5b-9) [96]. The formation of glomerular sub-epithelial immune complex deposits in the IMN is mediated by specific intrinsic podocyte antigens and their corresponding autoantibodies in humans. These include compounds, such as neutral endopeptidase (NEP), type M receptor for secretory phospholipase A2 (PLA2R1), and type 1 7A thrombospondin (THSD7A) (containing domain 8–10) [94–96]. The above-mentioned markers constitute the core of the research into the pathogenesis of membranous nephropathy. However, there are reports of a genetic susceptibility to idiopathic membranous nephropathy. This type of study was conducted in a high-prevalence area in Taiwan [97]. In these studies, the association of the *IL-6, NPHS1 (nephrin), TLR-4, TLR-9, STAT4 (signal transducer and activator of transcription)* and *MYH (mutY DNA glycosylase)*, genes with susceptibility to primary membranous nephropathy in Taiwan was established. In the case of the TLR4 receptor gene, the gene polymorphism indicated a significant single nucleotide difference in the rs10983755 A/G region ($p < 0.001$) and rs1927914 A/G ($p < 0.05$) between the control group and MN patients. In addition, the distributions of rs10759932 C/T and rs11536889 C/T polymorphisms differed significantly [97].

6.4. *IgA Nephropathy (IgAN)*

The development of IgA nephropathy consists of many mechanisms not yet fully understood. Literature data breaks down biomarkers for IgA nephropathy into a diagnostic and prognostic marker. The first group includes biomarkers detected in serum and urine, such as uromodulin, CD71, IL-6, complement components, and serum BAFF (B-cell activating factor) [98]. However, the group of prognostic markers includes urine kidney injury molecule-1, fractional excretion of IgG, soluble CD89, urinary angiotensinogen, and inflammatory cytokines (Figure 6). The above markers may indicate or predict the main cause of nephropathy development, which is the overproduction of anti-IgA complexes. One of the reasons for stimulating the body to produce IgA-related complexes may be signaling disorders associated with TLRs [99–101]. Ligands of bacterial or viral origin are recognized by toll-like receptors that trigger the process of chemokine release and recruitment of macrophages and neutrophils at the site of infection [102]. In numerous studies on IgAN pathogenesis, various types of receptors that could influence the development of this disease have been analyzed. These receptors were TLR3, mainly recognizing viral dsDNA [103]; TLR7 receptor [104]; binding to ssRNA viruses and TLR4 [105,106]; and binding of a variety of ligands, including LPS Gram-negative bacteria and DAMP (Table 2). Numerous observations of patients with diagnosed IgAN suggest the involvement of pathogens of viral origin, which is also confirmed by experimental models. There is an unexpected increase in the level of TLR4 activation, which is involved in the diagnosis of exogenous bacterial factors (LPS from Gram-negative bacteria, *Chlamydia pneumoniae*, HSP (heat shock proteins) proteins) and endogenous origin (HSP-60, additional fibronectin A domain, low-molecular LDL fractions, acid oligosaccharides hyaluronic acid, heparan sulphate), as well as factors derived from the breakdown of host cells [107–113]. To fully explain kidney damage in IgAN, it is necessary to fully understand the effects of TLR4 in the development of glomerulopathy, involving both glomerular cells and circulating leukocytes. Studies have shown that the administration of LPS activates TLR4 receptors on mesangial cells, and causes the release of chemokines (CXCs), which promotes neutrophil infusion and the development of glomerulonephritis [114–116]. In addition, the IFN-γ and IFN-α responses induced by TLR activation induce overexpression of the B-cell activation factor (BAFF) in dendritic cells, favoring the expansion of B-cells and increasing IgA synthesis [117–121]. It was also shown that in kidney biopsies of patients with IgAN, CD19+/CD5+ B cell infiltration is present, which in the progressive forms of this disease produce significant amounts of IFN-γ and IgA and are more resistant to apoptosis compared to cells obtained from healthy donors [122,123]. Moreover, Hitoshi Suzuki et al. [101] showed that there is an association between gene polymorphisms for TLR-9 and disease progression. Stimulation with ligands for TLR-9 led to the deterioration of kidney function in mice and influenced the shift of the balance towards Th1 lymphocytes. These findings led to the conclusion that activation of pathways related to this particular type of receptor may influence the severity of IgA nephropathy [101]. Moreover, Coppo et al. [124] showed that in patients diagnosed with IgA nephropathy, higher levels of TLR-4 in mononuclear cells and transcriptional mRNA were observed than in the control group. An important fact is that there is a statistical difference in the level of the above markers in patients with severe disease and those who do not have proteinuria and hematuria [124]. TLR-4 can be activated by many ligands, such as HLPs and LPS and DAMPs [106].

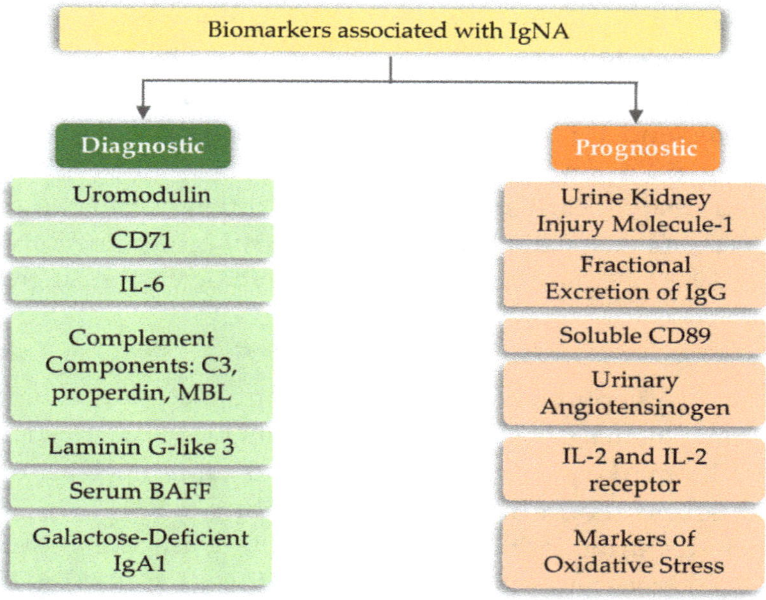

Figure 6. Biomarkers in IgA (immunoglobulin A) nephropathy.

7. The Role of TLR Receptors in Secondary Nephropathies

7.1. Lupus Nephritis

Systemic lupus erythematosus (SLE) is one example of systemic autoimmune diseases. SLE relies on the loss of tolerance to autoantigens, which is caused by the malfunctioning of acquired immunity cells [109,125–127]. In the case of SLE, clinical studies indicate that the most common source of biomarker searches is a urine sample. Due to this, numerous proteins, such as cytokines, chemokines, complement proteins, adhesive molecules, and autoantibodies, have been identified as potential biomarkers of disease activity in cross-sectional studies (Figure 7) [128].

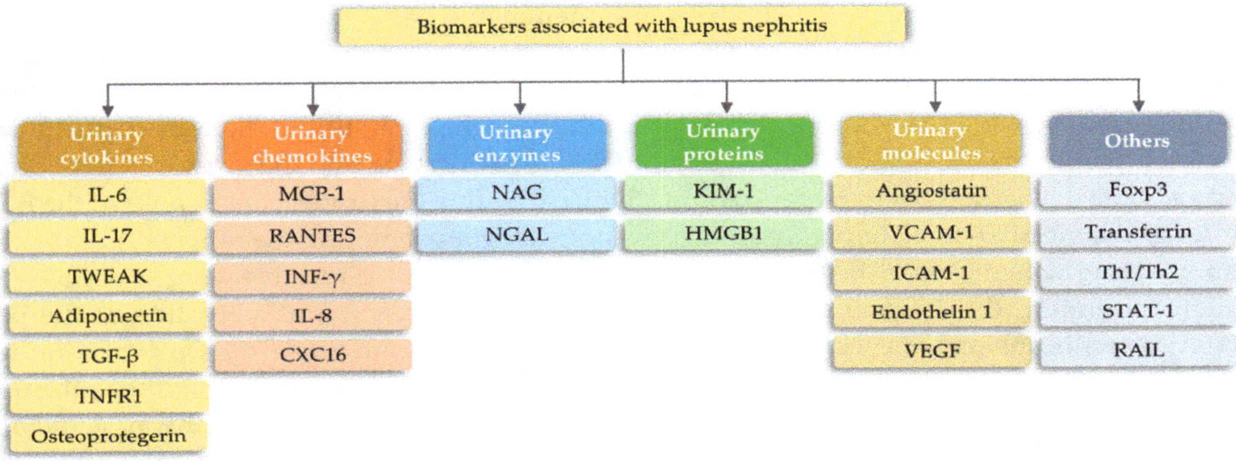

Figure 7. Biomarkers associated with lupus nephritis [128]; CXC16—C-X-C motif chemokine 16; FOXP3—forkhead box protein P3; HMGB1—High mobility group box 1; ICAM—Intercellular Adhesion Molecule 1; IL-6—Urinary Interleukin 6; IL-8—Interleukin 8; IL-17—Urinary Interleukin 17; KIM-1—Urinary kidney injury molecule-1; MCP-1—Monocyte chemoattractant protein-1; NAG—N-Acetyl-β-D Glucosaminidase; NGAL—neutrophil gelatinase-associated lipocalin; RAIL—Renal Activity Index for Lupus; RANTES—Regulated upon Activation, Normal T-cell Expressed, and Secreted; STAT-1—Signal transducer and activator of transcription 1; TGF-β—transforming growth factor beta; Th1—T helper 1; Th2—T helper 2; TNFR1—Tumor necrosis factor receptor 1; TWEAK—Urinary TNF-like weak inducer of apoptosis; VCAM—vascular cell adhesion molecule 1; VEGF—Vascular Endothelial Growth Factor.

Literature data of recent years indicate a special contribution to the etiopathogenesis of this disease of innate immunity elements, mainly TLR. External and endogenous ligands may interact with TLRs present on monocytes, dendritic cells, and B lymphocytes, infiltrating the glomeruli, and resulting in increased cytokine secretion [129,130]. In addition, mesangial cells and other cells of the parenchyma express TLR1-4 and TLR6 receptors and secrete interleukins and chemokines [15,129,131–134]. Studies show that most deposits of immune complexes contain TLR agonists that have the ability to activate mesangial cells and contribute to the development of lupus nephropathy [135]. Pawar et al. [136] summarized the literature data, indicating that microbial nucleic acids can constitute a universal PAMP. As a result, it is possible to activate various mechanisms, such as lymphoproliferation, production of autoantibodies, type I interferon, secretion of numerous cytokines, and promotion of lupus development, in genetically predisposed individuals [136].

TLR2 and TLR4 are expressed not only in parenchymal cells but also in infiltrating neutrophils and mononuclear phagocytes, including macrophages and dendritic cells [137]. The HMGB1 (high mobility group box 1) protein, which binds DNA and the lupus autoantigen released under inflammation, can induce the activation of NF-κB in a TLR2-dependent and TLR4-RAGE-dependent manner in mononuclear phagocytes and neutrophils [138–143] as well as in mesangial cells [144]. Mesangial cells and podocytes in humans are characterized by the expression of TLR4 [145]. Mesangial cells isolated from mice with autoimmune diseases have significantly higher TLR4 expression and produce much more proinflammatory chemokines both after LPS stimulation and spontaneously [146]. Other studies also indicate that the necrotic cell debris-enhanced endogenous TLR ligands stimulate cytokine release by TLR2/MyD88 from mesangial cells, which implies the expression of TLR2 in different cell populations, and kidney-building structure [147–150]. Intracellular expression of TLR2 and TLR4 is multiplied in the kidneys of CD32b receptor-deficient mice suffering from glomerulonephritis associated with cryoglobulinemia [145,151,152].

7.2. Diabetic Nephropathy (DN)

One of the most serious complications for patients diagnosed with type I or II diabetes is diabetic nephropathy, which can be caused by both environmental and genetic factors [18,153]. The diabetic nephropathy is important to the inflammatory process in which, besides an increase in the activity of macrophages and overproduction of adhesion molecules of leukocyte cells, the proximal tubular kidney releases cytokine chemoattractant protein matrix to the interstitium, thereby contributing to the development of the disease [154–156]. Literature studies indicate that the greatest risk of diabetic nephropathy is the occurrence of hyperglycemia, which disrupts the proper functioning of the human body. On the molecular level, hyperglycemia is responsible for promoting the mitochondrial electron transport chain, which causes the formation of excessive amounts of reactive oxygen species (ROS) (through formation of the advanced glycation end products (AGEs) and activation of the polyol pathway, hexosamine pathway, protein kinase C (PKC), and angiotensin II). ROS occurring in the cell initiate or also intensify the formation of oxidative stress, which causes the intensification of inflammation and formation of fibrosis. Abnormalities in the lipid metabolism pathway, activation of the renin-angiotensin-aldosterone system (RAAS), as well as systemic and glomerular hypertension are also involved in the progression of this disease. Impairment of insulin signaling, an increase in growth factors and proinflammatory cytokines, and activation of the intracellular signaling pathway also play a role in the development of this disease [157]. Therefore, the currently known DN biomarkers focus on three areas: Detection of oxidative stress, the occurrence of inflammation, and activation of the RAAS system (Figure 8).

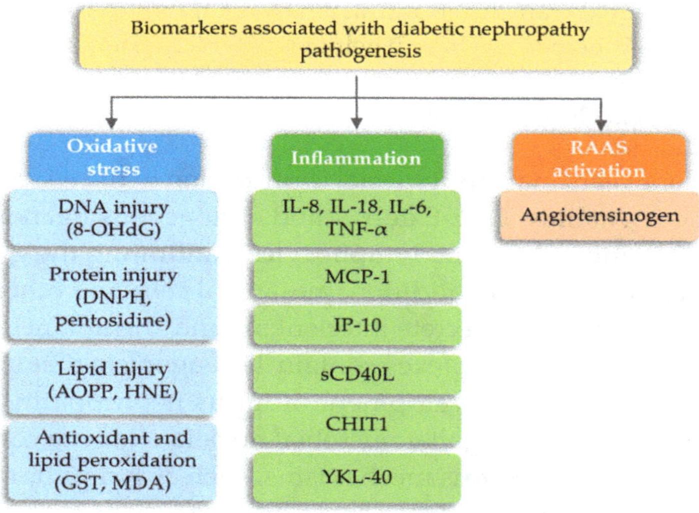

Figure 8. Biomarkers associated with diabetic nephropathy pathogenesis (based on [157]). 8-OHdG—8-hydroxy-2′-deoxyguanine; AOPP—advanced oxidation protein product; CHIT1—chitotriosidase; DNPH—2,4-dinitrophenylhydrazine; GS—Glutathione s-transferase; HNE—4-hydroxy-nonenal; IL-6—interleukin 6; IL-8—interleukin 8; IL-18—interleukin 18; IP-10—interferon-inducible protein-10; MCP-1—Monocyte chemoattractant protein-1; MDA—malondialdehyde; sCD40L—soluble CD40 ligand; TNF-α—Tumor necrosis factor alpha; YKL-40—cartilage glycoprotein 40.

Literature data from recent years indicate that an important role in diabetic nephropathy etiopathogenesis may be played by signal transduction pathways that are dependent on TLR2, TLR9, and TLR4 receptors. However, it is not clear which receptor is more pathogenic [154,158–160]. Studies of many research teams indicate increased expression of TLR2 and the presence of endogenous ligands HMGB1 [161,162] and HSP70 [107,122,163], detected on the basis of research conducted on diabetic-induced rats. In addition, the expression of MyD88 and MCP-1, NF-κB, and infiltration of macrophages has been demonstrated [164–167]. High TLR2 expression was also observed in the glomeruli and renal tubules of people with diabetes. The results were confirmed in vitro in cultures of NRK-52E cell lines in which a high glucose concentration induced TLR2 mRNA expression [168–170]. The pathogenic role of TLR4 in diabetic nephropathy has also been found. In vitro studies have shown that activation of NF-κB and the expression of proinflammatory cytokines was reduced when TLR4 expression was silenced or its signaling was inhibited. During mouse studies, higher TLR4 activity and expression of the NF-κB p65 subunit in the kidney cortex of mice with experimental diabetes was demonstrated [171]. In vitro, researchers also observed increased TLR4 expression and proinflammatory cytokine synthesis when podocytes and adipocytes were exposed to both high glucose and NEFA (non-esterified "free" fatty acids), suggesting a key role of TLR4 in supporting inflammation in diabetic nephropathy [171–173]. In addition, another research team [174] showed an increase in the expression of TLR4 and signaling proteins for this receptor along with the activation of NF-κB, but not TLR2, in a mouse mesangium that was exposed to high glucose concentrations. It was also observed that hyperglycemia stimulated the expression of TLR4 in glomerular renal endothelial cells in a mouse model of type 1 and type 2 diabetes, which underlines the relationship of the discussed receptor with diabetic nephropathy [174,175]. In addition, clinical data indicate that in patients with type 1 diabetes, ligands, endotoxins, heat shock proteins 60 (Hsp60), and high mobility groups 1 (HMGB1) of both TLR2 and TLR4 [176,177] are increased. Increased expression of mRNA was also observed. TLR2, MyD88, and proinflammatory cytokines in leukocytes of patients with type 1 diabetes mellitus suggests that the inflammatory process is mediated by TLR2 [176]. However, in patients with type 2 diabetes and confirmed biopsy, diabetic kidney disease has been found to increase TLR4 expression on renal tubules as opposed to TLR2. In addition, in patients with type II diabetes and confirmed diabetic kidney disease, microalbuminuria, mRNA, and TLR4 protein were overexpressed 4 to 10 times more in glomeruli and tubules compared to the control group. However, both TLR2 and TLR4 expression was increased on monocytes in patients with type II diabetes [176]. Although the literature data indicate a key role of TLR2 and TLR4 in the pathophysiology of diabetic nephropathy, the participation of other receptors is not excluded. There is evidence to suggest the involvement of TLR3, TLR7, and TLR9 receptors in the pathogenesis of type 1 diabetes by destroying pancreatic islets induced by viral infection [114,178,179].

7.3. Acute Kidney Injury (AKI) to Chronic Kidney Disease (CKD) Development

The 2019 definition published by Ronco in The Lancet says that AKI: "is defined by a rapid increase in serum creatinine, decrease in urine output, or both". The authors indicate that acute kidney injury accounts for up to 15% of the reasons for admission to hospital and occurs in as much as 50% of patients treated in intensive care units [180]. Therefore, it is argued that AKI is still associated with high morbidity and mortality [181]. There are many causes of AKI, including acute ischemia, analgesic nephropathy, sepsis, and severe glomerulopathies. Meta-analyses and cohort studies confirm the role of acute kidney injury in the development of chronic kidney disease and, as a complication of AKI, the more frequent need for chronic renal replacement therapy in the form of dialysis therapy [182–184]. The literature does not indicate clear causes and markers of the transition of acute kidney injury to chronic kidney disease, although it is known that this process involves numerous immune mechanisms. Inflammation, induced death, and fibrosis are likely contributors to the progression of AKI to CKD [185]. The renal epithelium plays an important role in promoting inflammation after damage by attracting leukocytes to the site of damage, which is seen as a strong role for TLR-4 [186]. The role of TLR2 and TLR4 in reperfusion after ischemic kidney injury is significant, where their expression increases significantly and enhances the proinflammatory response of tissues, with the participation of numerous cytokines and chemokines [187,188]. It is also noteworthy that the TLR-3 receptor system is involved in ischemia/reperfusion injury in the kidney. Studies have been carried out that showed rapid activation of these receptors, resulting in significant kidney damage, which was associated with elevated rates of apoptosis and necrosis in the renal tubes of mice [189]. Both TLR2 and TLR4 are also involved in sepsis-induced kidney damage [190], caused by Gram-positive and G-negative bacteria; nevertheless, the roles of single TLRs are differing [191]. There is also the TLR4-IL-22 pathway, which probably has regenerative functions in opposition to the above, and more research is needed on this topic [192]. After the action of a harmful factor, the repair process takes place, the element of which is sterile ignition [193]. In the first stage of inflammation, neutrophilic exudate appears, which over time is replaced by a monocytic-lymphocytic infiltrate [194,195]. The presence of monocytes is regarded as a mechanism promoting fibrosis and fibroblast proliferation [196]. The influx of cells of the immune system leads to cell apoptosis and the formation of a large amount of breakdown products and other substances that act as DAMPs, which can activate receptors, including TLRs [78,197]. It then promotes and strengthens the inflammatory response, attracting more cells of the immune system and subsequent fibrosis. Kidney infiltration by monocytes is recognized as a feature of chronic kidney disease [198] and the degree of monocyte infiltration correlates with the severity of kidney damage [199]. The above data indicate that it is the intensified process of fibrosis, mediated largely by the elements of the immune system, that can lead to permanent damage to the kidney function and the progression of AKI to CKD.

8. Conclusions

The innate immunity system in which TLRs participate, among others, cells, such as monocytes, macrophages, and NK (natural killer) cells, expressing TLR and lectin receptors are the body's first line of defense. TLRs identify the pathogen based on the specific pattern of the molecule and therefore stimulate the immune system acquired, including T and B lymphocytes to fight pathogens [15]. Long-term continuous antigenic stimulation, increasing the work of TLRs, can lead to the development of serious diseases, organ specific or systemic. In an increasing number of studies, the role of TLRs has become more important. Recognition receptors are certainly of importance in the pathogenesis of diseases associated with nephropathy, for example, glomerulopathy, diabetic, lupus IgA, or FSGS [1,16]. However, further research is necessary to clarify the possible involvement of TLR in the development of other disease entities associated with kidney damage.

Author Contributions: S.M., P.L., E.G., W.Z.; conceptualization, S.M., P.L., D.B., I.M., P.N.-R., E.G., R.H.; writing—original draft preparation; S.M., P.L., D.B., I.M., P.N.-R., E.G., R.H., W.Z., J.R.; writing—review and editing. All authors have read and agreed to the published version of the manuscript.

Abbreviations

8-OHdG	8-hydroxy-2′-deoxyguanine
ABCB1 Glycoprotein-P	ATP-binding cassette subfamily B member 1 Glycoprotein-P
AKI	Acute kidney injury
AOPP	Advanced oxidation protein product
AR	Androgen Receptor
BAFF	B-cell activation factor
CD80	Cluster of differentiation 80
CHIT1	Chitotriosidase; DNPH-2,4-dinitrophenylhydrazine
CKD	Chronic kidney disease

CXC16	C-X-C motif chemokine 16
DAMP	Damage-associated molecular patterns
DN	Diabetic nephropathy
FOXP3	Forkhead box protein P3
FSGS	Focal segmental glomerulosclerosis
GST	Glutathione s-transferase
HMGB1	High mobility group box 1
HNE	4-hydroxy-nonenal
HSP70	Heat shock proteins 70
ICAM	Intercellular Adhesion Molecule 1
IFN-α	Interferon alpha
IFN-γ	Interferon gamma
IgAN	IgA nephropathy
IL-17	Interleukin 13
IL-13	Interleukin 13
IL-2	Interleukin 2
IL-6	Interleukin 6
IL-7	Interleukin 7
IL-8	Interleukin 8
IP-10	Interferon-inducible protein-10
KIM-1	Urinary kidney injury molecule-1
LPS	Lipopolysaccharides
LRRs	Leucine-rich tandem repeats
MCN	Minimal change nephropathy
MCP-1	Monocyte chemoattractant protein-1
MDA	Malondialdehyde
MN	Membranous nephropathy
NAG	N-Acetyl-β-D Glucosaminidase
NAG	N-Acetyl-β-D Glucosaminidase
NF-κB	Nuclear factor kappa-light-chain-enhancer of activated B cells
NGAL	Neutrophil gelatinase-associated lipocalin
NK cells	Natural killer cells
PAMP	Pathogen-associated molecular patterns
PKC	Protein kinase C
PLA2R	M-type phospholipase A2 receptor
PRRs	Pattern recognition receptors
RAAS	Renin-angiotensin-aldosterone system
RAIL	Renal Activity Index for Lupus
RANTES	Regulated upon Activation, Normal T cell Expressed, and Secreted
ROS	Reactive oxygen species
sCD40L	Soluble CD40 ligand
sIL-2R	Soluble IL-2 receptor
SLE	Systemic lupus erythematosus
SOD2	manganese superoxide-dismutase 2
STAT-1	Signal transducer and activator of transcription 1
suPAR	Soluble urokinase-type plasminogen activator receptor
TGF-β1	Transforming growth factor beta 1
TLR	Toll-like receptor
TNF-a	Tumor necrosis factor alpha
TNFR1	Tumor necrosis factor receptor 1
TWEAK	Urinary TNF-like weak inducer of apoptosis
VCAM	Vascular cell adhesion molecule 1
VEGF	Vascular Endothelial Growth Factor
YKL-40	Cartilage glycoprotein 40

References

1. World Health Organization; International Programme on Chemical Safety. *Biomarkers in Risk Assessment: Validity and Validation*; World Health Organization: Geneva, Switzerland, 2001; ISBN 978-92-4-157222-4.
2. Fuentes-Arderiu, X. What is a biomarker? It's time for a renewed definition. *Clin. Chem. Lab. Med.* **2013**, *51*, 1689–1690. [CrossRef] [PubMed]
3. Goerlich, N.; Brand, H.A.; Langhans, V.; Tesch, S.; Schachtner, T.; Koch, B.; Paliege, A.; Schneider, W.; Grützkau, A.; Reinke, P.; et al. Kidney transplant monitoring by urinary flow cytometry: Biomarker combination of T cells, renal tubular epithelial cells, and podocalyxin-positive cells detects rejection. *Sci. Rep.* **2020**, *10*, 796. [CrossRef] [PubMed]
4. Kasurinen, A.; Hagström, J.; Laitinen, A.; Kokkola, A.; Böckelman, C.; Haglund, C. Evaluation of toll-like receptors as prognostic biomarkers in gastric cancer: High tissue TLR5 predicts a better outcome. *Sci. Rep.* **2019**, *9*, 12553. [CrossRef] [PubMed]
5. Darrabie, M.D.; Cheeseman, J.; Limkakeng, A.T.; Borawski, J.; Sullenger, B.A.; Elster, E.A.; Kirk, A.D.; Lee, J. Toll-like receptor activation as a biomarker in traumatically injured patients. *J. Surg. Res.* **2018**, *231*, 270–277. [CrossRef]
6. Webster, A.C.; Nagler, E.V.; Morton, R.L.; Masson, P. Chronic Kidney Disease. *Lancet* **2017**, *389*, 1238–1252. [CrossRef]
7. Dobrică, E.-C.; Găman, M.-A.; Cozma, M.-A.; Bratu, O.G.; Pantea Stoian, A.; Diaconu, C.C. Polypharmacy in Type 2 Diabetes Mellitus: Insights from an Internal Medicine Department. *Medicina* **2019**, *55*, 436. [CrossRef]
8. O'Shaughnessy, M.M.; Hogan, S.L.; Thompson, B.D.; Coppo, R.; Fogo, A.B.; Jennette, J.C. Glomerular disease frequencies by race, sex and region: Results from the International Kidney Biopsy Survey. *Nephrol. Dial. Transplant.* **2018**, *33*, 661–669. [CrossRef]
9. Naylor, S. Biomarkers: Current perspectives and future prospects. *Expert Rev. Mol. Diagn.* **2003**, *3*, 525–529. [CrossRef]
10. Sahu, P.; Pinkalwar, N.; Dubey, R.D.; Paroha, S.; Chatterjee, S.; Chatterjee, T. Biomarkers: An Emerging Tool for Diagnosis of a Disease and Drug Development. *Asian J. Res. Pharm. Sci.* **2011**, *1*, 9–16.
11. Drucker, E.; Krapfenbauer, K. Pitfalls and limitations in translation from biomarker discovery to clinical utility in predictive and personalised medicine. *EPMA J.* **2013**, *4*, 7. [CrossRef]
12. Mayeux, R. Biomarkers: Potential Uses and Limitations. *NeuroRx* **2004**, *1*, 182–188. [CrossRef] [PubMed]
13. FDA. About Biomarkers and Qualification. Available online: https://www.fda.gov/drugs/cder-biomarker-qualification-program/about-biomarkers-and-qualification (accessed on 10 August 2020).
14. Levin, A.; Tonelli, M.; Bonventre, J.; Coresh, J.; Donner, J.-A.; Fogo, A.B.; Fox, C.S.; Gansevoort, R.T.; Heerspink, H.J.L.; Jardine, M.; et al. Global kidney health 2017 and beyond: A roadmap for closing gaps in care, research, and policy. *Lancet* **2017**, *390*, 1888–1917. [CrossRef]
15. Devarapu, S.K.; Anders, H. Toll-like receptors in lupus nephritis. *J. Biomed. Sci.* **2018**, *25*, 35. [CrossRef]
16. Luyckx, V.A.; Tonelli, M.; Stanifer, J.W. The global burden of kidney disease and the sustainable development goals. *Bull. World Health Organ.* **2018**, *96*, 414–422D. [CrossRef] [PubMed]
17. Yeo, S.C.; Cheung, C.K.; Barratt, J. New insights into the pathogenesis of IgA nephropathy. *Pediatr. Nephrol.* **2018**, *33*, 763–777. [CrossRef] [PubMed]
18. Zheng, Z.; Zheng, F. Immune Cells and Inflammation in Diabetic Nephropathy. *J. Diabetes Res.* **2016**, *2016*, 1841690. [CrossRef]
19. Mohammad Hosseini, A.; Majidi, J.; Baradaran, B.; Yousefi, M. Toll-Like Receptors in the Pathogenesis of Autoimmune Diseases. *Adv. Pharm. Bull.* **2015**, *5*, 605–614. [CrossRef] [PubMed]
20. Imig, J.D.; Ryan, M.J. Immune and Inflammatory Role in Renal Disease. *Compr. Physiol.* **2013**, *3*, 957–976. [CrossRef]
21. Berger, S.P.; Daha, M.R. Complement in glomerular injury. *Semin. Immunopathol.* **2007**, *29*, 375–384. [CrossRef]
22. Kawasaki, T.; Kawai, T. Toll-Like Receptor Signaling Pathways. *Front. Immunol.* **2014**, *5*, 461. [CrossRef]
23. Eleftheriadis, T.; Lawson, B.R. Toll-like receptors and kidney diseases. *Inflamm. Allergy Drug Targets* **2009**, *8*, 191–201. [CrossRef] [PubMed]
24. Liu, Y.; Xue, G.; Li, S.; Fu, Y.; Yin, J.; Zhang, R.; Li, J. Effect of Intermittent and Mild Cold Stimulation on the Immune Function of Bursa in Broilers. *Animals* **2020**, *10*, 1275. [CrossRef] [PubMed]

25. Botos, I.; Segal, D.M.; Davies, D.R. The Structural Biology of Toll-Like Receptors. *Structure* **2011**, *19*, 447–459. [CrossRef] [PubMed]
26. UniProt. Toll-Like Receptor 1. Available online: https://www.uniprot.org/uniprot/Q15399 (accessed on 10 August 2020).
27. Protein Data Bank in Europe. Crystal Structure of the TLR1-TLR2 Heterodimer Induced by Binding of a tri-Acylatedlipopeptide. Available online: https://www.ebi.ac.uk/pdbe/entry/pdb/2z7x (accessed on 10 August 2020).
28. UniProt. Toll-Like Receptor 2. Available online: https://www.uniprot.org/uniprot/O60603 (accessed on 10 August 2020).
29. Protein Data Bank in Europe. Crystal Structure of TLR2-TLR6-Pam2CSK4 Complex. Available online: https://www.ebi.ac.uk/pdbe/entry/pdb/3a79 (accessed on 10 August 2020).
30. UniProt. Toll-Like Receptor 3. Available online: https://www.uniprot.org/uniprot/O15455 (accessed on 10 August 2020).
31. Protein Data Bank in Europe. Crystal Structure of the Complex of TLR3 and bi-Specific Diabody. Available online: https://www.ebi.ac.uk/pdbe/entry/pdb/5gs0 (accessed on 10 August 2020).
32. UniProt. Toll-Like Receptor 4. Available online: https://www.uniprot.org/uniprot/O00206 (accessed on 10 August 2020).
33. Protein Data Bank in Europe. The Crystal Structure of Mouse TLR4/MD-2/neoseptin-3. Available online: https://www.ebi.ac.uk/pdbe/entry/pdb/5ijc (accessed on 10 August 2020).
34. UniProt. Toll-Like Receptor 5. Available online: https://www.uniprot.org/uniprot/O60602 (accessed on 10 August 2020).
35. Protein Data Bank in Europe. Homology Model of Human Toll-Like Receptor 5 Fitted into an Electron Microscopy Single Particle Reconstruction. Available online: https://www.ebi.ac.uk/pdbe/entry/pdb/3j0a (accessed on 10 August 2020).
36. UniProt. Toll-Like Receptor 6. Available online: https://www.uniprot.org/uniprot/Q9Y2C9 (accessed on 10 August 2020).
37. Protein Data Bank in Europe. Crystal Structure of TIR Domain TLR6. Available online: https://www.ebi.ac.uk/pdbe/entry/pdb/4om7 (accessed on 10 August 2020).
38. UniProt. Toll-Like Receptor 7. Available online: https://www.uniprot.org/uniprot/Q9NYK1 (accessed on 10 August 2020).
39. UniProt. Toll-Like Receptor 8. Available online: https://www.uniprot.org/uniprot/Q9NR97 (accessed on 10 August 2020).
40. Protein Data Bank in Europe. Crystal Structure of Human TLR8 in Complex with XG-1-236. Available online: https://www.ebi.ac.uk/pdbe/entry/pdb/4qc0 (accessed on 10 August 2020).
41. UniProt. Toll-Like Receptor 9. Available online: https://www.uniprot.org/uniprot/Q9NR96 (accessed on 10 August 2020).
42. UniProt. Toll-Like Receptor 10. Available online: https://www.uniprot.org/uniprot/Q9BXR5 (accessed on 10 August 2020).
43. Protein Data Bank in Europe. The TIR Domain of Human Toll-Like Receptor 10 (TLR10). Available online: https://www.ebi.ac.uk/pdbe/entry/pdb/2j67 (accessed on 10 August 2020).
44. UniProt. Toll-Like Receptor 11. Available online: https://www.uniprot.org/uniprot/Q6R5P0 (accessed on 10 August 2020).
45. UniProt. Toll-Like Receptor 12. Available online: https://www.uniprot.org/uniprot/Q6QNU9 (accessed on 10 August 2020).
46. UniProt. Toll-Like Receptor 13. Available online: https://www.uniprot.org/uniprot/Q6R5N8 (accessed on 10 August 2020).
47. Farhat, K.; Riekenberg, S.; Heine, H.; Debarry, J.; Lang, R.; Mages, J.; Buwitt-Beckmann, U.; Röschmann, K.; Jung, G.; Wiesmüller, K.-H.; et al. Heterodimerization of TLR2 with TLR1 or TLR6 expands the ligand spectrum but does not lead to differential signaling. *J. Leukoc. Biol.* **2008**, *83*, 692–701. [CrossRef] [PubMed]
48. Zhao, S.; Zhang, Y.; Zhang, Q.; Wang, F.; Zhang, D. Toll-like receptors and prostate cancer. *Front. Immunol.* **2014**, *5*, 352. [CrossRef]
49. Goulopoulou, S.; McCarthy, C.G.; Clinton Webb, R. Toll-like receptors in the vascular system: Sensing the dangers within. *Pharmacol. Rev.* **2016**, *68*, 142–167. [CrossRef]

50. Schaefer, L. Complexity of danger: The diverse nature of damage-associated molecular patterns. *J. Biol. Chem.* **2014**, *289*, 35237–35245. [CrossRef]
51. Brubaker, S.W.; Bonham, K.S.; Zanoni, I.; Kagan, J.C. Innate immune pattern recognition: A cell biological perspective. *Annu. Rev. Immunol.* **2015**, *33*, 257–290. [CrossRef]
52. Miao, E.A.; Andersen-Nissen, E.; Warren, S.E.; Aderem, A. TLR5 and Ipaf: Dual sensors of bacterial flagellin in the innate immune system. *Semin. Immunopathol.* **2007**, *29*, 275–288. [CrossRef]
53. Takeuchi, O.; Kawai, T.; Sanjo, H.; Copeland, N.G.; Gilbert, D.J.; Jenkins, N.A.; Takeda, K.; Akira, S. TLR6: A novel member of an expanding Toll-like receptor family. *Gene* **1999**, *231*, 59–65. [CrossRef]
54. Oosting, M.; Cheng, S.C.; Bolscher, J.M.; Vestering-Stenger, R.; Plantinga, T.S.; Verschueren, I.C.; Arts, P.; Garritsen, A.; van Eenennaam, H.; Sturm, P.; et al. Human TLR10 is an anti-inflammatory pattern-recognition receptor. *Proc. Natl. Acad. Sci. USA* **2014**, *111*, E4478–E4484. [CrossRef] [PubMed]
55. Raetz, M.; Kibardin, A.; Sturge, C.R.; Pifer, R.; Li, H.; Burstein, E.; Ozato, K.; Larin, S.; Yarovinsky, F. Cooperation of TLR12 and TLR11 in the IRF8-Dependent IL-12 Response to Toxoplasma gondii Profilin. *J. Immunol.* **2013**, *191*, 4818–4827. [CrossRef] [PubMed]
56. Yarovinsky, F.; Zhang, D.; Andersen, J.F.; Bannenberg, G.L.; Serhan, C.N.; Hayden, M.S.; Hieny, S.; Sutterwala, F.S.; Flavell, R.A.; Ghosh, S.; et al. Immunology: TLR11 activation of dendritic cells by a protozoan profilin-like protein. *Science* **2005**, *308*, 1626–1629. [CrossRef] [PubMed]
57. Xiao, X.; Zhao, P.; Rodriguez-Pinto, D.; Qi, D.; Henegariu, O.; Alexopoulou, L.; Flavell, R.A.; Wong, F.S.; Wen, L. Inflammatory Regulation by TLR3 in Acute Hepatitis. *J. Immunol.* **2009**, *183*, 3712–3719. [CrossRef] [PubMed]
58. Negishi, H.; Osawa, T.; Ogami, K.; Ouyang, X.; Sakaguchi, S.; Koshiba, R.; Yanai, H.; Seko, Y.; Shitara, H.; Bishop, K.; et al. A critical link between Toll-like receptor 3 and type II interferon signaling pathways in antiviral innate immunity. *Proc. Natl. Acad. Sci. USA* **2008**, *105*, 20446–20451. [CrossRef]
59. Hemmi, H.; Kaisho, T.; Takeuchi, O.; Sato, S.; Sanjo, H.; Hoshino, K.; Horiuchi, T.; Tomizawa, H.; Takeda, K.; Akira, S. Small-antiviral compounds activate immune cells via the TLR7 MyD88-dependent signaling pathway. *Nat. Immunol.* **2002**, *3*, 196–200. [CrossRef] [PubMed]
60. Peng, G.; Guo, Z.; Kiniwa, Y.; Voo, K.S.; Peng, W.; Fu, T.; Wang, D.Y.; Li, Y.; Wang, H.Y.; Wang, R.F. Immunology: Toll-like receptor 8-mediated reversal of CD4+ regulatory T cell function. *Science* **2005**, *309*, 1380–1384. [CrossRef]
61. Notley, C.A.; Jordan, C.K.; McGovern, J.L.; Brown, M.A.; Ehrenstein, M.R. DNA methylation governs the dynamic regulation of inflammation by apoptotic cells during efferocytosis. *Sci. Rep.* **2017**, *7*, 1–10. [CrossRef]
62. Kanherkar, R.R.; Bhatia-Dey, N.; Csoka, A.B. Epigenetics across the human lifespan. *Front. Cell Dev. Biol.* **2014**, *2*, 49. [CrossRef]
63. Anders, H.-J.; Banas, B.; Schlöndorff, D. Signaling Danger: Toll-Like Receptors and their Potential Roles in Kidney Disease. *J. Am. Soc. Nephrol.* **2004**, *15*, 854–867. [CrossRef]
64. Verstak, B.; Stack, J.; Ve, T.; Mangan, M.; Hjerrild, K.; Jeon, J.; Stahl, R.; Latz, E.; Gay, N.; Kobe, B.; et al. The TLR signaling adaptor TRAM interacts with TRAF6 to mediate activation of the inflammatory response by TLR4. *J. Leukoc. Biol.* **2014**, *96*, 427–436. [CrossRef] [PubMed]
65. Kayagaki, N.; Phung, Q.; Chan, S.; Chaudhari, R.; Quan, C.; O'Rourke, K.M.; Eby, M.; Pietras, E.; Cheng, G.; Bazan, J.F.; et al. DUBA: A deubiquitinase that regulates type I interferon production. *Science* **2007**, *318*, 1628–1632. [CrossRef] [PubMed]
66. Han, C.; Jin, J.; Xu, S.; Liu, H.; Li, N.; Cao, X. Integrin CD11b negatively regulates TLR-triggered inflammatory responses by activating Syk and promoting degradation of MyD88 and TRIF via Cbl-b. *Nat. Immunol.* **2010**, *11*, 734–742. [CrossRef] [PubMed]
67. Skaug, B.; Chen, J.; Du, F.; He, J.; Ma, A.; Chen, Z.J. Direct, noncatalytic mechanism of IKK inhibition by A20. *Mol. Cell* **2011**, *44*, 559–571. [CrossRef] [PubMed]
68. Yuk, J.M.; Shin, D.M.; Lee, H.M.; Kim, J.J.; Kim, S.W.; Jin, H.S.; Yang, C.S.; Park, K.A.; Chanda, D.; Kim, D.K.; et al. The orphan nuclear receptor SHP acts as a negative regulator in inflammatory signaling triggered by Toll-like receptors. *Nat. Immunol.* **2011**, *12*, 742–751. [CrossRef] [PubMed]
69. Kondo, T.; Kawai, T.; Akira, S. Dissecting negative regulation of Toll-like receptor signaling. *Trends Immunol.* **2012**, *33*, 449–458. [CrossRef] [PubMed]

70. Saitoh, T.; Tun-Kyi, A.; Ryo, A.; Yamamoto, M.; Finn, G.; Fujita, T.; Akira, S.; Yamamoto, N.; Lu, K.P.; Yamaoka, S. Negative regulation of interferon-regulatory factor 3-dependent innate antiviral response by the prolyl isomerase Pin1. *Nat. Immunol.* **2006**, *7*, 598–605. [CrossRef]
71. Kawai, T.; Akira, S. The role of pattern-recognition receptors in innate immunity: Update on Toll-like receptors. *Nat. Immunol.* **2010**, *11*, 373–384. [CrossRef]
72. Kawai, T.; Akira, S. Signaling to NF-kappaB by Toll-like receptors. *Trends Mol. Med.* **2007**, *13*, 460–469. [CrossRef]
73. Liu, T.; Zhang, L.; Joo, D.; Sun, S.C. NF-κB signaling in inflammation. *Signal Transduct. Target. Ther.* **2017**, *2*, 1–9. [CrossRef]
74. Couser, W.G.; Johnson, R.J. The etiology of glomerulonephritis: Roles of infection and autoimmunity. *Kidney Int.* **2014**, *86*, 905–914. [CrossRef] [PubMed]
75. Rock, K.L.; Latz, E.; Ontiveros, F.; Kono, H. The sterile inflammatory response. *Annu. Rev. Immunol.* **2010**, *28*, 321–342. [CrossRef] [PubMed]
76. Yamanishi, Y.; Kitaura, J.; Izawa, K.; Kaitani, A.; Komeno, Y.; Nakamura, M.; Yamazaki, S.; Enomoto, Y.; Oki, T.; Akiba, H.; et al. TIM1 is an endogenous ligand for LMIR5/CD300b: LMIR5 deficiency ameliorates mouse kidney ischemia/reperfusion injury. *J. Exp. Med.* **2010**, *207*, 1501–1511. [CrossRef] [PubMed]
77. Anders, H.J. Toll-Like Receptors and Danger Signaling in Kidney Injury. *J. Am. Soc. Nephrol.* **2010**, *21*, 1270–1274. [CrossRef]
78. Rosin, D.L.; Okusa, M.D. Dangers Within: DAMP Responses to Damage and Cell Death in Kidney Disease. *J. Am. Soc. Nephrol.* **2011**, *22*, 416–425. [CrossRef] [PubMed]
79. Mertowski, S.; Grywalska, E.; Gosik, K.; Smarz-Widelska, I.; Hymos, A.; Dworacki, G.; Niedźwiedzka-Rystwej, P.; Drop, B.; Roliński, J.; Załuska, W. TLR2 Expression on Select Lymphocyte Subsets as a New Marker in Glomerulonephritis. *J. Clin. Med.* **2020**, *9*, 541. [CrossRef]
80. Rosenberg, A.Z.; Kopp, J.B. Focal Segmental Glomerulosclerosis. *Clin. J. Am. Soc. Nephrol.* **2017**, *12*, 502–517. [CrossRef]
81. Reggiani, F.; Ponticelli, C. Focal segmental glomerular sclerosis: Do not overlook the role of immune response. *J. Nephrol.* **2016**, *29*, 525–534. [CrossRef]
82. Eardley, K.S.; Kubal, C.; Zehnder, D.; Quinkler, M.; Lepenies, J.; Savage, C.O.; Howie, A.J.; Kaur, K.; Cooper, M.S.; Adu, D.; et al. The role of capillary density, macrophage infiltration and interstitial scarring in the pathogenesis of human chronic kidney disease. *Kidney Int.* **2008**, *74*, 495–504. [CrossRef]
83. Wu, X.; Dolecki, G.J.; Sherry, B.; Zagorski, J.; Lefkowith, J.B. Chemokines are expressed in a myeloid cell-dependent fashion and mediate distinct functions in immune complex glomerulonephritis in rat. *J. Immunol.* **1997**, *158*, 3917–3924.
84. Wang, H.; Zheng, C.; Xu, X.; Zhao, Y.; Lu, Y.; Liu, Z. Fibrinogen links podocyte injury with Toll-like receptor 4 and is associated with disease activity in FSGS patients. *Nephrology* **2018**, *23*, 418–429. [CrossRef] [PubMed]
85. Gaman, A.M.; Moisa, C.; Diaconu, C.C.; Gaman, M.A. Crosstalk between Oxidative Stress, Chronic Inflammation and Disease Progression in Essential Thrombocythemia. *Rev. Chim.* **2019**, *70*, 3486–3489. [CrossRef]
86. Găman, M.A.; Epîngeac, M.E.; Diaconu, C.C.; Găman, A.M. Evaluation of oxidative stress levels in obesity and diabetes by the free oxygen radical test and free oxygen radical defence assays and correlations with anthropometric and laboratory parameters. *World J. Diabetes* **2020**, *11*, 193–201. [CrossRef] [PubMed]
87. Yacov, N.; Feldman, B.; Volkov, A.; Ishai, E.; Breitbart, E.; Mendel, I. Treatment with lecinoxoids attenuates focal and segmental glomerulosclerosis development in nephrectomized rats. *Basic Clin. Pharmacol. Toxicol.* **2019**, *124*, 131–143. [CrossRef]
88. Segarra-Medrano, A.; Carnicer-Cáceres, C.; Arbós-Via, M.A.; Quiles-Pérez, M.T.; Agraz-Pamplona, I.; Ostos-Roldán, E. Biological markers of nephrotic syndrome: A few steps forward in the long way. *Nefrología* **2012**, *32*, 558–572. [CrossRef] [PubMed]
89. Shah, S.R.; Choi, M. Minimal Change Disease in Adults. In *Glomerulonephritis*; Trachtman, H., Herlitz, L.C., Lerma, E.V., Hogan, J.J., Eds.; Springer International Publishing: Cham, Switzerland, 2019; pp. 97–114. ISBN 978-3-319-49379-4.
90. Uwaezuoke, S.N. Biomarkers of Common Childhood Renal Diseases. In *Biomarker—Indicator of Abnormal Physiological Process*; IntechOpen: London, UK, 2018. [CrossRef]

91. Srivastava, T.; Sharma, M.; Yew, K.H.; Sharma, R.; Duncan, R.S.; Saleem, M.A.; McCarthy, E.T.; Kats, A.; Cudmore, P.A.; Alon, U.S.; et al. LPS and PAN-induced podocyte injury in an in vitro model of minimal change disease: Changes in TLR profile. *J. Cell Commun. Signal.* **2013**, *7*, 49–60. [CrossRef]
92. Mishra, O.P.; Kumar, R.; Narayan, G.; Srivastava, P.; Abhinay, A.; Prasad, R.; Singh, A.; Batra, V.V. Toll-like receptor 3 (TLR-3), TLR-4 and CD80 expression in peripheral blood mononuclear cells and urinary CD80 levels in children with idiopathic nephrotic syndrome. *Pediatr. Nephrol.* **2017**, *32*, 1355–1361. [CrossRef] [PubMed]
93. Ishimoto, T.; Shimada, M.; Araya, C.E.; Huskey, J.; Garin, E.H.; Johnson, R.J. Minimal Change Disease: A CD80 podocytopathy? *Semin. Nephrol.* **2011**, *31*, 320–325. [CrossRef]
94. Lai, W.L.; Yeh, T.H.; Chen, P.M.; Chan, C.K.; Chiang, W.C.; Chen, Y.M.; Wu, K.D.; Tsai, T.J. Membranous nephropathy: A review on the pathogenesis, diagnosis, and treatment. *J. Formos. Med. Assoc.* **2015**, *114*, 102–111. [CrossRef]
95. Couser, W.G. Primary Membranous Nephropathy. *Clin. J. Am. Soc. Nephrol.* **2017**, *12*, 983–997. [CrossRef]
96. Liu, W.; Gao, C.; Dai, H.; Zheng, Y.; Dong, Z.; Gao, Y.; Liu, F.; Zhang, Z.; Liu, Z.; Liu, W.; et al. Immunological Pathogenesis of Membranous Nephropathy: Focus on PLA2R1 and Its Role. *Front. Immunol.* **2019**, *10*, 1809. [CrossRef] [PubMed]
97. Chen, S.Y.; Chen, C.H.; Huang, Y.C.; Chan, C.J.; Chen, D.C.; Tsai, F.J. Genetic susceptibility to idiopathic membranous nephropathy in high-prevalence Area, Taiwan. *Biomedicine* **2014**, *4*, 9. [CrossRef] [PubMed]
98. Nafar, M.; Samavat, S. Biomarkers in IgA Nephropathy. In *Biomarkers in Kidney Disease*; Patel, V.B., Ed.; Springer: Dordrecht, The Netherlands, 2015; pp. 1–29. ISBN 978-94-007-7743-9.
99. Liu, Y.; Ma, X.; Lv, J.; Shi, S.; Liu, L.; Chen, Y.; Zhang, H. Risk factors for pregnancy outcomes in patients with IgA nephropathy: A matched cohort study. *Am. J. Kidney Dis.* **2014**, *64*, 730–736. [CrossRef] [PubMed]
100. Coppo, R.; Camilla, R.; Amore, A.; Peruzzi, L. Oxidative Stress in IgA Nephropathy. *Nephron Clin. Pract.* **2010**, *116*, c196–c199. [CrossRef]
101. Suzuki, H.; Suzuki, Y.; Narita, I.; Aizawa, M.; Kihara, M.; Yamanaka, T.; Kanou, T.; Tsukaguchi, H.; Novak, J.; Horikoshi, S.; et al. Toll-Like Receptor 9 Affects Severity of IgA Nephropathy. *J. Am. Soc. Nephrol.* **2008**, *19*, 2384–2395. [CrossRef]
102. Rollino, C.; Vischini, G.; Coppo, R. IgA nephropathy and infections. *J. Nephrol.* **2016**, *29*, 463–468. [CrossRef]
103. Merkle, M.; Ribeiro, A.; Köppel, S.; Pircher, J.; Mannell, H.; Roeder, M.; Wörnle, M. TLR3-dependent immune regulatory functions of human mesangial cells. *Cell. Mol. Immunol.* **2012**, *9*, 334–340. [CrossRef]
104. Coppo, R.; Amore, A.; Peruzzi, L.; Vergano, L.; Camilla, R. Innate immunity and IgA nephropathy. *J. Nephrol.* **2010**, *23*, 626–632.
105. Sheng, X.; Zuo, X.; Liu, X.; Zhou, Y.; Sun, X. Crosstalk between TLR4 and Notch1 signaling in the IgA nephropathy during inflammatory response. *Int. Urol. Nephrol.* **2018**, *50*, 779–785. [CrossRef]
106. Lim, B.J.; Lee, D.; Hong, S.W.; Jeong, H.J. Toll-Like Receptor 4 Signaling is Involved in IgA-Stimulated Mesangial Cell Activation. *Yonsei Med. J.* **2011**, *52*, 610–615. [CrossRef]
107. Chebotareva, N.; Bobkova, I.; Shilov, E. Heat shock proteins and kidney disease: Perspectives of HSP therapy. *Cell Stress Chaperones* **2017**, *22*, 319–343. [CrossRef] [PubMed]
108. Kaneko, T.; Mii, A.; Fukui, M.; Nagahama, K.; Shimizu, A.; Tsuruoka, S. IgA Nephropathy and Psoriatic Arthritis that Improved with Steroid Pulse Therapy and Mizoribine in Combination with Treatment for Chronic Tonsillitis and Epipharyngitis. *Intern. Med.* **2015**, *54*, 1085–1090. [CrossRef] [PubMed]
109. Brown, H.J.; Lock, H.R.; Wolfs, T.G.A.M.; Buurman, W.A.; Sacks, S.H.; Robson, M.G. Toll-like receptor 4 ligation on intrinsic renal cells contributes to the induction of antibody-mediated glomerulonephritis via CXCL1 and CXCL2. *J. Am. Soc. Nephrol.* **2007**, *18*, 1732–1739. [CrossRef] [PubMed]
110. Myllymäki, J.; Syrjänen, J.; Helin, H.; Pasternack, A.; Kattainen, A.; Mustonen, J. Vascular diseases and their risk factors in IgA nephropathy. *Nephrol. Dial. Transplant.* **2006**, *21*, 1876–1882. [CrossRef] [PubMed]
111. Feehally, J.; Barratt, J. The Genetics of IgA Nephropathy: An Overview from Western Countries. *Kidney Dis.* **2015**, *1*, 33–41. [CrossRef]
112. Takeda, K.; Kaisho, T.; Akira, S. Toll-Like Receptors. *Annu. Rev. Immunol.* **2003**, *21*, 335–376. [CrossRef] [PubMed]
113. Sano, N.; Kitazawa, K.; Sugisaki, T. Localization and roles of CD44, hyaluronic acid and osteopontin in IgA nephropathy. *Nephron* **2001**, *89*, 416–421. [CrossRef]

114. Zhang, Y.-M.; Zhou, X.-J.; Zhang, H. What Genetics Tells Us About the Pathogenesis of IgA Nephropathy: The Role of Immune Factors and Infection. *Kidney Int. Rep.* **2017**, *2*, 318–331. [CrossRef]
115. Cui, Y.; Liu, S.; Cui, W.; Gao, D.; Zhou, W.; Luo, P. Identification of potential biomarkers and therapeutic targets for human IgA nephropathy and hypertensive nephropathy by bioinformatics analysis. *Mol. Med. Rep.* **2017**, *16*, 3087–3094. [CrossRef]
116. Tycová, I.; Hrubá, P.; Maixnerová, D.; Girmanová, E.; Mrázová, P.; Straňavová, L.; Zachoval, R.; Merta, M.; Slatinská, J.; Kollár, M.; et al. Molecular profiling in IgA nephropathy and focal and segmental glomerulosclerosis. *Physiol. Res.* **2018**, *67*, 93–105. [CrossRef]
117. Wardle, E.N. B Lymphocyte Stimulator and Autoimmune Disease. *Saudi J. Kidney Dis. Transplant.* **2004**, *15*, 155.
118. Li, W.; Peng, X.; Liu, Y.; Liu, H.; Liu, F.; He, L.; Liu, Y.; Zhang, F.; Guo, C.; Chen, G.; et al. TLR9 and BAFF: Their expression in patients with IgA nephropathy. *Mol. Med. Rep.* **2014**, *10*, 1469–1474. [CrossRef] [PubMed]
119. Gao, R.; Wu, W.; Wen, Y.; Li, X. Hydroxychloroquine alleviates persistent proteinuria in IgA nephropathy. *Int. Urol. Nephrol.* **2017**, *49*, 1233–1241. [CrossRef] [PubMed]
120. Wu, M.Y.; Chen, C.S.; Yiang, G.T.; Cheng, P.W.; Chen, Y.L.; Chiu, H.C.; Liu, K.H.; Lee, W.C.; Li, C.J. The Emerging Role of Pathogenesis of IgA Nephropathy. *J. Clin. Med.* **2018**, *7*, 225. [CrossRef] [PubMed]
121. Coppo, R. Treatment of IgA nephropathy: Recent advances and prospects. *Nephrol. Ther.* **2018**, *14*, S13–S21. [CrossRef]
122. Yuling, H.; Ruijing, X.; Xiang, J.; Yanping, J.; Lang, C.; Li, L.; Dingping, Y.; Xinti, T.; Jingyi, L.; Zhiqing, T.; et al. CD19+CD5+ B Cells in Primary IgA Nephropathy. *J. Am. Soc. Nephrol.* **2008**, *19*, 2130–2139. [CrossRef]
123. Wang, Y.Y.; Zhang, L.; Zhao, P.W.; Ma, L.; Li, C.; Zou, H.B.; Jiang, Y.F. Functional implications of regulatory B cells in human IgA nephropathy. *Scand. J. Immunol.* **2014**, *79*, 51–60. [CrossRef]
124. Coppo, R.; Camilla, R.; Amore, A.; Peruzzi, L.; Daprà, V.; Loiacono, E.; Vatrano, S.; Rollino, C.; Sepe, V.; Rampino, T.; et al. Toll-like receptor 4 expression is increased in circulating mononuclear cells of patients with immunoglobulin A nephropathy. *Clin. Exp. Immunol.* **2010**, *159*, 73–81. [CrossRef]
125. Almaani, S.; Meara, A.; Rovin, B.H. Update on Lupus Nephritis. *Clin. J. Am. Soc. Nephrol.* **2017**, *12*, 825–835. [CrossRef]
126. Ruiz Irastorza, G.; Espinosa, G.; Frutos, M.A.; Jiménez Alonso, J.; Praga, M.; Pallarés, L.; Rivera, F.; Robles Marhuenda, A.; Segarra, A.; Quereda, C.; et al. Diagnosis and treatment of lupus nephritis. Consensus document from the systemic auto-immune disease group (GEAS) of the Spanish Society of Internal Medicine (SEMI) and Spanish Society of Nephrology (S.E.N.). *Nefrologia* **2012**, *32* (Suppl. 1), 1–35. [CrossRef]
127. Klonowska-Szymczyk, A.; Kulczycka-Siennicka, L.; Robak, T.; Smolewski, P.; Cebula-Obrzut, B.; Robak, E. The impact of agonists and antagonists of TLR3 and TLR9 on concentrations of IL-6, IL10 and sIL-2R in culture supernatants of peripheral blood mononuclear cells derived from patients with systemic lupus erythematosus. *Adv. Hyg. Exp. Med.* **2017**, *71*, 867–875. [CrossRef] [PubMed]
128. Aragón, C.C.; Tafúr, R.A.; Suárez-Avellaneda, A.; Martínez, M.D.T.; de las Salas, A.; Tobón, G.J. Urinary biomarkers in lupus nephritis. *J. Transl. Autoimmun.* **2020**, *3*, 100042. [CrossRef] [PubMed]
129. Patole, P.S.; Pawar, R.D.; Lech, M.; Zecher, D.; Schmidt, H.; Segerer, S.; Ellwart, A.; Henger, A.; Kretzler, M.; Anders, H.-J. Expression and regulation of Toll-like receptors in lupus-like immune complex glomerulonephritis of MRL-Fas(lpr) mice. *Nephrol. Dial. Transplant.* **2006**, *21*, 3062–3073. [CrossRef] [PubMed]
130. Pawar, R.D.; Patole, P.S.; Zecher, D.; Segerer, S.; Kretzler, M.; Schlöndorff, D.; Anders, H.J. Toll-Like Receptor-7 Modulates Immune Complex Glomerulonephritis. *J. Am. Soc. Nephrol.* **2006**, *17*, 141–149. [CrossRef] [PubMed]
131. Gao, R.; Yu, W.; Wen, Y.; Li, H. Beta2-glycoprotein I Expression in Lupus Nephritis Patients with Antiphospholipid-associated Nephropathy. *J. Rheumatol.* **2016**, *43*, 2026–2032. [CrossRef]
132. Kwok, S.K.; Tsokos, G.C. New insights into the role of renal resident cells in the pathogenesis of lupus nephritis. *Korean J. Intern. Med.* **2018**, *33*, 284–289. [CrossRef]
133. Urbonaviciute, V.; Starke, C.; Pirschel, W.; Pohle, S.; Frey, S.; Daniel, C.; Amann, K.; Schett, G.; Herrmann, M.; Voll, R.E. Toll-like Receptor 2 Is Required for Autoantibody Production and Development of Renal Disease in Pristane-Induced Lupus. *Arthritis Rheum.* **2013**, *65*, 1612–1623. [CrossRef]

134. Conti, F.; Spinelli, F.R.; Truglia, S.; Miranda, F.; Alessandri, C.; Ceccarelli, F.; Bombardieri, M.; Giannakakis, K.; Valesini, G. Kidney Expression of Toll Like Receptors in Lupus Nephritis: Quantification and Clinicopathological Correlations. *Mediat. Inflamm.* **2016**, *2016*, 7697592. [CrossRef]
135. Lorenz, G.; Lech, M.; Anders, H.J. Toll-like receptor activation in the pathogenesis of lupus nephritis. *Clin. Immunol.* **2017**, *185*, 86–94. [CrossRef]
136. Pawar, R.D.; Patole, P.S.; Ellwart, A.; Lech, M.; Segerer, S.; Schlondorff, D.; Anders, H.J. Ligands to Nucleic Acid–Specific Toll-Like Receptors and the Onset of Lupus Nephritis. *J. Am. Soc. Nephrol.* **2006**, *17*, 3365–3373. [CrossRef]
137. Lorenz, G.; Anders, H.J. Neutrophils, Dendritic Cells, Toll-Like Receptors, and Interferon-α in Lupus Nephritis. *Semin. Nephrol.* **2015**, *35*, 410–426. [CrossRef]
138. Chen, D.N.; Fan, L.; Wu, Y.X.; Zhou, Q.; Chen, W.; Yu, X.Q. A Predictive Model for Estimation Risk of Proliferative Lupus Nephritis. *Chin. Med. J.* **2018**, *131*, 1275–1281. [CrossRef] [PubMed]
139. Pisetsky, D.S. HMGB1: A smoking gun in lupus nephritis? *Arthritis Res. Ther.* **2012**, *14*, 112. [CrossRef] [PubMed]
140. Sun, F.; Teng, J.; Yu, P.; Li, W.; Chang, J.; Xu, H. Involvement of TWEAK and the NF-κB signaling pathway in lupus nephritis. *Exp. Ther. Med.* **2018**, *15*, 2611–2619. [CrossRef] [PubMed]
141. Watanabe, H.; Watanabe, K.S.; Liu, K.; Hiramatsu, S.; Zeggar, S.; Katsuyama, E.; Tatebe, N.; Akahoshi, A.; Takenaka, F.; Hanada, T.; et al. Anti-high Mobility Group Box 1 Antibody Ameliorates Albuminuria in MRL/lpr Lupus-Prone Mice. *Mol. Ther. Meth. Clin. Dev.* **2017**, *6*, 31–39. [CrossRef]
142. Ma, K.; Li, J.; Fang, Y.; Lu, L. Roles of B Cell-Intrinsic TLR Signals in Systemic Lupus Erythematosus. *Int. J. Mol. Sci.* **2015**, *16*, 13084–13105. [CrossRef] [PubMed]
143. Wirestam, L.; Schierbeck, H.; Skogh, T.; Gunnarsson, I.; Ottosson, L.; Erlandsson-Harris, H.; Wetterö, J.; Sjöwall, C. Antibodies against High Mobility Group Box protein-1 (HMGB1) versus other anti-nuclear antibody fine-specificities and disease activity in systemic lupus erythematosus. *Arthritis Res. Ther.* **2015**, *17*, 338. [CrossRef]
144. Qing, X.; Pitashny, M.; Thomas, D.B.; Barrat, F.J.; Hogarth, M.P.; Putterman, C. Pathogenic anti-DNA antibodies modulate gene expression in mesangial cells: Involvement of HMGB1 in anti-DNA antibody-induced renal injury. *Immunol. Lett.* **2008**, *121*, 61–73. [CrossRef]
145. Banas, M.C.; Banas, B.; Hudkins, K.L.; Wietecha, T.A.; Iyoda, M.; Bock, E.; Hauser, P.; Pippin, J.W.; Shankland, S.J.; Smith, K.D.; et al. TLR4 Links Podocytes with the Innate Immune System to Mediate Glomerular Injury. *J. Am. Soc. Nephrol.* **2008**, *19*, 704–713. [CrossRef]
146. Jończyk, M.; Kuliczkowska-Płaksej, J.; Mierzwicka, A.; Bolanowski, M. The polycystic ovarian syndrome and chronic inflammation: The role of Toll-like receptors. *Postepy Hig. Med. Dosw.* **2018**, *72*, 1199–1207. [CrossRef]
147. Lartigue, A.; Colliou, N.; Calbo, S.; François, A.; Jacquot, S.; Arnoult, C.; Tron, F.; Gilbert, D.; Musette, P. Critical role of TLR2 and TLR4 in autoantibody production and glomerulonephritis in lpr mutation-induced mouse lupus. *J. Immunol.* **2009**, *183*, 6207–6216. [CrossRef] [PubMed]
148. Horton, C.G.; Pan, Z.; Farris, A.D. Targeting toll-like receptors for treatment of SLE. *Mediat. Inflamm.* **2010**, *2010*, 498980. [CrossRef] [PubMed]
149. Wardle, E.N. Toll-Like Receptors and Glomerulonephritis. *Saudi J. Kidney Dis. Transpl.* **2007**, *18*, 159–172.
150. Lichtnekert, J.; Vielhauer, V.; Zecher, D.; Kulkarni, O.; Clauss, S.; Hornung, V.; Mayadas, T.; Beutler, B.; Akira, S.; Anders, H.-J. Trif is not required for immune complex glomerulonephritis: Dying cells activate mesangial cells via Tlr2/Myd88 rather than Tlr3/Trif. *Am. J. Physiol. Renal. Physiol.* **2009**, *296*, F867–F874. [CrossRef]
151. Pradhan, V.; Patwardhan, M.; Ghosh, K. Fc gamma receptor polymorphisms in systemic lupus erythematosus and their correlation with the clinical severity of the disease. *Indian J. Hum. Genet.* **2008**, *14*, 77–81. [CrossRef] [PubMed]
152. Mackay, M.; Stanevsky, A.; Wang, T.; Aranow, C.; Li, M.; Koenig, S.; Ravetch, J.V.; Diamond, B. Selective dysregulation of the FcγIIB receptor on memory B cells in SLE. *J. Exp. Med.* **2006**, *203*, 2157–2164. [CrossRef] [PubMed]
153. Lim, A.K. Diabetic nephropathy—Complications and treatment. *Int. J. Nephrol. Renovasc. Dis.* **2014**, *7*, 361–381. [CrossRef] [PubMed]

154. Mudaliar, H.; Pollock, C.; Panchapakesan, U. Role of Toll-like receptors in diabetic nephropathy. *Clin. Sci.* **2014**, *126*, 685–694. [CrossRef] [PubMed]
155. Conserva, F.; Gesualdo, L.; Papale, M. A Systems Biology Overview on Human Diabetic Nephropathy: From Genetic Susceptibility to Post-Transcriptional and Post-Translational Modifications. *J. Diabetes Res.* **2016**, *2016*, 7934504. [CrossRef] [PubMed]
156. Umanath, K.; Lewis, J.B. Update on Diabetic Nephropathy: Core Curriculum 2018. *Am. J. Kidney Dis.* **2018**, *71*, 884–895. [CrossRef]
157. Zhang, J.; Liu, J.; Qin, X.; Zhang, J.; Liu, J.; Qin, X. Advances in early biomarkers of diabetic nephropathy. *Rev. Assoc. Med. Bras.* **2018**, *64*, 85–92. [CrossRef] [PubMed]
158. Mansour, I.; Thajudeen, B. Overview of Diabetic Nephropathy. *J. R. Soc. Med.* **2017**, 1–21. [CrossRef]
159. Wifi, M.-N.A.; Assem, M.; Elsherif, R.H.; El-Azab, H.A.-F.; Saif, A. Toll-like receptors-2 and -9 (TLR2 and TLR9) gene polymorphism in patients with type 2 diabetes and diabetic foot. *Medicine* **2017**, *96*, e6760. [CrossRef] [PubMed]
160. Eknoyan, G. A Historical Overview of Diabetic Nephropathy. In *Diabetic Nephropathy*; Springer: Cham, Switzerland, 2019; pp. 3–19. [CrossRef]
161. Chen, X.; Ma, J.; Kwan, T.; Stribos, E.G.D.; Messchendorp, A.L.; Loh, Y.W.; Wang, X.; Paul, M.; Cunningham, E.C.; Habib, M.; et al. Blockade of HMGB1 Attenuates Diabetic Nephropathy in Mice. *Sci. Rep.* **2018**, *8*, 8319. [CrossRef]
162. Shi, H.; Che, Y.; Bai, L.; Zhang, J.; Fan, J.; Mao, H. High mobility group box 1 in diabetic nephropathy (Review). *Exp. Ther. Med.* **2017**, *14*, 2431–2433. [CrossRef]
163. Bellini, S.; Barutta, F.; Mastrocola, R.; Imperatore, L.; Bruno, G.; Gruden, G. Heat Shock Proteins in Vascular Diabetic Complications: Review and Future Perspective. *Int. J. Mol. Sci.* **2017**, *18*, 2709. [CrossRef]
164. Guo, C.; Zhang, L.; Nie, L.; Zhang, N.; Xiao, D.; Ye, X.; Ou, M.; Liu, Y.; Zhang, B.; Wang, M.; et al. Association of polymorphisms in the MyD88, IRAK4 and TRAF6 genes and susceptibility to type 2 diabetes mellitus and diabetic nephropathy in a southern Han Chinese population. *Mol. Cell. Endocrinol.* **2016**, *429*, 114–119. [CrossRef]
165. Wang, Y.; Li, Y.; Zhang, T.; Chi, Y.; Liu, M.; Liu, Y. Genistein and Myd88 Activate Autophagy in High Glucose-Induced Renal Podocytes In Vitro. *Med. Sci. Monit.* **2018**, *24*, 4823–4831. [CrossRef]
166. Murea, M.; Register, T.C.; Divers, J.; Bowden, D.W.; Carr, J.J.; Hightower, C.R.; Xu, J.; Smith, S.C.; Hruska, K.A.; Langefeld, C.D.; et al. Relationships between serum MCP-1 and subclinical kidney disease: African American-Diabetes Heart Study. *BMC Nephrol.* **2012**, *13*, 148. [CrossRef]
167. Suryavanshi, S.V.; Kulkarni, Y.A. NF-κβ: A Potential Target in the Management of Vascular Complications of Diabetes. *Front. Pharmacol.* **2017**, *8*, 798. [CrossRef]
168. Lu, Q.; Wang, W.-W.; Zhang, M.-Z.; Ma, Z.-X.; Qiu, X.-R.; Shen, M.; Yin, X.-X. ROS induces epithelial-mesenchymal transition via the TGF-β1/PI3K/Akt/mTOR pathway in diabetic nephropathy. *Exp. Ther. Med.* **2019**, *17*, 835–846. [CrossRef]
169. Tong, Y.; Chuan, J.; Bai, L.; Shi, J.; Zhong, L.; Duan, X.; Zhu, Y. The protective effect of shikonin on renal tubular epithelial cell injury induced by high glucose. *Biomed. Pharmacother.* **2018**, *98*, 701–708. [CrossRef]
170. Li, F.; Yang, N.; Zhang, L.; Tan, H.; Huang, B.; Liang, Y.; Chen, M.; Yu, X. Increased Expression of Toll-Like Receptor 2 in Rat Diabetic Nephropathy. *Am. J. Nephrol.* **2010**, *32*, 179–186. [CrossRef]
171. Cha, J.J.; Hyun, Y.Y.; Lee, M.H.; Kim, J.E.; Nam, D.H.; Song, H.K.; Kang, Y.S.; Lee, J.E.; Kim, H.W.; Han, J.Y.; et al. Renal protective effects of toll-like receptor 4 signaling blockade in type 2 diabetic mice. *Endocrinology* **2013**, *154*, 2144–2155. [CrossRef]
172. Stadler, K.; Goldberg, I.J.; Susztak, K. The Evolving Understanding of the Contribution of Lipid Metabolism to Diabetic Kidney Disease. *Curr. Diabetes Rep.* **2015**, *15*, 40. [CrossRef]
173. Cao, A.; Wang, L.; Chen, X.; Guo, H.; Chu, S.; Zhang, X.; Peng, W. Ursodeoxycholic Acid Ameliorated Diabetic Nephropathy by Attenuating Hyperglycemia-Mediated Oxidative Stress. *Biol. Pharm. Bull.* **2016**, *39*, 1300–1308. [CrossRef]
174. Kaur, H.; Chien, A.; Jialal, I. Hyperglycemia induces Toll like receptor 4 expression and activity in mouse mesangial cells: Relevance to diabetic nephropathy. *Am. J. Physiol. Renal Physiol.* **2012**, *303*, F1145–F1150. [CrossRef]
175. Takata, S.; Sawa, Y.; Uchiyama, T.; Ishikawa, H. Expression of Toll-Like Receptor 4 in Glomerular Endothelial Cells under Diabetic Conditions. *Acta Histochem. Cytochem.* **2013**, *46*, 35–42. [CrossRef]

176. Panchapakesan, U.; Pollock, C. The role of toll-like receptors in diabetic kidney disease. *Curr. Opin. Nephrol. Hypertens.* **2018**, *27*, 30–34. [CrossRef]
177. Aluksanasuwan, S.; Sueksakit, K.; Fong-Ngern, K.; Thongboonkerd, V. Role of HSP60 (HSPD1) in diabetes-induced renal tubular dysfunction: Regulation of intracellular protein aggregation, ATP production, and oxidative stress. *FASEB J.* **2017**, *31*, 2157–2167. [CrossRef]
178. Zyzak, J.; Matuszyk, J.; Siednienko, J. Multilevel maturation of Toll-like receptor 9. *Postepy Hig. Med. Dosw.* **2013**, *67*, 1034–1046. [CrossRef] [PubMed]
179. Zipris, D. Toll-like receptors and type 1 diabetes. *Adv. Exp. Med. Biol.* **2010**, *654*, 585–610. [CrossRef]
180. Ronco, C.; Bellomo, R.; Kellum, J.A. Acute kidney injury. *Lancet* **2019**, *394*, 1949–1964. [CrossRef]
181. Baer, P.C.; Koch, B.; Geiger, H. Kidney Inflammation, Injury and Regeneration. *Int. J. Mol. Sci.* **2020**, *21*, 1164. [CrossRef] [PubMed]
182. Coca, S.G.; Yusuf, B.; Shlipak, M.G.; Garg, A.X.; Parikh, C.R. Long-term risk of mortality and other adverse outcomes after acute kidney injury: A systematic review and meta-analysis. *Am. J. Kidney Dis.* **2009**, *53*, 961–973. [CrossRef]
183. Hsu, C.; Chertow, G.M.; McCulloch, C.E.; Fan, D.; Ordoñez, J.D.; Go, A.S. Nonrecovery of kidney function and death after acute on chronic renal failure. *Clin. J. Am. Soc. Nephrol.* **2009**, *4*, 891–898. [CrossRef]
184. Wald, R.; Quinn, R.R.; Luo, J.; Li, P.; Scales, D.C.; Mamdani, M.M.; Ray, J.G.; University of Toronto Acute Kidney Injury Research Group. Chronic dialysis and death among survivors of acute kidney injury requiring dialysis. *JAMA* **2009**, *302*, 1179–1185. [CrossRef]
185. Dong, Y.; Zhang, Q.; Wen, J.; Chen, T.; He, L.; Wang, Y.; Yin, J.; Wu, R.; Xue, R.; Li, S.; et al. Ischemic Duration and Frequency Determines AKI-to-CKD Progression Monitored by Dynamic Changes of Tubular Biomarkers in IRI Mice. *Front. Physiol.* **2019**, *10*, 153. [CrossRef]
186. Leemans, J.C.; Stokman, G.; Claessen, N.; Rouschop, K.M.; Teske, G.J.D.; Kirschning, C.J.; Akira, S.; van der Poll, T.; Weening, J.J.; Florquin, S. Renal-associated TLR2 mediates ischemia/reperfusion injury in the kidney. *J. Clin. Investig.* **2005**, *115*, 2894–2903. [CrossRef]
187. Kim, B.S.; Lim, S.W.; Li, C.; Kim, J.S.; Sun, B.K.; Ahn, K.O.; Han, S.W.; Kim, J.; Yang, C.W. Ischemia-reperfusion injury activates innate immunity in rat kidneys. *Transplantation* **2005**, *79*, 1370–1377. [CrossRef]
188. Wolfs, T.G.A.M.; Buurman, W.A.; van Schadewijk, A.; de Vries, B.; Daemen, M.A.R.C.; Hiemstra, P.S.; van't Veer, C. In vivo expression of Toll-like receptor 2 and 4 by renal epithelial cells: IFN-gamma and TNF-alpha mediated up-regulation during inflammation. *J. Immunol.* **2002**, *168*, 1286–1293. [CrossRef]
189. Paulus, P.; Rupprecht, K.; Baer, P.; Obermüller, N.; Penzkofer, D.; Reissig, C.; Scheller, B.; Holfeld, J.; Zacharowski, K.; Dimmeler, S.; et al. The early activation of toll-like receptor (TLR)-3 initiates kidney injury after ischemia and reperfusion. *PLoS ONE* **2014**, *15*, e94366. [CrossRef] [PubMed]
190. Good, D.W.; George, T.; Watts, B.A. Toll-like Receptor 2 Is Required for LPS-induced Toll-like Receptor 4 Signaling and Inhibition of Ion Transport in Renal Thick Ascending Limb. *J. Biol. Chem.* **2012**, *287*, 20208–20220. [CrossRef] [PubMed]
191. Good, D.W.; George, T.; Watts, B.A. Toll-like receptor 2 mediates inhibition of HCO_3^- absorption by bacterial lipoprotein in medullary thick ascending limb. *Am. J. Physiol. Renal Physiol.* **2010**, *299*, F536–F544. [CrossRef] [PubMed]
192. Vallés, P.G.; Lorenzo, A.G.; Bocanegra, V.; Vallés, R. Acute kidney injury: What part do toll-like receptors play? *Int. J. Nephrol. Renovasc. Dis.* **2014**, *7*, 241–251. [CrossRef]
193. Bonventre, J.V.; Yang, L. Cellular pathophysiology of ischemic acute kidney injury. *J. Clin. Investig.* **2011**, *121*, 4210–4221. [CrossRef]
194. Devarajan, P. Update on Mechanisms of Ischemic Acute Kidney Injury. *J. Am. Soc. Nephrol.* **2006**, *17*, 1503–1520. [CrossRef]
195. Kinsey, G.R.; Li, L.; Okusa, M.D. Inflammation in acute kidney injury. *Nephron Exp. Nephrol.* **2008**, *109*, e102–e107. [CrossRef]
196. Venkatachalam, M.A.; Griffin, K.A.; Lan, R.; Geng, H.; Saikumar, P.; Bidani, A.K. Acute kidney injury: A springboard for progression in chronic kidney disease. *Am. J. Physiol. Renal Physiol.* **2010**, *298*, F1078–F1094. [CrossRef]
197. Lee, S.; Huen, S.; Nishio, H.; Nishio, S.; Lee, H.K.; Choi, B.-S.; Ruhrberg, C.; Cantley, L.G. Distinct macrophage phenotypes contribute to kidney injury and repair. *J. Am. Soc. Nephrol.* **2011**, *22*, 317–326. [CrossRef]

198. Wang, Y.; Harris, D.C.H. Macrophages in Renal Disease. *J. Am. Soc. Nephrol.* **2011**, *22*, 21–27. [CrossRef] [PubMed]

199. Lan, H.Y.; Paterson, D.J.; Atkins, R.C. Initiation and evolution of interstitial leukocytic infiltration in experimental glomerulonephritis. *Kidney Int.* **1991**, *40*, 425–433. [CrossRef] [PubMed]

4

Biomarker Development for Metastatic Renal Cell Carcinoma: Omics, Antigens, T-cells and Beyond

Benjamin Miron, David Xu and Matthew Zibelman *

Department of Hematology/Oncology, Fox Chase Cancer Center, Philadelphia, PA 19111, USA; benjamin.miron@tuhs.temple.edu (B.M.); david.xu@tuhs.temple.edu (D.X.)
* Correspondence: Matthew.Zibelman@fccc.edu.

Abstract: The treatment of metastatic renal cell carcinoma has evolved quickly over the last few years from a disease managed primarily with sequential oral tyrosine kinase inhibitors (TKIs) targeting the vascular endothelial growth factor (VEGF) pathway, to now with a combination of therapies incorporating immune checkpoint blockade (ICB). Patient outcomes have improved with these innovations, however, controversy persists regarding optimal sequence and patient selection amongst the available combinations. Ideally, predictive biomarkers would aid in guiding treatment decisions and personalizing care. However, clinically-actionable biomarkers have remained elusive. We aim to review the available evidence regarding biomarkers for both TKIs and ICB and will present where the field may be headed in the years to come.

Keywords: biomarkers; renal cell carcinoma; clear cell; VEGF; immunotherapy; PD-L1; immune checkpoint inhibitors; immune checkpoint blockade; tyrosine-kinase inhibitors

---

1. Introduction

Renal cell carcinoma (RCC) is traditionally classified according to its histology. Clear cell (ccRCC) is the most common subtype, accounting for 75–85% of all RCCs. Current first-line standard of care therapies for metastatic ccRCC involve the use of vascular endothelial growth factor (VEGF) inhibitors, checkpoint inhibitors, anti-CTLA4 agents, or a combination of these drugs. Choice of therapy is guided by whether the patient's disease falls under favorite or intermediate/poor risk based on validated prognostic models. Within each risk category, there are several acceptable alternatives, including VEGF inhibitor monotherapy, combination immunotherapy (e.g., ipilimumab/nivolumab), or a combination of a VEGF inhibitor and a checkpoint inhibitor (e.g., axitinib/pembrolizumab). Given the increasing number of available treatment options for mRCC there is also a growing need for predictive biomarkers to help guide clinicians (Figure 1). We aim to review the literature regarding the evidence for selecting one type of regimen over another and determining who would benefit more from either angiogenesis antagonism or immune checkpoint blockade (ICB).

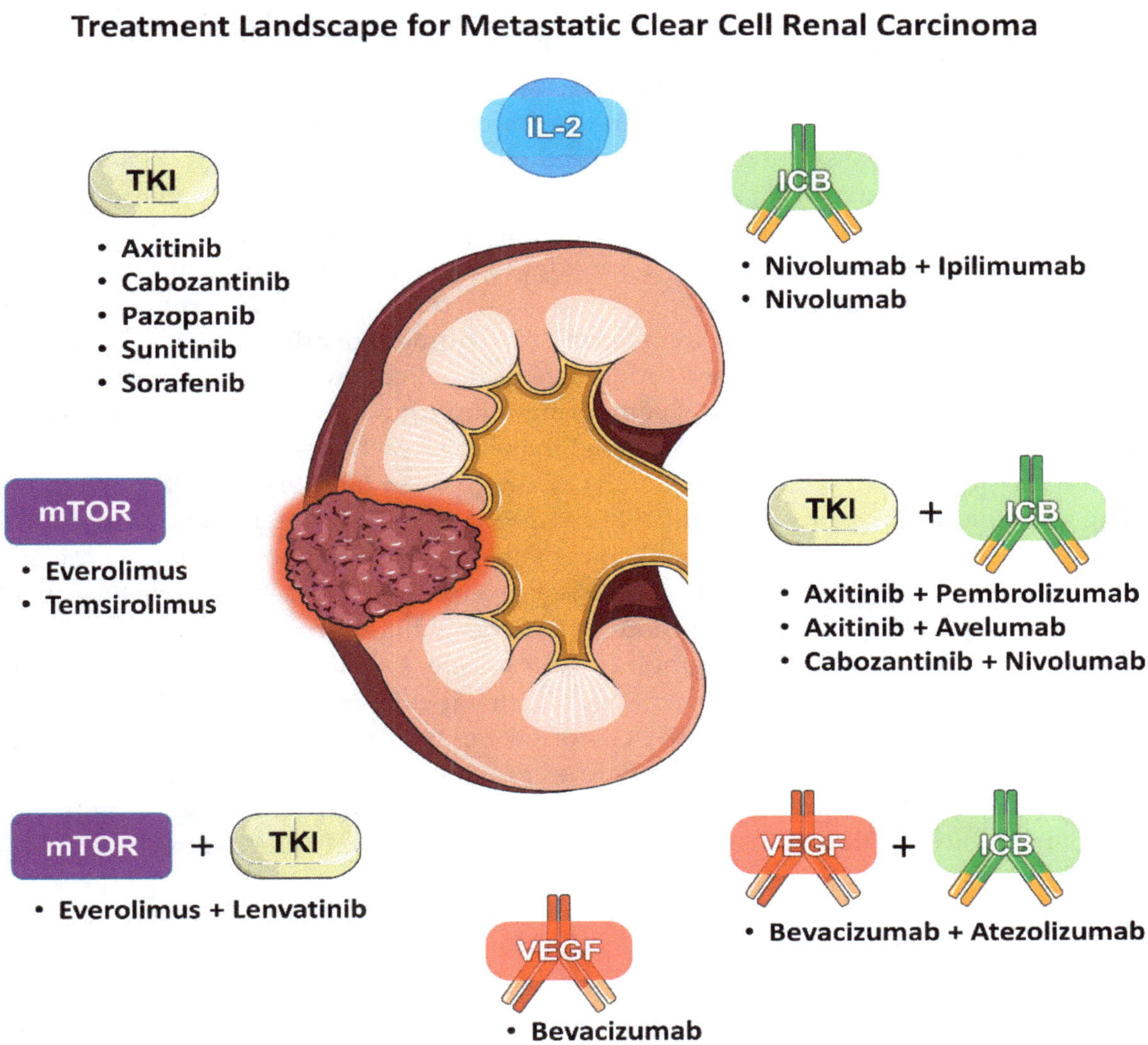

Figure 1. Treatment landscape for metastatic clear cell renal carcinoma.

2. Biomarkers for Angiogenesis Inhibitors

2.1. International Metastatic Renal Cell Carcinoma Database Consortium Score

Past attempts to create clinical prognostication tools to risk stratify patients treated with molecularly-targeted agents include the International Metastatic Renal Cell Carcinoma Database Consortium (IMDC) score. This was a model based on a multicenter study of 645 patients with metastatic RCC (mRCC) who were treated with VEGF pathway-targeted therapies, such as sunitinib, sorafenib, or bevacizumab (plus interferon-alfa) for mRCC [1]. Six factors were noted to be associated with worse survival: Karnofsky Performance Status (KPS) score < 80, time from diagnosis to initiation of targeted therapy < 1 year, hemoglobin less than lower limit of normal, corrected calcium greater than the upper limit of normal, absolute neutrophil count greater than upper limit of normal, and platelet count greater than the upper limit of normal. Scoring was binary with each factor assigned a score of 0 or 1, and a total sum was taken. A total score of 0 corresponded to a favorable risk group with a median overall survival (mOS) of 43.2 months; a score of 1–2 indicated intermediate risk with a mOS of 22.5 months; and a score ≥ 3 represented a poor risk group with a mOS of 7.8 months. This clinical prediction tool was subsequently externally validated in a study of 849 patients with mRCC who were treated with first-line anti-VEGF therapies [2]. Another study found that the IMDC score can be applied to patients who progressed after first-line anti-VEGF therapy [3]. Although there have been other risk models that have been developed, including the MSKCC model, Cleveland Clinic

Foundation model, French model, and International Kidney Cancer Working Group, the IMDC model has become the one most widely utilized in contemporary clinical trials.

While clinical tools such as the IMDC score were originally developed to estimate patients' prognoses regardless of the treatment early in the era of VEGF-targeted therapy, there has been a gradual evolution toward assuming a role in predicting response to therapy. The IMDC criteria has been used to retrospectively risk stratify patients who underwent ICB combination therapies (e.g., ipilimumab/nivolumab vs. axitinib + pembrolizumab/avelumab) or anti-VEGF agents in first-line or second-line settings [4]. There is growing evidence that using the risk score may be useful in guiding the selection of a particular therapy. For example, in KEYNOTE-426, there was a benefit for pembrolizumab/axitinib over sunitinib in the first-line treatment of advanced ccRCC in an updated analysis [5]. However, this effect was less pronounced for patients who fell into the IMDC favorable risk category. Similarly, a prospective trial comparing ipilimumab/nivolumab (ipi/nivo) combination vs. sunitinib in untreated advanced ccRCC showed that patients who were at intermediate or poor risk and treated with ipi/nivo had superior 18-month OS, progression free survival (PFS), overall response rate (ORR), and complete response (CR) rates as compared to patients treated with sunitinib alone [6]. However, an exploratory analysis of favorable risk patients, who were found to have a lower baseline PD-L1 expression level when compared to higher risk groups, failed to demonstrate the same benefits of ipi/nivo over sunitinib. In fact, the 18-month OS trended higher for sunitinib, and the ORR was lower and mPFS shorter for the ipi/nivo group in a statistically significant manner, although there was no OS advantage for sunitinib. Given such a disparate therapeutic response to ICB vs. sunitinib based on the risk profile, it is conceivable that IMDC scoring can be used to predict treatment response in addition to estimating the prognosis. That higher risk group patients with advanced ccRCC responded better to ICB-based therapies suggests that there may be differences in the underlying tumor and/or microenvironment biology that influence response to the current available treatments.

2.2. Genomic Alterations

Earlier studies on biomarkers focused on driver mutations, epigenetic modifications, or chromosomal aberrations associated with ccRCC to evaluate their potential in clinical prognostication. An obvious candidate was the *von Hippel-Lindau* (*VHL*) gene, which is inactivated in RCC via a point mutation or through epigenetic silencing. This mutation is present in about 60–90% of cases of ccRCC. Inactivation of the protein product of *VHL* leads to abnormal stabilization of hypoxia-inducible factor (HIF), which drives oncogene transcription. However, no clear relationship between *VHL* abnormalities and patient outcome exists [7]. A meta-analysis from 2017 revealed that *VHL* was not a predictive marker in patients treated with anti-VEGF-targeted agents, as abnormal *VHL* failed to show a relationship with ORR, PFS, or OS [8]. *Polybromo 1*, (*PBRM1*), also known as BAF180, is encoded in a gene locus near *VHL* and is a component of the PBAF complex, a mammalian SWItch/Sucrose Non-Fermentable (SWI/SNF) complex, which is a tumor suppressor protein that is thought to become mutated early in RCC pathogenesis [9]. Older studies evaluating its role as a prognostic marker did not include targeted agents and failed to predict cancer-specific survival [9,10]. However, a study published in 2016 showed that among 31 metastatic ccRCC patients, the vast majority of whom received anti-VEGF therapy, those who were maintained for longer durations of therapy were more likely to harbor a *PBRM1* mutation [11]. A separate study found that a group of so-called "extreme responders," defined as partial response (PR) or complete response (CR) for ≥3 years in mRCC on either first-line sunitinib or pazopanib, was enriched for *PBRM1* mutations [12]. A third biomarker that has been studied is *SETD2*, which is sometimes co-mutated with *PBRM1*. It encodes for a histone-lysine N-methyltransferase and acts as a chromatin regulator. It does not appear to have a definite correlation with survival but is associated with higher risk of disease recurrence after surgery for localized disease. Its mutation status did not seem to correlate with PFS in mRCC patients treated with sunitinib [13].

2.3. Targets of Tumor-Driven Angiogenesis

With growing evidence that tumor and microenvironmental biology could impact clinical factors and lead to differential outcomes depending on the type of systemic therapy, identifying predictive biomarkers became an increasing focus. Earlier studies acknowledged the hyperangiogenic state of ccRCC and the mechanism of action of VEGF-targeted tyrosine kinase inhibitors (TKIs) as a rationale for studying the components of the VEGF signaling cascade. One study looked at whether VEGF expression in tumor and endothelial cells was predictive and/or prognostic in 41 patients with metastatic RCC (mRCC) treated with radical nephrectomy and sunitinib [14]. In this study, higher VEGF expression within the tumor cells correlated with the MSKCC group and was associated with higher tumor stage and inferior OS. There was no correlation between intratumoral VEGF expression and PFS or OS on first-line sunitinib, suggesting that the VEGF level may be prognostic but not predictive. A different study evaluated the role of serum VEGF levels in predicting treatment response to sunitinib in 85 patients with advanced RCC (mostly clear cell) who overwhelmingly fell into the favorable or intermediate categories based on the MSKCC model; these patients were undergoing systemic treatment in the second line and beyond [15]. The patients who had serum VEGF levels higher than reference value of 707 pg/mL had a longer PFS by about six months. A third small, single-institution study of 23 mRCC patients attempted to associate tumor expression of 16 selected biomarkers with treatment response to second-line sunitinib after the failure of first-line interferon-α. They quantified biomarker expression using qRT-PCR and categorized tumor response using the RECIST criteria. The authors noted that specific soluble VEGF isoforms, $VEGF_{121}$ and $VEGF_{165}$ in particular, were associated with partial response, and they proposed that a ratio of $VEGF_{121}/VEGF_{165}$ of <1.25 predicted superior OS [16]. Despite these studies, neither peritumoral nor serum VEGF is routinely measured in clinical practice.

2.4. Gene Expression Signatures

More recent studies have investigated gene expression signatures as potential guides for the tailoring of therapy. A study published in 2013 found that tumor upregulation of the so-called VEGF-dependent vascular gene profile appeared to predict improved PFS when bevacizumab was added to standard oxaliplatin-based systemic therapy for treatment-naïve metastatic colorectal cancer [17]. To see if such a phenomenon was also applicable to mRCC, an exploratory analysis of the IMmotion150 study looked at tumor mutation burden as well as angiogenesis and immune gene expression signatures in previously untreated mRCC patients who were treated with sunitinib vs. atezolizumab with or without bevacizumab [18]. The Angio gene signature consisted of the following genes: *VEGFA*, *KDR*, *ESM1*, *PECAM1*, *ANGPTL4*, and *CD34*. In the IMmotion150 study, increased the expression of the Angio signature correlated with a higher ORR and longer PFS among the group of patients treated with sunitinib, including a 7% CR rate as compared to 0% in the low Angio expression group. If the Angio expression level was low, the combination arm had better PFS as compared to that of sunitinib monotherapy. Although the angiogenesis gene signature tended to have upregulation of *VHL* and *PBRM1* mutants, *VHL* status itself was not associated with differences in PFS [18]. Although these results were intriguing, they remain hypothesis-generating.

2.5. Association of Angiogenesis Signatures with Traditional Biomarkers

One group analyzed data from the phase III COMPARZ trial to associate tumor gene expression profiling with clinical endpoints in untreated metastatic ccRCC [19]. This trial randomized untreated mRCC patients to receive either pazopanib or sunitinib to assess for differences in efficacy, toxicity, and quality of life. In patients treated with an anti-VEGF TKI, such as sunitinib or pazopanib, increased expression of angiogenesis genes significantly correlated with better ORR, PFS, and OS as compared to those with lower expression. However, this benefit appeared to be abrogated in the group of patients that was enriched for *TP53* and *BAP1* mutations. The group of patients with higher frequency of *TP53* and *BAP1* mutations tended to have high immune infiltration and higher PD-L1 expression. Ultimately, there was no significant difference in the angiogenesis gene profile among the three different IMDC risk groups, suggesting that the prediction of enhanced response to TKIs was independent of previously established clinical prognostic markers. As was the case in IMmotion150 study, in the COMPARZ trial, mRCC tumors with *PBRM1* mutations were noted to have upregulated angiogenesis gene expression in contrast to tumors harboring *BAP1* mutations, which were associated with decreased expression of angiogenesis-related genes. There was no association between the angiogenesis gene signature expression level and *SETD2* mutation.

2.6. Pure VEGF Antagonism vs. Combination Anti-VEGF/ICB Therapy

Combination therapy with anti-angiogenic agents and ICB has become the standard of care for the majority of patients with mRCC. It would be clinically actionable to understand whether angiogenic or immune biomarkers could help predict the therapeutic response in order to better stratify patients to combination therapy versus a single agent strategy to minimize toxicity while optimizing efficacy. A study evaluated association between angiogenesis signatures and outcomes in the phase 3 JAVELIN Renal trial that enrolled patients with untreated mRCC and randomized them to avelumab/axitinib or sunitinib. High levels of expression of angiogenesis-related genes were associated with better PFS in patients treated with sunitinib. In patients whose tumors had low expression of an angiogenesis signature, there was improved PFS in patients treated with avelumab/axitinib in comparison to sunitinib [20]. All in all, several studies have shown evidence that upregulation of a set of angiogenesis-related genes seemed to help predict a better response to anti-VEGF therapy, which would be important information in guiding selection of therapy. Those who registered low in angiogenesis gene expression predictably did not benefit as much, and there is a suggestion that mRCC patients harboring low tumor angiogenesis gene expression signatures represent an immune-enriched subtype that is less likely to respond to anti-VEGF therapy alone and may benefit more from strategies involving ICB.

2.7. Predictive Value of Trends in Angiogenesis-Related Biomarkers during Treatment

A retrospective analysis of tumor samples or blood samples obtained from 52 mRCC patients treated with first-line axitinib/pembrolizumab in a phase Ib trial was assessed for angiogenesis-related biomarkers [21]. Angiopoietin-1 and 2 (Ang-1; Ang-2), VEGF, VEGFR-1, VEGFR-2, and VEGFR-3 were chosen for evaluation as serum biomarkers given their known roles in angiogenesis [22]. The study authors found that serum concentrations of Ang-1, Ang-2, VEGF, VEGFR2, and VEGFR3 at baseline had no correlation with PFS as a continuous variable. However, when patients were divided into two categories of PFS (<9 months vs. >20 months), the median Ang-2 protein level on treatment was lower in the PFS > 20 month group as compared to PFS < 9 months. The Ang-1 protein level was lower in patients with PFS > 20 months at the end of the treatment. The ratio of VEGF at the end of treatment to VEGF at baseline was also lower for patients who experienced PFS > 20 months [21]. This study suggested the potential that these biomarkers may have in assessing whether a patient on treatment is a responder, enabling earlier escalation of therapy for those with a lower chance of response. These results require prospective validation, however (Table 1).

Table 1. Summary of biomarkers for angiogenesis inhibitors.

Biomarker	Key Findings as a Predictive or Prognostic Biomarker
von Hippel-Lindau (VHL) [7]	• No correlation with patient outcome in general • No correlation with ORR, PFS, or OS in patients treated with anti-VEGF therapy
Polybromo-1 (PBRM1) [11,12]	• Associated with a longer duration of response to anti-VEGF therapy
SET domain containing 2, histone lysine methyltransferase (SETD2) [13]	• No definite association with overall survival • Does not predict response to sunitinib
BRCA1 Associated Protein 1 (BAP1) [19]	• Associated with lower expression of angiogenesis-related genes • Possibly blunts response to anti-VEGF therapy
Vascular Endothelial Growth Factor (VEGF) [14–16,21]	• Intratumoral overexpression associated with worse OS but does not predict response to first-line sunitinib • Lower ratio of soluble isoforms 121–165 (<1.25) may help to predict response to second-line sunitinib after progression on interferon-α • Lower ratio of serum levels at the end of treatment to baseline level associated with longer PFS with first-line axitinib/pembrolizumab
Angiopoietins (Ang-1, Ang-2) [21]	• Associated with longer PFS when treated with first-line axitinib/pembrolizumab when either of the following were observed: ○ Decrease in Ang-1 protein level at the end of treatment ○ Decrease in Ang-2 protein level mid-treatment
Angio gene signature (VEGFA, KDR, ESM1, PECAM1, ANGPTL4, and CD34) [18–20]	• More often upregulated in VHL and PBRM1 mutants • Increased expression correlated with higher ORR, PFS, and/or OS in patients treated with first-line sunitinib or pazopanib except when TP53 or BAP1 mutations were present • Improved PFS with first-line avelumab/axitinib as compared to sunitinib monotherapy if the Angio expression level was low

3. Biomarkers for Immunotherapy

Renal cell carcinoma is often considered an immunogenic tumor. This has been evidenced from pathologic examination of RCC tumor tissue showing significant infiltration by both T-cells and natural killer cells [23]. In addition, efficacy of early immunotherapy agents, like interleukin-2 (IL-2) and Interferon alpha (IFN-α), and more recently ICB in the treatment of RCC support this notion pragmatically [24–26]. ICB targeting the programmed death 1 (PD-1) and cytotoxic T-lymphocyte associated protein 4 (CTLA-4) pathways have demonstrated favorable outcomes, with ORRs of 25% for anti-PD-1 targeted single-agent therapy and up to 39% and 59% when combined with CTLA-4 or vascular endothelial growth factor (VEGF) inhibitors, respectively [5,6,27]. Consequently, combination strategies with ICB have become the standard of care for most eligible mRCC patients.

However, since both combination ICB/ICB and ICB/TKI regimens are approved as first-line therapy for mRCC, it would be beneficial to have clinical biomarkers to understand which tumors are more likely to benefit from an immunotherapy based regimen versus a combination regimen with VEGF inhibition.

3.1. PD-L1 Expression

The programmed death-ligand 1 (PD-L1), also known as B7 homolog 1 (B7-H1), is found on tumor and immune cells in the TME, and its receptor PD-1 on T-cells are the primary targets for this form of ICB. In the era of ICB, expression of PD-L1 by immunohistochemistry (IHC) has been a focus of much of biomarker research across tumor types but in the case of mRCC it has not borne out to be a very useful predictive biomarker.

When focusing specifically on registration studies for ICB in mRCC, patients without any measurable PD-L1 expression have benefited from these drugs. In a meta-analysis of six randomized controlled trials of ICB in mRCC an association was observed between PD-L1 expression and PFS, but the analysis failed to show significant correlation with OS [28]. The authors concluded from this data that the role of PD-L1 expression in selecting treatment for RCC was not well established, in line with FDA drug approvals and the NCCN guidelines which do not include or require PD-L1 expression [29,30]. This difference is likely multifactorial and could be due to the unique biology of RCC, related to the non-standardized testing utilized in for PD-L1 expression as a biomarker in earlier trials, including the use of different antibodies for various IHC assays and inconsistent cutoffs for positivity, tumor heterogeneity and the dynamic nature of PD-L1 expression on tumor cells [31].

Furthermore, prior to the era of immunotherapy, PD-L1 expression by IHC was studied in mRCC and was shown to be associated with poor prognosis [32]. The observation that PD-L1 positivity is linked to poor prognosis was again reported more recently in a post-hoc analysis of the COMPARZ trial (pazopinib vs. sunitinib) which showed that patients who were PD-L1 positive had significantly worse OS and PFS compared to the PD-L1 negative population. This is also supported by an analysis of CHECKMATE-214 study (nivolumab+ipilumimab vs. sunitinib) which demonstrated that PD-L1 positivity was more common in patients with intermediate and poor risk disease as defined by IMDC criteria compared to those with favorable risk disease [6]. It is possible that the prognostic implications of PD-L1 positivity in mRCC also have a negative impact on its usefulness as a predictive biomarker.

3.2. Genomic Markers

3.2.1. PBRM1 Mutations

Differences in the genomic landscape of RCC have also been the subject of much study in the search for clinical biomarkers for ICB treatment PBRM1 and PBAF complex mutations have drawn much attention in this regard and, as discussed above, have also been investigated as both a prognostic and predictive markers for VEGF TKIs. In relation to ICB, PBRM1 was first identified by Miao et al. in a set of 35 patients with mRCC who participated in a prospective clinical study of nivolumab. Whole-exome sequencing was performed on tissue samples and identified PBRM1 as being strongly enriched in the group who derived clinical benefit. This finding was then validated in a separate 63 patient cohort treated with PD-1 or PD-L1 inhibitions alone or in combination with anti-CTLA-4 therapies and replicated findings of association with clinical benefit [33].

However, after this initial publication, PBRM1 mutations were subsequently studied in several additional patient cohorts. An analysis by McDermott et al. of a first-line clinical trial of atezolizumab alone or in combination with bevacizumab vs. sunitinib failed to demonstrate an association with clinical benefit in patients with PBRM1 mutations in the atezolizumab monotherapy arm but instead favored benefit in the sunitinib arm [18]. A subsequent analysis from the Checkmate-025 study of patients with mRCC treated in the second-line or beyond and randomized to nivolumab or everolimus showed that there was enrichment of clinical benefit in the PBRM1 mutant group in nivolumab-treated patients, though this trial did not include a VEGF-targeted therapy. The effect of PBRM1 mutations on response and survival in this study was modest, with median PFS 5.6 vs. 2.9 months (HR, 0.67; 95% CI, 0.47–0.96; $p = 0.03$) and median OS 27.9 vs. 20.9 months (HR, 0.65; 95% CI, 0.44–0.96; $p = 0.03$) [34].

Finally, a large retrospective analysis ($n = 2936$) explored the interaction between PBRM1 mutations and immunotherapy across cancer types and failed to show a statistically significant association with

OS (HR 0.9, $p = 0.7$). Interestingly, this trial included 189 patients with mRCC treated with ICB and this subgroup did demonstrate an association with OS (HR 1.24, $p = 0.47$). It was previously hypothesized in the initial discovery study by Miao et al. that PBRM1 mutations increased interferon-gamma (IFNγ) gene expression and thereby modulated the immune response. However, this analysis explored the impact of IFNγ signaling in both the cohort studied by McDermott et al. and a cohort from the previously mentioned COMPARZ trial and showed unchanged or decreased IFNγ signaling in PBRM1 mutants compared to the wild-type, which conflicted with the hypothesized mechanism of action [35]. Due to the conflicting nature of these results, doubt has been cast on the potential use of PBRM1 as a biomarker for ICB [36].

3.2.2. TERT Promoter Mutations

Although much focus is in finding mutations associated with response, it is also useful to examine the opposite phenomenon and identify mutations that are associated with resistance to immunotherapy. This would help route patients to therapies more likely to be beneficial and avoid unnecessary toxicity. For example, in non-small cell lung cancer mutations in STK11 have been identified as predictors of poor responses to ICBs [37]. STK11 is not a useful biomarker for RCC since it is very rarely found in RCC on the order of 0.2% of patients based on data from cBioPortal [38]. A retrospective study of patients with mRCC ($n = 75$), the majority with clear cell histology (~80%), who received comprehensive genomic profiling (whole exome and RNA sequencing) as part of routine care, including both immunotherapy and targeted therapy, attempted to identify genomic and transcriptomic correlates of clinical benefit. The authors found that mutations in the TERT promoter were specifically associated with a lack of benefit from ICB. In this subgroup of TERT promoter mutated tumors the authors also found enrichment of transcription factor targets of MYC and KATA2, and kinase targets of CDK4, ATM, and MAPK14 [39].

3.2.3. Multi-gene Expression Signatures

Similar to approaches in VEGF TKI treated patients, researchers have investigated potential tumor genomic signatures that might serve as predictive biomarkers for ICB. In an exploratory analysis of the IMmotion150 study, the authors used gene signatures previously defined and representing angiogenesis, immune response (T-effector/IFNγ), and myeloid inflammatory gene expression to perform a subgroup analysis and investigate associations with response. They found that tumors with high expression of a T-effector gene signature (T_{eff}^{High}) was positively associated with expression of PD-L1 and CD8 T-cell infiltration. They also showed that within this group there was increased expression of the myeloid inflammation genes. The T_{eff}^{High} gene signature was also associated with improved ORR and PFS when compared to the T_{eff}^{Low} group within the atezolizumab/bevacizumab arm. They also showed that T_{eff}^{High} was associated with improved PFS when compared across groups to the sunitinib arm. High myeloid inflammation gene signature expression (Myeloid^{High}), which had previously been shown to be associated with suppressed T-cell responses, was shown to be associated with worse PFS in both the atezolizumab monotherapy and atezolizumab/bevacizumab arms [18].

A separate group utilized machine learning techniques to build upon the prior IMmotion150 gene signatures to define a specific 66-gene signature created for mRCC using RNA sequencing data from The Cancer Genome Atlas (TCGA) dataset in cBioPortal. They identified that the genes in the IMmotion150 gene signature were selected by analysis of the literature and citations which defined the three biological axes explored in the study and not based on an empirical analysis of the data, which they considered to be a limitation of the previous approach. To develop their signature, they first leveraged the gene signatures defined by the IMmotion150 study to perform unsupervised clustering to categorize patients into three groups and confirmed they separated into the same three categories; angiogenesis, T-effector and myeloid inflammation. They then utilized a separate featured selection machine learning technique to analyze the global gene expression profile of the sub-classified patients and selected the top 500 ranked and subsequently refined them using several different techniques to investigate the underlying biology and came up with their 66-gene signature. Using training and validation cohorts, they were able to show that this signature performed better with regards to association with OS and DFS than the original IMmotion150 signature. However, interpretation of this signature thus far is limited since annotation of treatments record and outcome are not available in the TCGA data and survival data was calculated prior to the approval of ICBs. The signature does, however, hold promise to be tested in cohorts who did receive ICB to test what they hypothesize as an improvement in the clustering of patients into unique groups defined by tumor biology [40].

In an analysis of the results of KEYNOTE-427 (pembrolizumab monotherapy) 11 separate gene signatures were analyzed for associations with response. They identified one signature, a T-cell inflamed gene expression profile (GEP), which stood out demonstrating a strong association with ORR to pembrolizumab. The same T-cell inflamed GEP signature, however, was not associated with longer PFS or OS in the same study and thus remains hypothesis generating [41] (Table 2).

3.2.4. DNA Damage Repair Mutations, Microsatellite Instability, and Tumor Mutational Burden

Although less common in some other tumor types, RCC can harbor alterations in DNA damage repair (DDR) pathways, including defects in DNA mismatch repair (dMMR). Loss of function of certain genes related to dMMR defects can lead to lead to high levels of microsatellite instability (MSI), which has been established as a biomarker for response to immunotherapy irrespective of tumor type [42]. MSI-Hi tumors are not a common finding in RCC and are estimated to be present in only 1–2% of cases [43]. As a result, MSI is not a practical biomarker in a broad sense for ICB in RCC since many non-MSI RCC tumors respond to immunotherapy.

Looking more broadly, mutations in genes involved in the various DDR pathways, which do not necessarily result in MSI, are relatively prevalent in RCC. In one cohort published by Ged et al., about 19% of patients (43/229) with mRCC harbor DDR mutations, with CHEK2 and ATM being the most frequently mutated. In this cohort, they were able to demonstrate a correlation between DDR mutation status and superior OS (HR 0.41; 95% CI: 0.14–1.14; p = 0.09) in patients treated with ICB [44]. This finding was also reported in a smaller cohort (n = 34) by Labriola et al. who showed that patients with DDR mutant tumors had improved disease control (defined as CR, PR, or SD) with ICB [45].

Table 2. Summary of gene expression signatures.

Gene Signature	Dataset	Genes	Key Findings
IMmotion150 Signature [18]	**Sample size:** 263 patients **Study Type:** Randomized phase 2 study of atezolizumab alone or combined with bevacizumab (anti-VEGF) versus sunitinib	**Angiogenesis (Angio)** • VEGFA • FLT1 • PECAM1 • CD34 • ANGPLT4 • KDR • ESM1 **Myeloid Inflammation** • CXCL1 • CXCL8 • CXCL2 • IL6 • CXCL3 • PTGS2 **T-effector (T_{eff})** • CD8A • CD274 • CD27 • CTLA4 • IFNG • FOXP3 • GZMA • TIGIT • GZMB • IDO1 • PRF1 • PSMB8 • EOMES • PSMB9 • CXCL9 • TAP1 • CXCL10 • TAP2 • CXCL11	• T_{eff}^{High} associated with PD-L1 expression and CD8 T-cell infiltration • T_{eff}^{High} vs. T_{eff}^{Low} in atezolizumab + bevacizumab associated with improved ORR (49% vs. 16%) and improved PFS (HR 0.50; CI 0.30–0.86) • T_{eff}^{High} atezolizumab + bevacizumab vs. sunitinib improved PFS (HR 0.55; CI 0.32–0.95) • Myeloid^{High} associated with worse PFS in immunotherapy arms • Distinct population of Myeloid^{High} tumors within the T_{eff}^{High} group • T_{eff}^{High}Myeloid^{High} vs. T_{eff}^{High}Myeloid^{low} associated with worse activity of atezolizumab (HR 3.82; CI 1.70–8.60)

Table 2. *Cont.*

Gene Signature	Dataset	Genes	Key Findings
66 Gene Signature [40]	**Sample Size:** *Training cohort* 469 patients *Validation cohort* 64 patients **Study Type:** Retrospective analysis of ccRCC patients from The Cancer Genome Atlas (TCGA)	**Angiogenesis** • VEGFA • EDN1 • KDR • FLT1 • EDNRB • CD34 • PECAM1 • STIM2 • ANGPLT4 • ESM1 • NOTCH1 **T-effector** • PSMB9 • CTLA4 • PSMB8 • CD8A • LTA • GZMB • SLA2 • GZMA • PYHIN1 • TIGIT • PDCD1 • PREF1 • EOMES **Ca2+-flux** • CD2 • LCP1 • CCL5 • CD38 • CCL4 • LAX1 • GK2 • CD7 • LCK • CD3E • LAT • ITK **Invasion** • XCL2 • FYB1 • FOXP3 • NES • FERMT3 • S1PR1 • SLC9A3R2 • TCF4 • FASLG • HEY1 • NFATC1 • ETS1 • CD72 • PTPRB • WAS • PPM1F • PTK2B • MCF2L • CXCR3 • GJA1 • CORO1A • VWF • CCR5 • MYCT1 • PDE2A • NOS3 • TBCA2R • IL16	• T-effector genes clustered with Ca2+-flux • Subclasified patients into 3 categories: Angio, T_{eff}, and Mixed • Mixed cohort expressed genes from all four pathways • Angio cohort had improved survival compared to T_{eff} and Mixed (median OS 90.4 vs. 62.8 vs. 62.8 months) • Angio cohort had better DFS as compared to T_{eff} (HR = 2.2091, p = 0.0201) and Mixed • (HR = 1.7433, p = 0.0386) • Not yet tested or validated in a cohort who was homogenously treated • Developed on data prior to ICB
T-cell Inflamed GEP [41]	**Sample Size:** 78 patients **Study Type:** Open-label, single-arm phase 2 study of first-line pembrolizumab	**T-cell Inflamed** • CXCR6 • PSMB10 • TIGIT • CMKLR1 • CD27 • CD274 (PD-L1) • LAG3 • PDCD1LG2 • NKG7 • (PD-L2) • STAT1 • CXCL9 • CD8A • HLA.DQA1 • IDO1 • CD276 • CCL5 • HLA.DRB1 • HLA.E	• T-cell-inflamed GEP associated with higher ORR • No association with PFS or OS

Another measure of disruption of genomic integrity is tumor mutational burden (TMB). TMB is defined by the total number of non-synonymous alterations (single-nucleotide variants or insertions/deletions) and is typically calculated from next-generation sequencing (NGS) data of either the whole exome or large targeted panels. A high TMB is thought to be integral in promoting increases in the expression of tumor neoantigens which promote T-cell mediated immune responses against tumors [46,47]. TMB, similarly to MSI, has been investigated independent of tumor histology and has been shown to enrich response to ICB [48,49]. This also led to an FDA approval on 16 June 2020 of pembrolizumab for all TMB-high tumors (defined as >10 mutations per megabase) regardless of histology.

However, this approval has been met with controversy because of concerns that cutoffs for TMB and its performance as a biomarker may differ between tumor types. This skepticism is supported in RCC based on some of the available data. For example, in the study discussed above by Labriola et al., which focused solely on RCC, there was no observed association between TMB and disease control in patients treated with ICB [45]. This was also seen in a separate and larger cohort of 592 patients treated with nivolumab (pooled analysis of checkmate 009, 010, and 025) showed no association with response to PD-1 blockade. Paradoxically, it also has been shown that high-TMB is actually associated with inhibition of immune cell infiltrates in RCC tumors, which supports and possibly explains these unexpected clinical observations on a cellular level [50].

Another interesting observation that may help explain why RCC is such an immunogenic tumor but has a characteristically low TMB is the distribution of mutations that comprise its TMB [51,52]. TMB high tumors traditionally have a predominance of many single nucleotide variants (SNVs) making up the majority of mutations, while RCC on the other hand has a uniquely high proportion of insertions and deletions (indels) relative to other tumors. This phenomenon was identified as part of an analysis of the Cancer Genome Atlas study of 5777 solid tumors which identified RCC tumors as having more than double the median proportion of indels to SNVs. The authors then hypothesized that indels are more efficient in the formation of immunogenic peptides serving as neoantigens and using in silico prediction models they were able to show an enrichment of high-affinity neoantigens from indels that was three times that of SNV [53]. This suggests that RCC may be a case of quality over quantity in regards to immunogenic mutations.

Another approach to improving performance of TMB as a biomarker is incorporating HLA correction. HLA correction is a computational method by which incorporation of loss of heterozygosity of HLA alleles is thought to improve upon TMB by predicting the proportion of functional neoantigens present. This has been studied in non-small cell lung cancer and shown to identify and reclassify tumors previously characterized as TMB-high and, in doing so, improve the association with the response to ICB, but has yet to be studied in RCC [54].

3.3. Analysis of Immune Cells

In the search for biomarkers predicting a response to ICB, the investigation has necessarily expanded beyond clinical- and tumor-dependent factors, such as performance status or genomics, and additionally focused on host-dependent components of the immune system. In order to study the cellular components of the immune system, including T-cells, neutrophils, NK cells, and antigen-presenting cells, a variety of techniques have been approached, ranging from simple analytes (like a complete blood count with differential) to more complex methods like flow cytometry and advanced staining techniques, like multiplex IHC.

3.3.1. Neutrophil Lymphocyte Ratio

One of the first biomarkers developed to attempt to quantify the immunologic milieu in patients with cancer is the neutrophil lymphocyte ratio (NLR). The biologic rationale for this biomarker is that it is a representation of cancer-related inflammation indicating more aggressive disease. Calculated simply by dividing the absolute neutrophil count by the absolute lymphocyte count on a complete blood count, this biomarker is essentially free and readily available for all patients. The NLR has been studied specifically in mRCC and a high pre-treatment NLR has been shown to have both prognostic and predictive implications. However, data in the specific context of treatment with ICB is limited [55–59]. One retrospective study of NLR in 42 patients with mRCC treated with ICB demonstrated that a pre-therapy NLR < 3 was associated with longer PFS (HR, 2.937; 95% CI, 1.44 to 5.97; $p = 0.003$) and OS (pre-therapy: HR, 3.977; 95% CI, 1.23 to 12.89; $p = 0.014$) [60]. A subsequent and larger study of 142 patients with mRCC treated with ICB showed that lower baseline NLR was only associated with a trend toward lower ORR, shorter PFS, and shorter OS. In this study they also looked at NLR at six weeks and showed that it was a significantly stronger predictor of all three outcomes than baseline NLR. They also, interestingly, showed that a $> 25\%$ decrease in NLR from baseline to six weeks was associated with significantly improved outcomes in mRCC patients treated with ICB [61]. Both of these were relatively small studies and larger prospective trials are needed to validate these findings before they could be incorporated more commonly into clinical practice.

3.3.2. Tumor Infiltrating Lymphocytes and Immune Microenvironment

Tumor infiltrating lymphocytes (TILs) and their role in the immune response against cancer has been investigated for decades and it is now understood that cytotoxic CD8+ T-cells, otherwise known as "T-killer cells," are essential components of a robust anti-tumor immune response. TILs are activated when presented an antigen via the class I major histocompatibility complex and release cytotoxins to kill the targeted cells [62]. RCC has long been understood to be one of the most immune-infiltrated tumors, as suggested as long as 30 years ago in a study characterizing samples from 120 different tumor histologies [63]. However, mere infiltration of a tumor with TILs does not prove that these immune cells have been properly activated to mount an anti-tumor response. The presence of PD-1 positive immune cells has been associated with worse outcomes as these tumors with large populations of PD-1-positive immune cells have evolved to promote quiescence of the immune system, which allows tumors to avoid detection and explains their more aggressive prognosis [64]. It has also been shown that changes in PD-1-positive immune cells were observed in response to surgical resection in a study of peripheral blood mononuclear cells (PBMC) from 90 patients with RCC before and after nephrectomy. This study showed that increased PD-1 expression on CD14 bright myelomonocytic cells, effector T cells, and natural killer (NK) cells correlated to disease stage, and expression was significantly reduced on all cell types soon after surgical resection of the primary tumor. This further suggests the association between PD-1 positivity of immune cells and the pathophysiology of this disease [65].

This phenomenon was further investigated with the incorporation of various known immune cell surface markers to better characterize the specific phenotype of ineffective TILs and the associated immune microenvironment. Giraldo et al. classified tumors into three basic categories defined by the phenotypic characteristics of their immune cells: immune-regulated, immune-activated, and immune silent. They showed in their study of 40 patients with mRCC that the immune-regulated tumors displayed aggressive histologic features and a high risk of disease progression in the year following nephrectomy for localized disease. The immune-regulated phenotype in this study was defined by CD8+PD-1+TIM-3+Lag-3+ TILs and CD4+ICOS+ helper T-cells in the presence of CD25+CD127-Foxp3+/Helios+GITR+ Tregs [66].

Understanding the importance of the immune infiltrate and microenvironment, new research has focused on the relationship between immune cell surface markers and response to immunotherapy. In an analysis of Checkmate-025 by Braun et al., they confirmed that RCC tumors tend to be heavily infiltrated with CD8+ TILs, but did not show an association between highly infiltrated tumors and ICB response. Interestingly, they noted that highly infiltrated tumors were less likely to carry PBRM1 mutations, which may help explain the association between PBRM1 mutations and favorable prognosis in RCC [67]. In a subsequent analysis of Checkmate-025 by the same group, subsets of the immune infiltrate were classified with methods similar to those used by Giraldo et al. They were able to show that having high levels of CD8+PD1+TIM3-LAG3- TILs was associated with benefit from nivolumab. They also showed that there was a linear association with the increased density of these cells and improvement in ORR, PFS, and OS. Furthermore, these observations were not seen in everolimus-treated patients suggesting a specific relationship to ICB response [68]. This data suggests specifically that TIM3 and LAG3 are important additional checkpoints, since their presence on TILs is associated with reduced benefit from ICB targeting the PD-1 pathway only. There are several inhibitors in development for both LAG3 and TIM3, including a bispecific antibody which targets both PD-L1 and LAG-3 and may be able to improve responses in these patients who express resistant immune phenotypes [69,70].

Lastly, there has been new research exploring the role of cancer-associated fibroblasts (CAFs) and their role in modulating the microenvironment in several tumor types, including mRCC. In mRCC models, CAFs have been shown to recruit macrophages leading to remodeling of the tumor microenvironment and, via signaling through fibroblast activation protein-a (FAP), may promote more aggressive tumor behavior [71]. FAP expression has also been shown to be associated with sarcomatoid features in mRCC, which have been shown, in a subgroup analysis of IMmotion151, to benefit from ICB in the first-line setting with atezolizumab and bevacizumab as compared to the VEGF TKI, sunitinib [18,72]. Finally, in lung cancer models CAFs have been shown to induce PD-L1 expression which further implies a specific role in modulating the immune response [73]. While they are not implicated directly as potential biomarkers for immunotherapy, the importance of CAFs in the immune milieu suggests they may have importance in biomarker development or become a potential target for future immunotherapy strategies.

4. Conclusions

Much progress has been made in the treatment of metastatic RCC since the early 2000s, first with the development of targeted therapies, and even more so with the addition of immunotherapy. Now, for the first time, clinicians are fortunate to have a dilemma of choice between equally efficacious first-line treatment for patients with this disease. Despite these advances, there is still ample room for improvement both in overcoming primary resistance and also in selecting the optimal treatment for each individual patient. Our review summarizes years of work and progress in both of these avenues but still few are validated for treatment selection with proven clinical utility. As a result, and in contrast to many other tumor types, there are still no biomarker-driven approvals for mRCC. However, we anticipate that as our understanding of the biology of mRCC and the molecular mechanisms that drive its evolution expands from studies like TRACERx Renal and large datasets, such as the TCGA, we will identify new biomarker-driven approaches to treatment [74]. Furthermore, as the treatment landscape of mRCC continues to evolve and more treatment options become available, the importance and need for clinically useful biomarkers will only increase. Given this growing need, we envision that a paradigm will be needed to guide clinicians to the best choice available to personalize treatment.

Author Contributions: B.M., D.X. and M.Z. performed data research, wrote, and edited this review. All authors have read and agreed to the published version of the manuscript.

References

1. Heng, D.Y.C.; Xie, W.; Regan, M.M.; Warren, M.A.; Golshayan, A.R.; Sahi, C.; Eigl, B.J.; Ruether, J.D.; Cheng, T.; North, S.; et al. Prognostic factors for overall survival in patients with metastatic renal cell carcinoma treated with vascular endothelial growth factor-targeted agents: Results from a large, multicenter study. *J. Clin. Oncol.* **2009**, *27*, 5794–5799. [CrossRef]
2. Heng, D.Y.C.; Xie, W.; Regan, M.M.; Harshman, L.C.; Bjarnason, G.A.; Vaishampayan, U.N.; Mackenzie, M.; Wood, L.; Donskov, F.; Tan, M.H.; et al. External validation and comparison with other models of the International Metastatic Renal-Cell Carcinoma Database Consortium prognostic model: A population-based study. *Lancet Oncol.* **2013**, *14*, 141–148. [CrossRef]
3. Ko, J.J.; Xie, W.; Kroeger, N.; Lee, J.; Rini, B.I.; Knox, J.J.; Bjarnason, G.A.; Srinivas, S.; Pal, S.K.; Yuasa, T.; et al. The International Metastatic Renal Cell Carcinoma Database Consortium model as a prognostic tool in patients with metastatic renal cell carcinoma previously treated with first-line targeted therapy: A population-based study. *Lancet Oncol.* **2015**, *16*, 293–300. [CrossRef]
4. Dudani, S.; Gan, C.L.; Wells, C.; Bakouny, Z.; Dizman, N.; Pal, S.K.; Wood, L.; Kollmannsberger, C.K.; Szabados, B.; Powles, T.; et al. Application of IMDC criteria across first-line (1L) and second-line (2L) therapies in metastatic renal-cell carcinoma (mRCC): New and updated benchmarks of clinical outcomes. *J. Clin. Oncol.* **2020**, *38*, 5063. [CrossRef]
5. Plimack, E.R.; Rini, B.I.; Stus, V.; Gafanov, R.; Waddell, T.; Nosov, D.; Pouliot, F.; Soulieres, D.; Melichar, B.; Vynnychenko, I.; et al. Pembrolizumab plus axitinib versus sunitinib as first-line therapy for advanced renal cell carcinoma (RCC): Updated analysis of KEYNOTE-426. *J. Clin. Oncol.* **2020**, *38*, 5001. [CrossRef]

6. Motzer, R.J.; Tannir, N.M.; McDermott, D.F.; Arén Frontera, O.; Melichar, B.; Choueiri, T.K.; Plimack, E.R.; Barthélémy, P.; Porta, C.; George, S.; et al. Nivolumab plus Ipilimumab versus Sunitinib in advanced renal-cell carcinoma. *N. Engl. J. Med.* **2018**, *378*, 1277–1290. [CrossRef]
7. Kondo, K.; Yao, M.; Yoshida, M.; Kishida, T.; Shuin, T.; Miura, T.; Moriyama, M.; Kobayashi, K.; Sakai, N.; Kaneko, S.; et al. Comprehensive mutational analysis of the VHL gene in sporadic renal cell carcinoma: Relationship to clinicopathological parameters. *Genes Chromosom. Cancer* **2002**, *34*, 58–68. [CrossRef]
8. Kim, B.J.; Kim, J.H.; Kim, H.S.; Zang, D.Y. Prognostic and predictive value of VHL gene alteration in renal cell carcinoma: A meta-analysis and review. *Oncotarget* **2017**, *8*, 13979–13985. [CrossRef]
9. Ricketts, C.J.; De Cubas, A.A.; Fan, H.; Smith, C.C.; Lang, M.; Reznik, E.; Bowlby, R.; Gibb, E.A.; Akbani, R.; Beroukhim, R.; et al. The Cancer Genome Atlas Comprehensive Molecular Characterization of Renal Cell Carcinoma. *Cell Rep.* **2018**, *23*, 313–326. [CrossRef]
10. Hakimi, A.A.; Chen, Y.B.; Wren, J.; Gonen, M.; Abdel-Wahab, O.; Heguy, A.; Liu, H.; Takeda, S.; Tickoo, S.K.; Reuter, V.E.; et al. Clinical and pathologic impact of select chromatin-modulating tumor suppressors in clear cell renal cell carcinoma. *Eur. Urol.* **2013**, *63*, 848–854. [CrossRef]
11. Ho, T.H.; Choueiri, T.K.; Wang, K.; Karam, J.A.; Chalmers, Z.; Frampton, G.; Elvin, J.A.; Johnson, A.; Liu, X.; Lin, Y.; et al. Correlation between Molecular Subclassifications of Clear Cell Renal Cell Carcinoma and Targeted Therapy Response. *Eur. Urol. Focus* **2016**, *2*, 204–209. [CrossRef]
12. Fay, A.P.; De Velasco, G.; Ho, T.H.; Van Allen, M.; Murray, B.; Albiges, L.; Signoretti, S.; Hakimi, A.A.; Stanton, M.L.; Bellmunt, J.; et al. Whole-exome sequencing in two extreme phenotypes of response to VEGF-targeted therapies in patients with metastatic clear cell renal cell carcinoma. *J. Natl. Compr. Cancer Netw.* **2016**, *14*, 820–824. [CrossRef]
13. Voss, M.H.; Reising, A.; Cheng, Y.; Patel, P.; Marker, M.; Kuo, F.; Chan, T.A.; Choueiri, T.K.; Hsieh, J.J.; Hakimi, A.A.; et al. Genomically annotated risk model for advanced renal-cell carcinoma: A retrospective cohort study. *Lancet Oncol.* **2018**, *19*, 1688–1698. [CrossRef]
14. Minardi, D.; Lucarini, G.; Santoni, M.; Mazzucchelli, R.; Burattini, L.; Pistelli, M.; Bianconi, M.; Di Primio, R.; Scartozzi, M.; Montironi, R.; et al. VEGF expression and response to sunitinib in patients with metastatic clear cell renal cell carcinoma. *Anticancer Res.* **2013**, *33*, 5017–5022. [PubMed]
15. Porta, C.; Paglino, C.; De Amici, M.; Quaglini, S.; Sacchi, L.; Imarisio, I.; Canipari, C. Predictive value of baseline serum vascular endothelial growth factor and neutrophil gelatinase-associated lipocalin in advanced kidney cancer patients receiving sunitinib. *Kidney Int.* **2010**, *77*, 809–815. [CrossRef] [PubMed]
16. Paule, B.; Bastien, L.; Deslandes, E.; Cussenot, O.; Podgorniak, M.P.; Allory, Y.; Naïmi, B.; Porcher, R.; de la Taille, A.; Menashi, S.; et al. Soluble isoforms of vascular endothelial growth factor are predictors of response to sunitinib in metastatic renal cell carcinomas. *PLoS ONE* **2010**, *5*, e10715. [CrossRef] [PubMed]
17. Brauer, M.J.; Zhuang, G.; Schmidt, M.; Yao, J.; Wu, X.; Kaminker, J.S.; Jurinka, S.S.; Kolumam, G.; Chung, A.S.; Jubb, A.; et al. Identification and analysis of in vivo VEGF downstream markers link VEGF pathway activity with efficacy of anti-VEGF therapies. *Clin. Cancer Res.* **2013**, *19*, 3681–3692. [CrossRef] [PubMed]
18. McDermott, D.F.; Huseni, M.A.; Atkins, M.B.; Motzer, R.J.; Rini, B.I.; Escudier, B.; Fong, L.; Joseph, R.W.; Pal, S.K.; Reeves, J.A.; et al. Clinical activity and molecular correlates of response to atezolizumab alone or in combination with bevacizumab versus sunitinib in renal cell carcinoma. *Nat. Med.* **2018**, *24*, 749–757. [CrossRef]
19. Hakimi, A.A.; Voss, M.H.; Kuo, F.; Sanchez, A.; Liu, M.; Nixon, B.G.; Vuong, L.; Ostrovnaya, I.; Chen, Y.B.; Reuter, V.; et al. Transcriptomic profiling of the tumor microenvironment reveals distinct subgroups of clear cell renal cell cancer: Data from a randomized phase III trial. *Cancer Discov.* **2019**, *9*, 510–525. [CrossRef] [PubMed]
20. Choueiri, T.K.; Albiges, L.; Haanen, J.B.A.G.; Larkin, J.M.G.; Uemura, M.; Pal, S.K.; Gravis, G.; Campbell, M.T.; Penkov, K.; Lee, J.-L.; et al. Biomarker analyses from JAVELIN Renal 101: Avelumab + axitinib (A+Ax) versus sunitinib (S) in advanced renal cell carcinoma (aRCC). *J. Clin. Oncol.* **2019**, *37*, 101. [CrossRef]
21. Martini, J.-F.; Plimack, E.R.; Choueiri, T.K.; McDermott, D.F.; Puzanov, I.; Fishman, M.N.; Cho, D.C.; Vaishampayan, U.; Rosbrook, B.; Fernandez, K.C.; et al. Angiogenic and immune-related biomarkers and outcomes following axitinib/pembrolizumab treatment in patients with advanced renal cell carcinoma. *Clin. Cancer Res.* **2020**, *26*, 5598–5608. [CrossRef] [PubMed]
22. Brindle, N.P.J.; Saharinen, P.; Alitalo, K. Signaling and functions of angiopoietin-1 in vascular protection. *Circ. Res.* **2006**, *98*, 1014–1023. [CrossRef]

23. Attig, S.; Hennenlotter, J.; Pawelec, G.; Klein, G.; Koch, S.D.; Pircher, H.; Feyerabend, S.; Wernet, D.; Stenzl, A.; Rammensee, H.G.; et al. Simultaneous infiltration of polyfunctional effector and suppressor T cells into renal cell carcinomas. *Cancer Res.* **2009**, *69*, 8412–8419. [CrossRef] [PubMed]
24. McDermott, D.F.; Regan, M.M.; Clark, J.I.; Flaherty, L.E.; Weiss, G.R.; Logan, T.F.; Kirkwood, J.M.; Gordon, M.S.; Sosman, J.A.; Ernstoff, M.S.; et al. Randomized phase III trial of high-dose interleukin-2 versus subcutaneous interleukin-2 and interferon in patients with metastatic renal cell carcinoma. *J. Clin. Oncol. Off. J. Am. Soc. Clin. Oncol.* **2005**, *23*, 133–141. [CrossRef] [PubMed]
25. Fyfe, G.; Fisher, R.I.; Rosenberg, S.A.; Sznol, M.; Parkinson, D.R.; Louie, A.C. Results of treatment of 255 patients with metastatic renal cell carcinoma who received high-dose recombinant interleukin-2 therapy. *J. Clin. Oncol. Off. J. Am. Soc. Clin. Oncol.* **1995**, *13*, 688–696. [CrossRef]
26. Negrier, S.; Escudier, B.; Lasset, C.; Douillard, J.Y.; Savary, J.; Chevreau, C.; Ravaud, A.; Mercatello, A.; Peny, J.; Mousseau, M.; et al. Recombinant human interleukin-2, recombinant human interferon alfa-2a, or both in metastatic renal-cell carcinoma. *N. Engl. J. Med.* **1998**, *338*, 1272–1278. [CrossRef]
27. Motzer, R.J.; Escudier, B.; McDermott, D.F.; George, S.; Hammers, H.J.; Srinivas, S.; Tykodi, S.S.; Sosman, J.A.; Procopio, G.; Plimack, E.R.; et al. Nivolumab versus Everolimus in Advanced Renal-Cell Carcinoma. *N. Engl. J. Med.* **2015**, *373*, 1803–1813. [CrossRef]
28. Carretero-González, A.; Lora, D.; Martín Sobrino, I.; Sáez Sanz, I.; Bourlon, M.T.; Anido Herranz, U.; Martínez Chanzá, N.; Castellano, D.; de Velasco, G. The Value of PD-L1 Expression as Predictive Biomarker in Metastatic Renal Cell Carcinoma Patients: A Meta-Analysis of Randomized Clinical Trials. *Cancers (Basel)* **2020**, *12*, 1945. [CrossRef]
29. National Comprehensive Cancer Network Kidney Cancer (Version 2.2020). Available online: https://www.nccn.org/professionals/physician_gls/pdf/kidney.pdf (accessed on 10 October 2020).
30. Nunes-Xavier, C.E.; Angulo, J.C.; Pulido, R.; López, J.I. A Critical Insight into the Clinical Translation of PD-1/PD-L1 Blockade Therapy in Clear Cell Renal Cell Carcinoma. *Curr. Urol. Rep.* **2019**, *20*, 1. [CrossRef]
31. López, J.I.; Pulido, R.; Cortés, J.M.; Angulo, J.C.; Lawrie, C.H. Potential impact of PD-L1 (SP-142) immunohistochemical heterogeneity in clear cell renal cell carcinoma immunotherapy. *Pathol. Res. Pract.* **2018**, *214*, 1110–1114. [CrossRef]
32. Thompson, R.H.; Kuntz, S.M.; Leibovich, B.C.; Dong, H.; Lohse, C.M.; Webster, W.S.; Sengupta, S.; Frank, I.; Parker, A.S.; Zincke, H.; et al. Tumor B7-H1 is associated with poor prognosis in renal cell carcinoma patients with long-term follow-up. *Cancer Res.* **2006**, *66*, 3381–3385. [CrossRef] [PubMed]
33. Miao, D.; Margolis, C.A.; Gao, W.; Voss, M.H.; Li, W.; Martini, D.J.; Norton, C.; Bossé, D.; Wankowicz, S.M.; Cullen, D.; et al. Genomic correlates of response to immune checkpoint therapies in clear cell renal cell carcinoma. *Science (80-)* **2018**, *359*, 801–806. [CrossRef] [PubMed]
34. Braun, D.A.; Ishii, Y.; Walsh, A.M.; Van Allen, E.M.; Wu, C.J.; Shukla, S.A.; Choueiri, T.K. Clinical Validation of PBRM1 Alterations as a Marker of Immune Checkpoint Inhibitor Response in Renal Cell Carcinoma. *JAMA Oncol.* **2019**, *5*, 1631. [CrossRef] [PubMed]
35. Hakimi, A.A.; Attalla, K.; DiNatale, R.G.; Ostrovnaya, I.; Flynn, J.; Blum, K.A.; Ged, Y.; Hoen, D.; Kendall, S.M.; Reznik, E.; et al. A pan-cancer analysis of PBAF complex mutations and their association with immunotherapy response. *Nat. Commun.* **2020**, *11*, 4168. [CrossRef]
36. Mizuno, R.; Oya, M. Biomarkers Towards New Era of Therapeutics for Metastatic Renal Cell Carcinoma. *Kidney Cancer* **2020**, *4*, 61–69. [CrossRef]
37. Skoulidis, F.; Goldberg, M.E.; Greenawalt, D.M.; Hellmann, M.D.; Awad, M.M.; Gainor, J.F.; Schrock, A.B.; Hartmaier, R.J.; Trabucco, S.E.; Gay, L.; et al. STK11/LKB1 mutations and PD-1 inhibitor resistance in KRAS-mutant lung adenocarcinoma. *Cancer Discov.* **2018**, *8*, 822–835. [CrossRef]
38. Cerami, E.; Gao, J.; Dogrusoz, U.; Gross, B.E.; Sumer, S.O.; Aksoy, B.A.; Jacobsen, A.; Byrne, C.J.; Heuer, M.L.; Larsson, E.; et al. The cBio Cancer Genomics Portal: An open platform for exploring multidimensional cancer genomics data. *Cancer Discov.* **2012**, *2*, 401–404. [CrossRef]
39. Salgia, N.; Dizman, N.; Lyou, Y.; Bergerot, P.G.; Hsu, J.; Byron, S.A.; Trent, J.M.; Pal, S.K. Genomic and transcriptomic correlates of clinical benefit from immunotherapy and targeted therapy among patients with metastatic renal cell carcinoma (mRCC). *J. Clin. Oncol.* **2020**, *38*, 5076. [CrossRef]
40. D'Costa, N.M.; Cina, D.; Shrestha, R.; Bell, R.H.; Lin, Y.Y.; Asghari, H.; Monjaras-Avila, C.U.; Kollmannsberger, C.; Hach, F.; Chavez-Munoz, C.I.; et al. Identification of gene signature for treatment response to guide precision oncology in clear-cell renal cell carcinoma. *Sci. Rep.* **2020**, *10*, 2026. [CrossRef]

41. McDermott, D.F.; Lee, J.-L.; Donskov, F.; Tykodi, S.S.; Bjarnason, G.A.; Larkin, J.M.G.; Gafanov, R.; Kochenderfer, M.D.; Malik, J.; Poprach, A.; et al. Association of gene expression with clinical outcomes in patients with renal cell carcinoma treated with pembrolizumab in KEYNOTE-427. *J. Clin. Oncol.* **2020**, *38*, 5024. [CrossRef]
42. Brahmer, J.R.; Tykodi, S.S.; Chow, L.Q.M.; Hwu, W.J.; Topalian, S.L.; Hwu, P.; Drake, C.G.; Camacho, L.H.; Kauh, J.; Odunsi, K.; et al. Safety and activity of anti-PD-L1 antibody in patients with advanced cancer. *N. Engl. J. Med.* **2012**, *366*, 2455–2465. [CrossRef] [PubMed]
43. Bonneville, R.; Krook, M.A.; Kautto, E.A.; Miya, J.; Wing, M.R.; Chen, H.-Z.; Reeser, J.W.; Yu, L.; Roychowdhury, S. Landscape of Microsatellite Instability Across 39 Cancer Types. *JCO Precis. Oncol.* **2017**, *1*, 1–15. [CrossRef] [PubMed]
44. Ged, Y.; Chaim, J.L.; DInatale, R.G.; Knezevic, A.; Kotecha, R.R.; Carlo, M.I.; Lee, C.H.; Foster, A.; Feldman, D.R.; Teo, M.Y.; et al. DNA damage repair pathway alterations in metastatic clear cell renal cell carcinoma and implications on systemic therapy. *J. Immunother. Cancer* **2020**, *8*, e000230. [CrossRef] [PubMed]
45. Labriola, M.K.; Zhu, J.; Gupta, R.; McCall, S.; Jackson, J.; Kong, E.F.; White, J.R.; Cerqueira, G.; Gerding, K.; Simmons, J.K.; et al. Characterization of tumor mutation burden, PD-L1 and DNA repair genes to assess relationship to immune checkpoint inhibitors response in metastatic renal cell carcinoma. *J. Immunother. Cancer* **2020**, *8*, 1–10. [CrossRef] [PubMed]
46. Chen, L.; Flies, D.B. Molecular mechanisms of T cell co-stimulation and co-inhibition. *Nat. Rev. Immunol.* **2013**, *13*, 227–242. [CrossRef]
47. Gubin, M.M.; Artyomov, M.N.; Mardis, E.R.; Schreiber, R.D. Tumor neoantigens: Building a framework for personalized cancer immunotherapy. *J. Clin. Investig.* **2015**, *125*, 3413–3421. [CrossRef]
48. Goodman, A.M.; Kato, S.; Bazhenova, L.; Patel, S.P.; Frampton, G.M.; Miller, V.; Stephens, P.J.; Daniels, G.A.; Kurzrock, R. Tumor mutational burden as an independent predictor of response to immunotherapy in diverse cancers. *Mol. Cancer Ther.* **2017**, *16*, 2598–2608. [CrossRef]
49. Marabelle, A.; Fakih, M.G.; Lopez, J.; Shah, M.; Shapira-Frommer, R.; Nakagawa, K.; Chung, H.C.; Kindler, H.L.; Lopez-Martin, J.A.; Miller, W.; et al. Association of tumour mutational burden with outcomes in patients with select advanced solid tumours treated with pembrolizumab in KEYNOTE-158. *Ann. Oncol.* **2019**, *30*, v477–v478. [CrossRef]
50. Zhang, C.; Li, Z.; Qi, F.; Hu, X.; Luo, J. Exploration of the relationships between tumor mutation burden with immune infiltrates in clear cell renal cell carcinoma. *Ann. Transl. Med.* **2019**, *7*, 648. [CrossRef]
51. Havel, J.J.; Chowell, D.; Chan, T.A. The evolving landscape of biomarkers for checkpoint inhibitor immunotherapy. *Nat. Rev. Cancer* **2019**, *19*, 133–150. [CrossRef]
52. McGrail, D.J.; Federico, L.; Li, Y.; Dai, H.; Lu, Y.; Mills, G.B.; Yi, S.; Lin, S.Y.; Sahni, N. Multi-omics analysis reveals neoantigen-independent immune cell infiltration in copy-number driven cancers. *Nat. Commun.* **2018**, *9*, 1–13. [CrossRef]
53. Turajlic, S.; Litchfield, K.; Xu, H.; Rosenthal, R.; McGranahan, N.; Reading, J.L.; Wong, Y.N.S.; Rowan, A.; Kanu, N.; Al Bakir, M.; et al. Insertion-and-deletion-derived tumour-specific neoantigens and the immunogenic phenotype: A pan-cancer analysis. *Lancet Oncol.* **2017**, *18*, 1009–1021. [CrossRef] [PubMed]
54. Shim, J.H.; Kim, H.S.; Cha, H.; Kim, S.; Kim, T.M.; Anagnostou, V.; Choi, Y.L.; Jung, H.A.; Sun, J.M.; Ahn, J.S.; et al. HLA-corrected tumor mutation burden and homologous recombination deficiency for the prediction of response to PD-(L)1 blockade in advanced non-small-cell lung cancer patients. *Ann. Oncol.* **2020**, *31*, 902–911. [CrossRef] [PubMed]
55. Hu, K.; Lou, L.; Ye, J.; Zhang, S. Prognostic role of the neutrophil-lymphocyte ratio in renal cell carcinoma: A meta-analysis. *BMJ Open* **2015**, *5*, e006404. [CrossRef]
56. Baum, Y.S.; Patil, D.; Huang, J.H.; Spetka, S.; Torlak, M.; Nieh, P.T.; Alemozaffar, M.; Ogan, K.; Master, V.A. Elevated preoperative neutrophil-tolymphocyte ratio may be associated with decreased overall survival in patients with metastatic clear cell renal cell carcinoma undergoing cytoreductive nephrectomy. *Asian J. Urol.* **2016**, *3*, 20–25. [CrossRef]
57. Pichler, M.; Hutterer, G.C.; Stoeckigt, C.; Chromecki, T.F.; Stojakovic, T.; Golbeck, S.; Eberhard, K.; Gerger, A.; Mannweiler, S.; Pummer, K.; et al. Validation of the pre-treatment neutrophil-lymphocyte ratio as a prognostic factor in a large European cohort of renal cell carcinoma patients. *Br. J. Cancer* **2013**, *108*, 901–907. [CrossRef]

58. Park, Y.H.; Ku, J.H.; Kwak, C.; Kim, H.H. Post-treatment neutrophil-to-lymphocyte ratio in predicting prognosis in patients with metastatic clear cell renal cell carcinoma receiving sunitinib as first line therapy. *Springerplus* **2014**, *3*, 1–6. [CrossRef]
59. Keizman, D.; Ish-Shalom, M.; Huang, P.; Eisenberger, M.A.; Pili, R.; Hammers, H.; Carducci, M.A. The association of pre-treatment neutrophil to lymphocyte ratio with response rate, progression free survival and overall survival of patients treated with sunitinib for metastatic renal cell carcinoma. *Eur. J. Cancer* **2012**, *48*, 202–208. [CrossRef]
60. Jeyakumar, G.; Kim, S.; Bumma, N.; Landry, C.; Silski, C.; Suisham, S.; Dickow, B.; Heath, E.; Fontana, J.; Vaishampayan, U. Neutrophil lymphocyte ratio and duration of prior anti-angiogenic therapy as biomarkers in metastatic RCC receiving immune checkpoint inhibitor therapy. *J. Immunother. Cancer* **2017**, *5*, 1–8. [CrossRef]
61. Lalani, A.K.A.; Xie, W.; Martini, D.J.; Steinharter, J.A.; Norton, C.K.; Krajewski, K.M.; Duquette, A.; Bossé, D.; Bellmunt, J.; Van Allen, E.M.; et al. Change in Neutrophil-to-lymphocyte ratio (NLR) in response to immune checkpoint blockade for metastatic renal cell carcinoma. *J. Immunother. Cancer* **2018**, *6*, 1–9. [CrossRef]
62. Lanzavecchla, A. Licence to kill. *Nature* **1998**, *393*, 413–414. [CrossRef]
63. Balch, C.M.; Riley, L.B.; Bae, Y.J.; Salmeron, M.A.; Platsoucas, C.D.; Von Eschenbach, A.; Itoh, K. Patterns of Human Tumor-Infiltrating Lymphocytes in 120 Human Cancers. *Arch. Surg.* **1990**, *125*, 200–205. [CrossRef] [PubMed]
64. Thompson, R.H.; Dong, H.; Lohse, C.M.; Leibovich, B.C.; Blute, M.L.; Cheville, J.C.; Kwon, E.D. PD-1 is expressed by tumor-infiltrating immune cells and is associated with poor outcome for patients with renal cell carcinoma. *Clin. Cancer Res.* **2007**, *13*, 1757–1761. [CrossRef] [PubMed]
65. MacFarlane, A.W.; Jillab, M.; Plimack, E.R.; Hudes, G.R.; Uzzo, R.G.; Litwin, S.; Dulaimi, E.; Al-Saleem, T.; Campbell, K.S. PD-1 expression on peripheral blood cells increases with stage in renal cell carcinoma patients and is rapidly reduced after surgical tumor resection. *Cancer Immunol. Res.* **2014**, *2*, 320–331. [CrossRef] [PubMed]
66. Giraldo, N.A.; Becht, E.; Vano, Y.; Petitprez, F.; Lacroix, L.; Validire, P.; Sanchez-Salas, R.; Ingels, A.; Oudard, S.; Moatti, A.; et al. Tumor-infiltrating and peripheral blood T-cell immunophenotypes predict early relapse in localized clear cell renal cell carcinoma. *Clin. Cancer Res.* **2017**, *23*, 4416–4428. [CrossRef] [PubMed]
67. Braun, D.A.; Hou, Y.; Bakouny, Z.; Ficial, M.; Sant' Angelo, M.; Forman, J.; Ross-Macdonald, P.; Berger, A.C.; Jegede, O.A.; Elagina, L.; et al. Interplay of somatic alterations and immune infiltration modulates response to PD-1 blockade in advanced clear cell renal cell carcinoma. *Nat. Med.* **2020**, *26*. [CrossRef] [PubMed]
68. Ficial, M.; Jegede, O.; Sant'Angelo, M.; Moreno, S.; Braun, D.A.; Wind-Rotolo, M.; Pignon, J.-C.; Catalano, P.J.; Sun, M.; Van Allen, E.M.; et al. Evaluation of predictive biomarkers for nivolumab in patients (pts) with metastatic clear cell renal cell carcinoma (mccRCC) from the CheckMate-025 (CM-025) trial. *J. Clin. Oncol.* **2020**, *38*, 5023. [CrossRef]
69. Kraman, M.; Faroudi, M.; Allen, N.L.; Kmiecik, K.; Gliddon, D.; Seal, C.; Koers, A.; Wydro, M.M.; Batey, S.; Winnewisser, J.; et al. FS118, a Bispecific Antibody Targeting LAG-3 and PD-L1, Enhances T-Cell Activation Resulting in Potent Antitumor Activity. *Clin. Cancer Res.* **2020**, *26*, 3333–3344. [CrossRef]
70. Long, L.; Zhang, X.; Chen, F.; Pan, Q.; Phiphatwatchara, P.; Zeng, Y.; Chen, H. The promising immune checkpoint LAG-3: From tumor microenvironment to cancer immunotherapy. *Genes Cancer* **2018**, *9*, 176–189. [CrossRef]
71. Errarte, P.; Larrinaga, G.; López, J.I. The role of cancer-associated fibroblasts in renal cell carcinoma. An example of tumor modulation through tumor/non-tumor cell interactions. *J. Adv. Res.* **2020**, *21*, 103–108. [CrossRef]
72. Errarte, P.; Guarch, R.; Pulido, R.; Blanco, L.; Nunes-Xavier, C.E.; Beitia, M.; Gil, J.; Angulo, J.C.; Lopez, J.I.; Larrinaga, G. The expression of fibroblast activation protein in clear cell renal cell carcinomas is associated with synchronous lymph node metastases. *PLoS ONE* **2016**, *11*, e169105. [CrossRef] [PubMed]
73. Inoue, C.; Miki, Y.; Saito, R.; Hata, S.; Abe, J.; Sato, I.; Okada, Y.; Sasano, H. PD-L1 induction by cancer-associated fibroblast-derived factors in lung adenocarcinoma cells. *Cancers (Basel)* **2019**, *11*, 1257. [CrossRef] [PubMed]
74. Turajlic, S.; Xu, H.; Litchfield, K.; Rowan, A.; Horswell, S.; Chambers, T.; O'Brien, T.; Lopez, J.I.; Watkins, T.B.K.; Nicol, D.; et al. Deterministic Evolutionary Trajectories Influence Primary Tumor Growth: TRACERx Renal. *Cell* **2018**, *173*, 595–610. [CrossRef] [PubMed]

5

Trichostatin A Alleviates Renal Interstitial Fibrosis through Modulation of the M2 Macrophage Subpopulation

Wei-Cheng Tseng [1,2,3,4], **Ming-Tsun Tsai** [1,2,3], **Nien-Jung Chen** [5] **and Der-Cherng Tarng** [1,2,3,4,6,7,*]

1 Division of Nephrology, Department of Medicine, Taipei Veterans General Hospital, Taipei 11217, Taiwan; wctseng@gmail.com (W.-C.T.); mingtsun74@gmail.com (M.-T.T.)
2 Faculty of Medicine, School of Medicine, National Yang-Ming University, Taipei 11221, Taiwan
3 Institute of Clinical Medicine, School of Medicine, National Yang-Ming University, Taipei 11221, Taiwan
4 Center for Intelligent Drug Systems and Smart Bio-devices (IDS2B), National Chiao-Tung University, Hsinchu 30010, Taiwan
5 Institute of Microbiology and Immunology, School of Life Sciences, National Yang-Ming University, Taipei 11221, Taiwan; njchen@ym.edu.tw
6 Department and Institute of Physiology, School of Medicine, National Yang-Ming University, Taipei 11221, Taiwan
7 Department of Biological Science and Technology, College of Biological Science and Technology, National Chiao-Tung University, Hsinchu 30010, Taiwan
* Correspondence: dctarng@vghtpe.gov.tw

Abstract: Mounting evidence indicates that an increase in histone deacetylation contributes to renal fibrosis. Although inhibition of histone deacetylase (HDAC) can reduce the extent of fibrosis, whether HDAC inhibitors exert the antifibrotic effect through modulating the phenotypes of macrophages, the key regulator of renal fibrosis, remains unknown. Moreover, the functional roles of the M2 macrophage subpopulation in fibrotic kidney diseases remain incompletely understood. Herein, we investigated the role of HDAC inhibitors on renal fibrogenesis and macrophage plasticity. We found that HDAC inhibition by trichostatin A (TSA) reduced the accumulation of interstitial macrophages, suppressed the activation of myofibroblasts and attenuated the extent of fibrosis in obstructive nephropathy. Moreover, TSA inhibited M1 macrophages and augmented M2 macrophage infiltration in fibrotic kidney tissue. Interestingly, TSA preferentially upregulated M2c macrophages and suppressed M2a macrophages in the obstructed kidneys, which was correlated with a reduction of interstitial fibrosis. TSA also repressed the expression of proinflammatory and profibrotic molecules in cultured M2a macrophages and inhibited the activation of renal myofibroblasts. In conclusion, our study was the first to show that HDAC inhibition by TSA alleviates renal fibrosis in obstructed kidneys through facilitating an M1 to M2c macrophage transition.

Keywords: macrophage subpopulation; renal fibrosis; trichostatin A

---

1. Introduction

Chronic kidney disease (CKD) is an emerging global public health issue with a prevalence rate of 10% to 12% worldwide [1]. Regardless of the etiologies of renal diseases, unresolved renal insult engages an excessive deposition of extracellular matrix in the tubulointerstitium, thereby bringing about end-stage renal disease [2]. Tubulointerstitial fibrosis is the final common pathway of all kidney diseases and, also, represents the major determinant of renal function decline [2]. A wealth of studies has indicated that renal function decline correlates well with the increasing risks for all-cause mortality, cardiovascular events and hospitalization [1,3,4]. Despite that current available therapies have targeted traditional risk factors for renal function decline—namely, hypertension, hyperglycemia and hyperlipidemia, nearly half of CKD patients still experience progressive renal function decline and eventual end-stage renal disease [5]. Hence, a novel treatment modality to tackle renal fibrosis and halt the progression of CKD is urgently needed.

Infiltrated renal macrophages play pivotal roles in the homeostasis of renal fibrogenesis following initial renal insult, either ischemic, immunologic, mechanical or toxic damage [6]. Macrophages are highly plastic and differentiate into different phenotypes in response to the local environments. Macrophage phenotypes can be broadly categorized into the proinflammatory "M1" macrophages (characterized by inducible nitric oxide synthase (iNOS)) and the anti-inflammatory, reparative "M2" macrophages (characterized by arginase-1 (Arg1)) [6]. M2 macrophages can be further classified into M2a and M2c subpopulations by the presence of C-type lectin domain family 7 member A (CLEC7A) and signaling lymphocytic activation molecule (SLAM), respectively [7]. These macrophage subsets play distinct roles in the wound-healing process following tissue injury [8]. During the normal wound-healing process, the initial proinflammatory milieu recruits M1 macrophages to induce apoptosis and eliminate the pathogen and necrotic tissue. Thereafter, anti-inflammatory M2 macrophages predominate in the later tissue repair stage to activate re-epithelialization and neoangiogenesis in the injured area. Finally, a resolution stage ends the whole healing process by promoting the apoptosis of recruited immune cells, suppression of inflammation and tissue remodeling [8]. Nonetheless, dysregulation of the M1-to-M2 transition in a normal wound-healing process would lead to pathologic fibrosis and tissue scarring [8]. Recent studies further suggest that the excessive activation of M1 macrophages and certain profibrotic M2 macrophages both contribute to the development of fibrosis formation [9].

M2 macrophages may function as a double-edged sword in regulating renal fibrosis. M2 macrophages help control inflammation through releasing interleukin (IL)-10, Arg1, transforming growth factor-β (TGF-β) and heme oxygenase-1 [9]. On the other hand, the chronic activation of M2 macrophages can activate resident fibroblasts through the release of TGF-β, platelet-derived growth factor, vascular endothelium growth factor, insulin-like growth factor-1 and galactin-3 [9]. In this regard, M2 macrophages are proposed to be profibrotic in the renal fibrosis model of unilateral ureteral obstruction (UUO), and depletion of these M2 macrophages in UUO should be beneficial [9,10]. However, not all macrophage depletion strategies result in a reduction in fibrosis in UUO [10]. Inhibition of the c-fms kinase almost suppresses all infiltrating macrophage numbers in day 14 obstructed kidneys but does not change the course of fibrosis, suggesting some antifibrotic M2 macrophages are also depleted [11]. Until now, the functional roles of the M2 macrophage subpopulation in renal fibrogenesis remained unclear and conflicting. M2a and M2c macrophages are initially found to be anti-inflammatory and reparative in murine Adriamycin nephrosis [12]. Nonetheless, two recent studies indicate that M2a macrophages are upregulated in endometrial fibrosis and skeletal muscle fibrosis [13,14], suggesting M2a macrophages may exhibit a profibrotic feature in chronic fibrotic diseases. Therefore, further elucidating the roles of the M2a and M2c subsets may help delineate the complex fibrogenic process in UUO.

Emerging evidence indicates that epigenetic modulation of the chromatin state is crucial in determining the progression of CKD and macrophage polarization [15,16]. The histone acetylation status has recently been found to associate with certain kidney diseases and renal fibrogenesis [17]. Histone deacetylases (HDACs) are a group of enzymes that exert epigenetic effects by altering the acetylation status of histone and nonhistone proteins [18]. Although potential favorable effects of HDAC inhibitors have been found in animal models of acute kidney injury [19], diabetic nephropathy [20] and Adriamycin nephropathy [21], the roles of HDAC inhibitors in UUO and macrophage plasticity remain incompletely understood. Marumo et al. found that the expression of HDAC1 and HDAC2 are upregulated in obstructed kidneys and contribute to proinflammatory and fibrotic responses [22]. Nonetheless, whether HDAC inhibition regulates the phenotypic change of renal interstitial macrophages in UUO is still unclear. Previously, HDAC3-deficient bone marrow-derived macrophages displayed an M2-polarized IL-4-induced alternatively activated phenotype [11], implying HDAC inhibition may contribute to M2 macrophage polarization. Currently, there is no study exploring the interaction between histone acetylation and macrophage subsets in kidney diseases. Hence, we aimed to investigate whether HDAC inhibition attenuates renal fibrosis through modulating the phenotype of renal interstitial macrophages.

In this study, we found the distinct expression of M2a and M2c subset macrophages in obstructed kidneys. An increased M2a macrophage infiltrate correlated with a higher extent of renal interstitial fibrosis. Interestingly, the administration of trichostatin A (TSA), an HDAC inhibitor, suppressed M2a macrophage infiltration, enhanced M2c macrophage expression and attenuated renal fibrosis in UUO. TSA also repressed the expression of proinflammatory and profibrotic molecules in cultured M2a macrophages and inhibited the activation of renal myofibroblasts. Our study is the first to demonstrate that TSA modulates the renal macrophage M2 subpopulation to inhibit renal fibrosis.

2. Results

2.1. *Infiltration of Interstitial Macrophages Correlates with Fibrosis in Obstructed Kidneys*

To investigate the role of macrophage infiltration in renal fibrosis, we compared five mice kidneys harvested seven days after UUO to five mice kidneys harvested 14 days after UUO. Masson trichrome staining indicated that the area of renal tubulointerstitial fibrosis increased with the time of UUO. Moreover, immunohistochemistry showed α-smooth muscle actin (α-SMA)-positive myofibroblasts progressively increased in the day 14 obstructed kidneys as compared to the day 7 ones. Notably, the area of F4/80 (pan-macrophage marker)-positive macrophage infiltrate also correspondingly increased in the day 14 obstructed kidneys (Figure 1), indicating that interstitial macrophages did play an essential role in the development of renal fibrosis.

2.2. *Preferential Accumulation of M1 and M2a Macrophages in Obstructed Kidneys*

As macrophage plasticity is critical for regulating renal fibrosis [8], next, we analyzed the phenotypes of macrophages at different time points of UUO. Immunohistochemistry showed that both iNOS-positive M1 macrophages and Arg1-positive M2 macrophages progressively accumulated in the day 14 obstructed kidneys. Thereafter, we explored the M2 macrophage subpopulation in UUO. Interestingly, CLEC7A-positive M2a macrophages predominantly expressed in the day 14 obstructed kidneys. By contrast, the number of SLAM-positive M2c macrophages was only slightly increased over time (Figure 2A,B). Western blot analyses also showed the consistent results that the expression of M1 and M2a markers progressively increased with the time of UUO (Figure 2C,D). These data suggest that M1 and M2a macrophages are involved in the development of renal fibrosis.

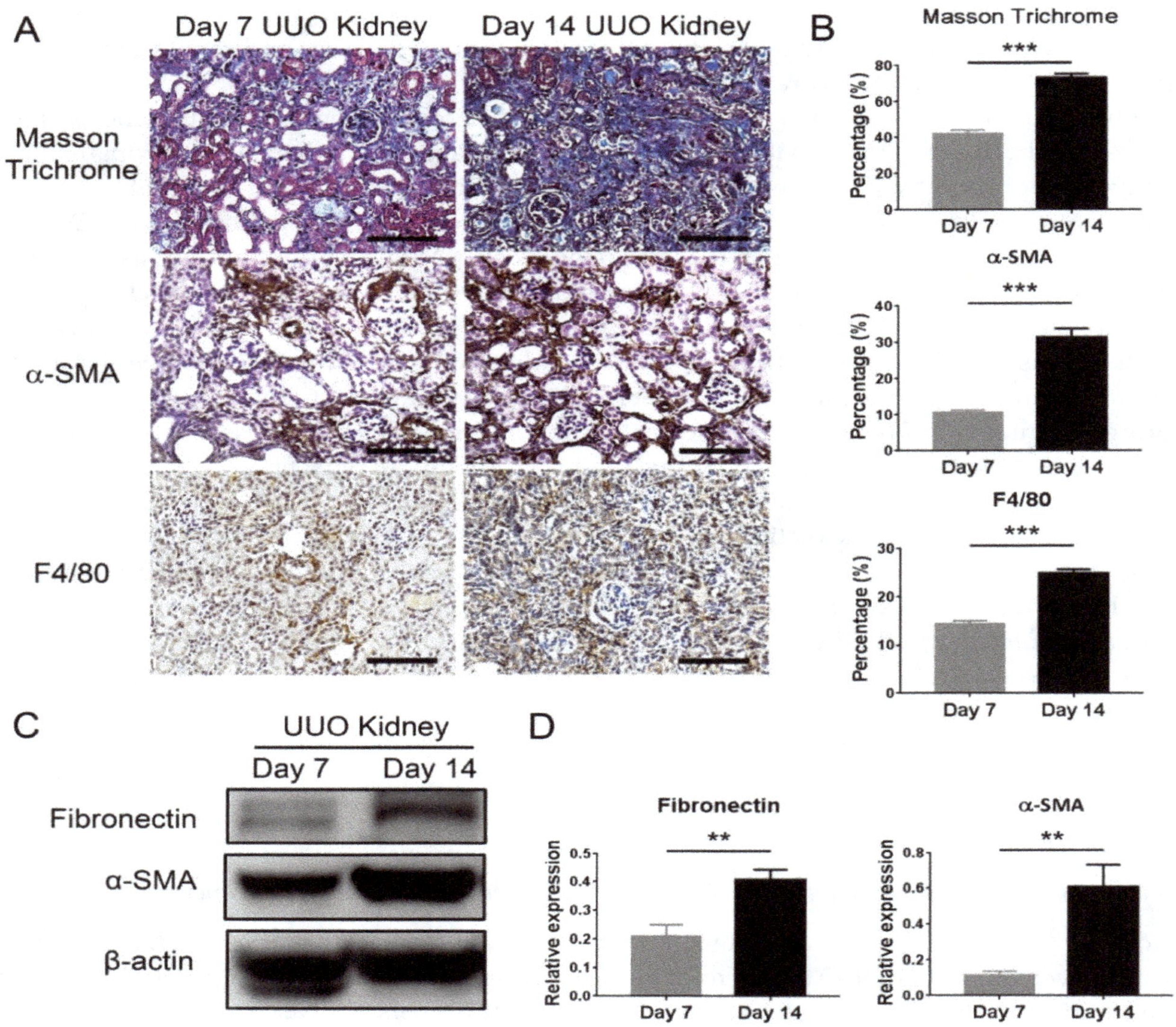

Figure 1. Macrophage infiltration correlates with renal interstitial fibrosis following a unilateral ureteral obstruction (UUO) injury. (**A**) Representative images of the Masson trichrome staining showed that the extent of fibrosis (blue staining) progressively increased in day 14 UUO kidneys as compared to day 7 ones. Immunohistochemistry demonstrated that more α-smooth muscle actin (α-SMA)-positive myofibroblasts and F4/80-positive macrophages accumulated in day 14 UUO kidneys. Scale bar = 100 μm. (**B**) Quantification of the fibrosis extent, α-SMA-positive and F4/80-positive areas. ** $p < 0.01$ and *** $p < 0.001$ by the unpaired Student's t-test; $n = 5$ for each group. (**C**) Western blot analysis of fibronectin and α-SMA expression in day 7 and day 14 obstructed kidneys. β-actin served as the loading control. (**D**) Quantification of the Western blot analyses. ** $p < 0.01$ and *** $p < 0.001$ by the unpaired Student's t-test; $n = 5$ for each group.

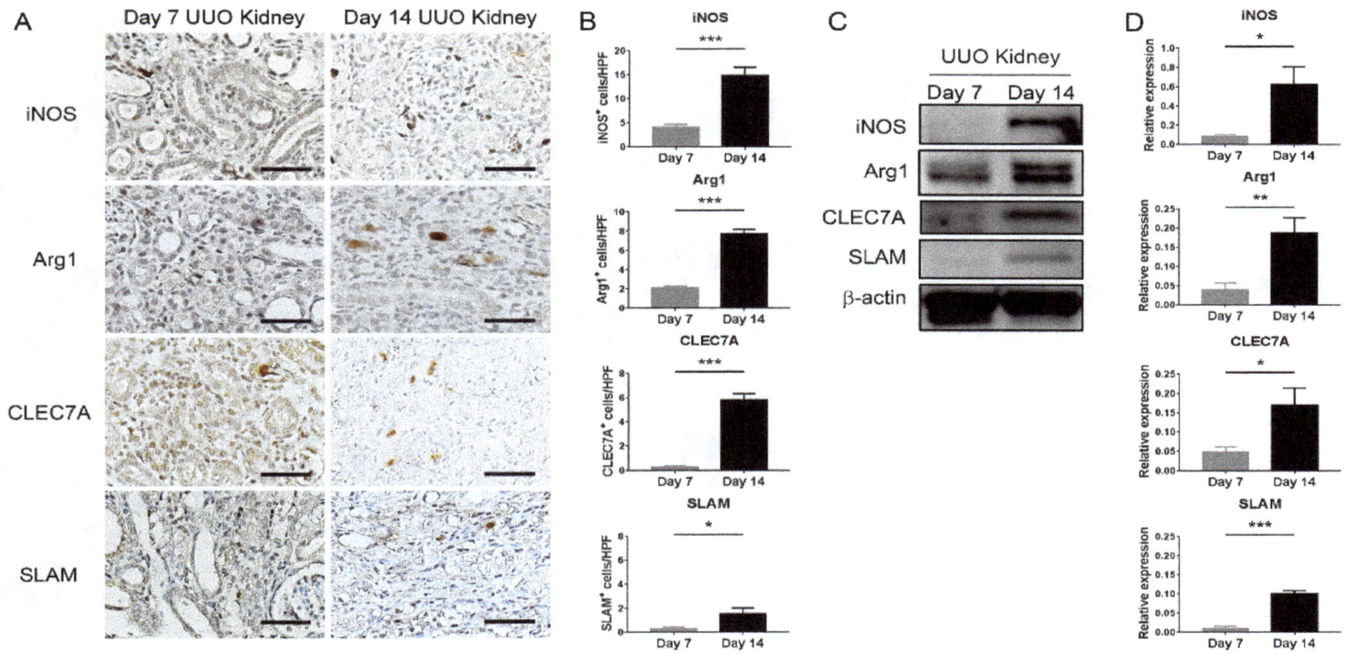

Figure 2. M1 and M2a macrophage infiltrates predominate in the late stage of unilateral ureteral obstruction (UUO). (**A**) Representative immunohistochemical photomicrographs of inducible nitric oxide synthase (iNOS), arginase-1 (Arg1), C-type lectin domain family 7 member A (CLEC7A) and signaling lymphocytic activation molecule (SLAM) in day 7 and day 14 obstructed kidneys. Scale bar = 25 μm. (**B**) Quantification of the iNOS-, Arg1-, CLEC7A- and SLAM-positive interstitial cells in day 7 and day 14 obstructed kidneys. * $p < 0.05$ and *** $p < 0.001$ by the unpaired Student's *t*-test; $n = 5$ for each group. (**C**) Western blot analyses of iNOS, Arg1, CLEC7A and SLAM expressions in day 7 and day 14 obstructed kidneys. β-actin served as the loading control. (**D**) Quantification of the Western blot analyses. * $p < 0.05$, ** $p < 0.01$ and *** $p < 0.001$ by the unpaired Student's *t*-test; $n = 5$ for each group.

2.3. *HDAC Inhibition Represses Renal Fibrosis and Macrophage Infiltration in UUO*

Given that increased histone deacetylation may be associated with renal fibrogenesis [17], we then investigated the therapeutic effect of TSA in UUO. The administration of TSA significantly reduced the extent of α-SMA-positive myofibroblasts and the area of renal interstitial fibrosis in UUO. Moreover, TSA also decreased the extent of interstitial macrophage infiltrate (Figure 3A,B). Western blot analysis also found that TSA reduced the expression of the extracellular matrix (fibronectin) and α-SMA in obstructed kidneys (Figure 3C,D).

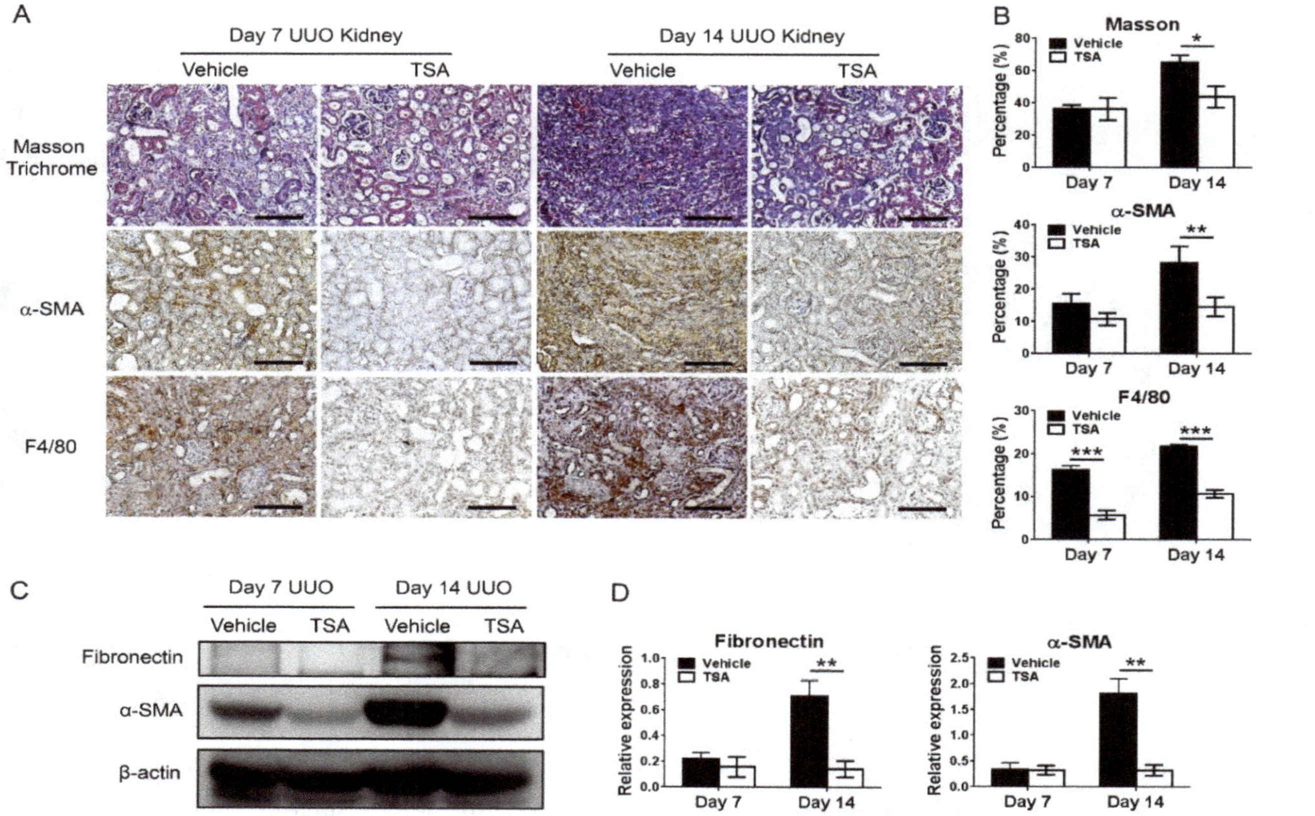

Figure 3. Trichostatin A (TSA) ameliorates renal inflammation and fibrosis in unilateral ureteral obstruction (UUO). (**A**) Representative images of Masson trichrome staining of obstructed kidneys at 7 days and 14 days following UUO in the vehicle and TSA groups. The TSA treatment markedly reduced the extent of interstitial fibrosis (blue area). Immunohistochemical staining for α-smooth muscle actin (α-SMA, myofibroblast marker) and F4/80 (pan-macrophage marker) in day 7 and day 14 obstructed kidneys. Scale bar = 100 μm. (**B**) Quantification of the fibrosis extent, α-SMA-positive and F4/80-positive areas. * $p < 0.05$, ** $p < 0.01$ and *** $p < 0.001$ by the unpaired Student's t-test; $n = 5$ for each group. (**C**) Western blots of fibronectin and α-SMA in day 7 and day 14 UUO kidneys treated with the vehicle or TSA. β-actin served as the loading control. (**D**) Quantification of fibronectin and α-SMA expression levels. ** $p < 0.01$ by the unpaired Student's t-test; $n = 5$ for each group.

2.4. HDAC Inhibition Promotes an M1-to-M2 Phenotypic Transition and Skews the M2 Macrophage Phenotype Towards an M2c Feature

To explore the role of HDAC inhibition on macrophage plasticity, we analyzed the phenotypes of interstitial macrophages in UUO after the administration of TSA. Upon treatment with TSA, immunohistochemistry showed that the infiltration of iNOS-positive M1 macrophages significantly decreased as compared to the vehicle group. Conversely, Arg1-positive macrophages were significantly upregulated in the TSA-treated kidneys following 14 days of obstruction (Figure 4A,B). Remarkably, TSA increased the number of SLAM-positive M2c macrophages but decreased the number of M2a macrophages. Immunofluorescent staining showed that both CLEC7A and SLAM colocalized with F4/80+CD206+ cells in obstructed kidneys, supporting that CLEC7A-positive and SLAM-positive cells represented M2a and M2c macrophages, respectively. Immunoblot confirmed that TSA downregulated the expression of iNOS and CLEC7A, as well as upregulated the expression of Arg1 and CLEC7A (Figure 4C–F). These data indicated that TSA suppressed the accumulation of proinflammatory M1 macrophages and profibrotic M2a macrophages in UUO. Instead, TSA increased the anti-inflammatory M2c macrophage infiltration, which limited the extent of inflammation and inhibited the activation of myofibroblasts and deposition of the extracellular matrix.

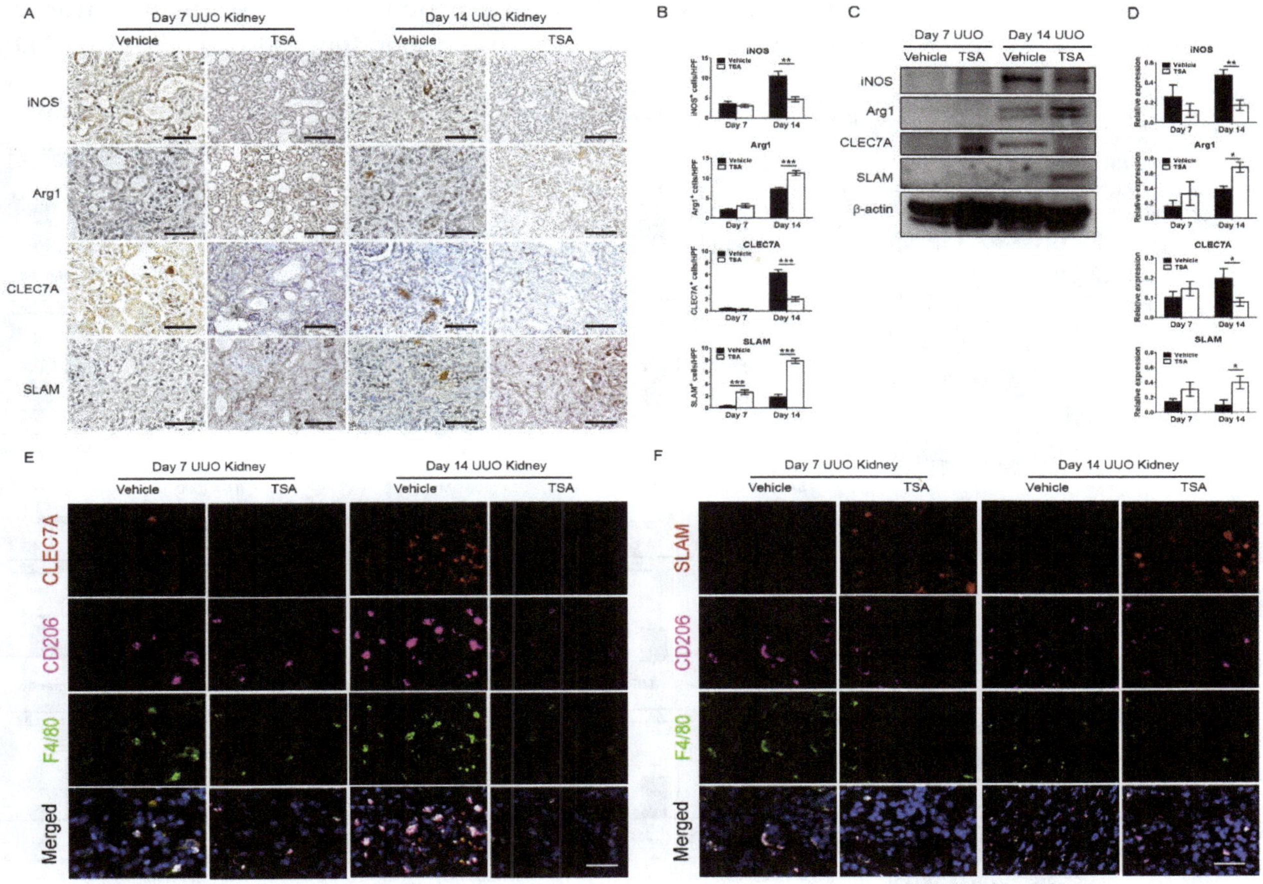

Figure 4. Trichostatin A (TSA) suppresses M1 and M2a macrophage infiltration but promotes M2c macrophage infiltration in unilateral ureteral obstruction (UUO). (**A**) Representative immunohistochemical images of inducible nitric oxide synthase (iNOS, M1 macrophage marker), arginase-1 (Arg1, pan-M2 macrophage marker), C-type lectin domain family 7 member A (CLEC7A, M2a macrophage marker) and signaling lymphocytic activation molecule (SLAM, M2c macrophage marker) in day 7 and day 14 obstructed kidneys either treated with the vehicle or TSA. Scale bar = 25 μm. (**B**) Quantification of the iNOS-, Arg1-, CLEC7A- and SLAM-positive interstitial cells in day 7 and day 14 obstructed kidneys treated with the vehicle or TSA. ** $p < 0.01$ and *** $p < 0.001$ by the unpaired Student's t-test; $n = 5$ for each group. (**C**) Western blots of iNOS, Arg1, CLEC7A and SLAM in day 7 and day 14 obstructed kidneys either treated with the vehicle or TSA. β-actin served as the loading control. (**D**) Quantification of iNOS, Arg1, CLEC7A and SLAM expression levels in obstructed kidneys. * $p < 0.05$ and ** $p < 0.01$ by the unpaired Student's t-test; $n = 5$ for each group. (**E**) Immunofluorescent staining of CLEC7A, CD206 and F4/80 in obstructed kidneys. Scale bar = 25 μm. (**F**) Immunofluorescent staining of SLAM, CD206 and F4/80 in obstructed kidneys. Scale bar = 25 μm. White color indicates colocalization in the merged panels.

2.5. HDAC Inhibition Suppresses Proinflammatory and Profibrotic Phenotypes in Cultured M2 Macrophages

To further clarify the effect of HDAC inhibition on the proinflammatory and profibrotic phenotypes of macrophages, J774A.1 macrophages were stimulated with IL-4/IL-13 or IL-10/TGF-b1 in the presence or absence of TSA for 24 h. IL-4/IL-13 induced the expression of Arg1 and CLEC7A in J774A.1 macrophages and polarized the cells towards an M2a phenotype. M2a J774A.1 macrophages increased the expression of profibrotic α-SMA and fibronectin, which were suppressed by TSA treatment. Furthermore, the amounts of proinflammatory tumor necrosis factor-α and iNOS in the M2a macrophages were also downregulated by TSA (Figure 5A,B). In contrast, IL-10/TGF-β1 induced the SLAM expression in J774A.1 macrophages and skewed the cells towards an M2c phenotype. The TSA treatment enhanced the SLAM expression in M2c J774A.1 macrophages and also further suppressed the amounts of TNF-α, iNOS, α-SMA and fibronectin in a dose-dependent manner (Figure 5C,D).

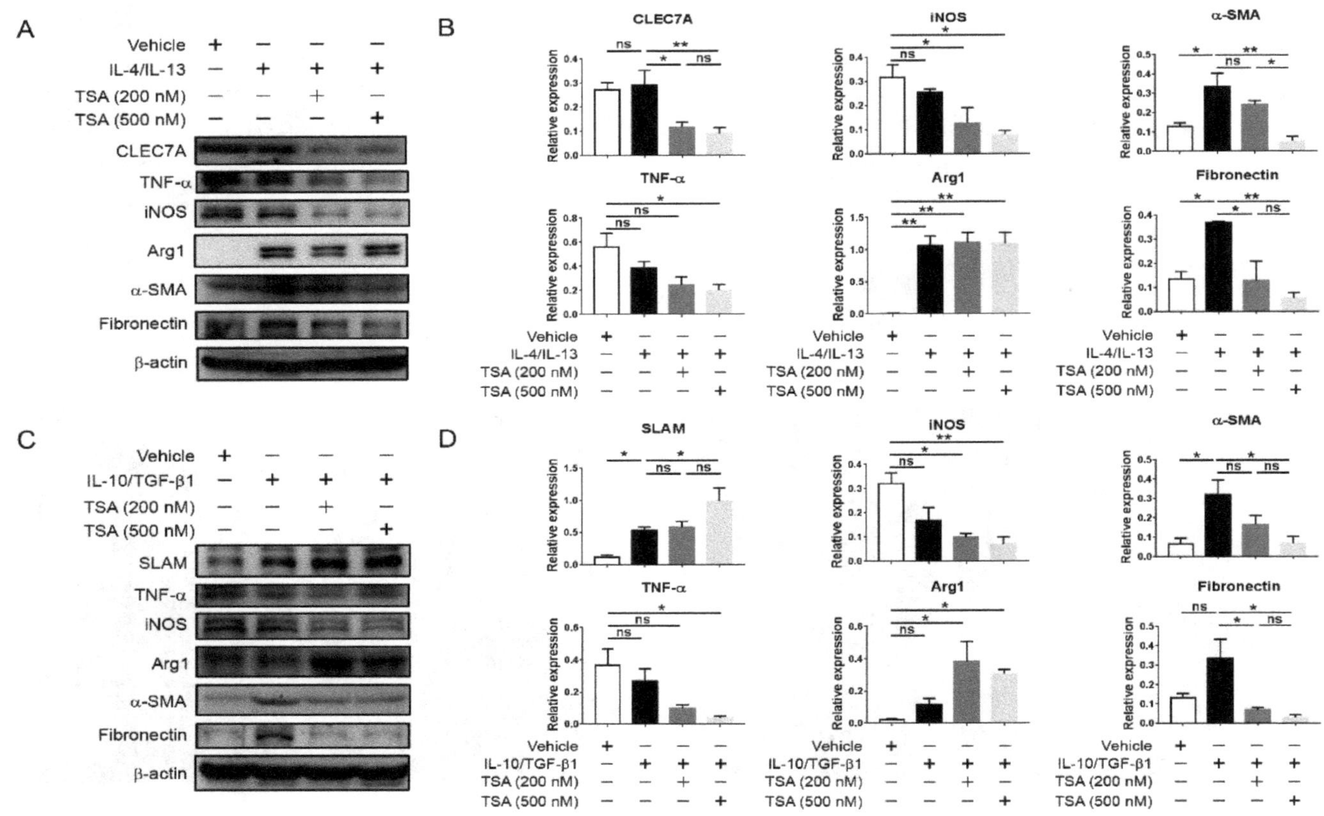

Figure 5. The effect of trichostatin A (TSA) on proinflammatory and profibrotic phenotypes of M2a and M2c macrophages. (**A**) Western blots of C-type lectin domain family 7 member A (CLEC7A), proinflammatory (tumor necrosis factor-α (TNF-α) and inducible nitric oxide synthase (iNOS)) and profibrotic (α-smooth muscle actin (α-SMA) and fibronectin) expressions in J774A.1 macrophages treated with the indicated conditions for 24 h. Concentrations of interleukin (IL)-4 and IL-13 were both 20 ng/mL. β-actin served as the loading control. (**B**) Quantification for the levels of indicated proteins. * $p < 0.05$ and ** $p < 0.01$ by ANOVA, followed by Tukey's post hoc multiple comparison test; $n = 3$ for each group. (**C**) Western blots of SLAM, proinflammatory (TNF-α and iNOS) and profibrotic (α-SMA and fibronectin) expressions in J774A.1 macrophages treated with the indicated conditions for 24 h. Concentrations of IL-10 and transforming growth factor (TGF)-β1 were both 20 ng/mL. β-actin served as the loading control. (**D**) Quantification for the levels of indicated proteins. * $p < 0.05$ and ** $p < 0.01$ by ANOVA, followed by Tukey's post hoc multiple comparison test; $n = 3$ for each group.

2.6. HDAC Inhibition Attenuates TGF-β1-Activated Renal Tubular Epithelial Cells and Fibroblasts

TGF-β1 is a well-known predominant mediator of the activation of renal myofibroblasts and resultant fibrogenesis in UUO [23]. To substantiate the role of HDAC inhibition on TGF-β1-induced renal fibrosis, renal tubular epithelial NRK-52E cells and renal NRK-49F fibroblasts were stimulated with TGF-β1 in the presence or absence of TSA. Western blotting revealed that TGF-β1 upregulated the expression of α-SMA and fibronectin in NRK-52E cells in a time-dependent manner. The treatment with TSA abrogated TGF-β1-induced fibrogenesis in NRK-52E cells (Figure 6A,B). These effects were further confirmed by immunofluorescent staining (Figure 6C,D). In NRK-49F fibroblasts, the TSA treatment also repressed TGF-β1-induced α-SMA expression (Supplementary Figure S1). These data indicate that TSA reduced renal fibrosis through attenuating the activation of myofibroblasts by TGF-β1.

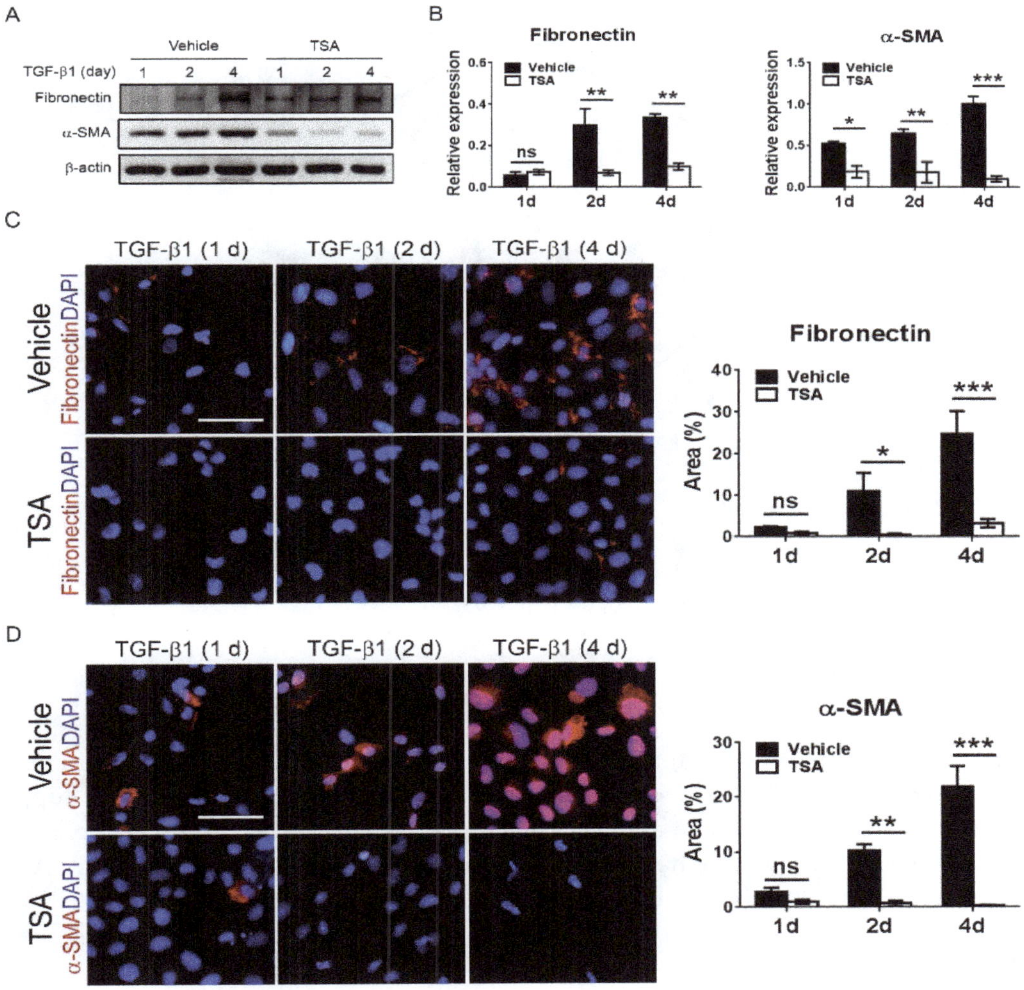

Figure 6. The effect of trichostatin A (TSA) on the activation of renal myofibroblasts. (**A**) Western blots of fibronectin and α-smooth muscle actin (a-SMA) expressions in transforming growth factor-β1 (TGF- β1, 20 ng/mL)-stimulated renal tubular epithelial NRK-52E cells at the indicated time. β-actin served as the loading control. (**B**) Quantification for the levels of indicated proteins. * $p < 0.05$, ** $p < 0.01$ and *** $p < 0.001$ by ANOVA, followed by Tukey's post hoc multiple comparison test. ns, nonsignificance. $n = 3$ for each group. (**C,D**) Immunofluorescent staining of fibronectin and α-SMA in the TGF-β1-treated NRK-52E cells at the indicated time. Scale bar = 50 μm. * $p < 0.05$, ** $p < 0.01$ and *** $p < 0.001$ by ANOVA, followed by Tukey's post hoc multiple comparison test. ns, nonsignificance. $n = 3$ for each group.

Our findings are summarized schematically in Figure 7. In renal fibrogenesis, the accumulation of M1 and M2a macrophages enhances inflammation and activates myofibroblasts. Trichostatin A suppresses the infiltration of proinflammatory M1 and M2a macrophages and increases the infiltration of anti-inflammatory M2c macrophages, thereby inhibiting the activation of renal myofibroblasts and resultant renal fibrosis.

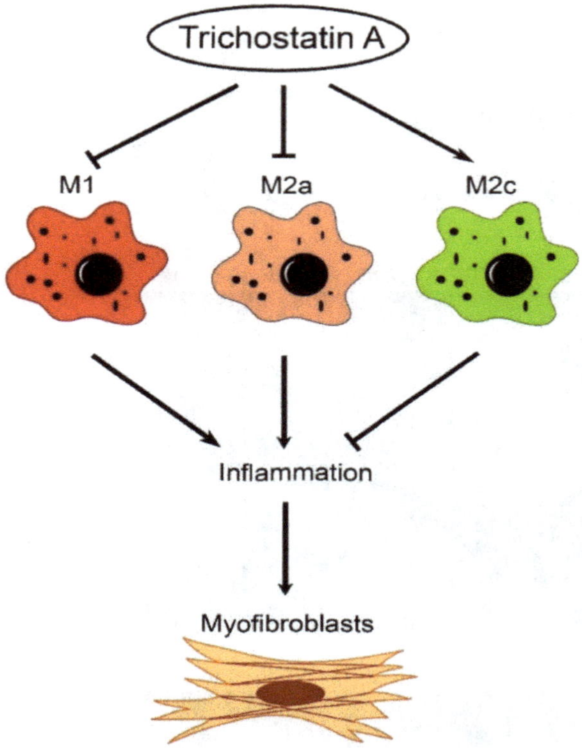

Figure 7. Proposed immunomodulatory and antifibrotic mechanism by trichostatin A in renal fibrosis. In a mice model of unilateral ureteral obstruction, the administration of trichostatin A suppresses the infiltration of proinflammatory M1a and M2a macrophages, as well as promotes the accumulation of anti-inflammatory M2c macrophages, thereby limiting excessive inflammation. Accordingly, the activation of myofibroblasts is limited, and renal fibrosis is attenuated.

3. Discussion

This present study showed that HDAC inhibition by TSA reduced renal fibrosis through modulating the M2 macrophage subpopulation. We found that a TSA treatment significantly decreased the extent of interstitial fibrosis, myofibroblast accumulation and macrophage infiltration in the obstructed kidneys. Interestingly, TSA downregulated iNOS expression and upregulated Arg1 expression in the whole kidney protein expression levels. Consistently, immunochemistry also found that TSA suppressed the infiltration of iNOS-positive M1 macrophages and promoted the accumulation of Arg1-positive M2 macrophages in the obstructed renal interstitial areas. Specifically, TSA suppressed the accumulation of CLEC7A-positive M2a macrophages but increased the number of SLAM-positive M2c macrophages. These data indicated that the increment of M2 macrophages by TSA in UUO was preferentially attributed to the increased accumulation of M2c macrophages. Consistently, we also found that TSA suppressed CLEC7A expression in M2a macrophages and enhanced SLAM expression in M2c macrophages in vitro. Notably, TSA further downregulated the expression of proinflammatory and profibrotic factors in M2a macrophages. Moreover, TSA attenuated the TGF-β1-induced expression of α-SMA and fibronectin in cultured renal tubular epithelial cells and fibroblasts, indicating that TSA also attenuated the activation of renal myofibroblasts through inhibiting the epithelial-mesenchymal transition. Collectively, our findings indicated that TSA suppressed renal fibrogenesis through increasing the anti-inflammatory and antifibrotic M2 subpopulation.

Conflicting results exist regarding the role of M2 macrophages on renal fibrosis in UUO [9], probably related to the heterogeneity of the M2 subpopulation. Previously, M2 macrophages were proposed to be profibrotic, because the macrophage infiltrate in the UUO-kidney has a predominant M2 phenotype and the percentage of M2 macrophages increases along with the duration of obstruction [10]. If this is the case, the depletion of all macrophages in the later stage of UUO should mitigate renal fibrosis. However, not all macrophage ablation strategies result in the improvement of renal fibrosis in UUO [10]. The depletion of infiltrating macrophages through targeting the c-fms kinase fails to attenuate the extent of renal fibrosis in day 14 obstructed kidneys [11], suggesting certain antifibrotic M2 macrophages are also depleted and also highlighting the complex functional heterogeneity of the M2 macrophage population [24]. Our study found that the TSA treatment resulted in fibrosis reduction, the downregulation of iNOS-positive M1 macrophages and CLEC7A-positive M2a macrophages and the upregulation of SLAM-positive M2c macrophages. In line with our observations, Wang et al. found that M2a macrophages are associated with the accumulation of collagen and muscle fibrosis [14]. Moreover, Duan et al. showed that the adoptive transfer of M2a macrophages significantly increased the extent of fibrosis in endometriosis [13], suggesting that M2a macrophages are profibrotic and critically involved in fibrogenesis. The controversy regarding the profibrotic or antifibrotic roles of M2 macrophages may be reconciled by the balance of distinct M2a and M2c macrophages in chronic fibrotic disorders.

Recent attention has focused on the significance of post-translational histone modifications in determining the progression of CKD and macrophage polarization [15,16]. Nonetheless, the role of epigenetic regulation on macrophage phenotypes in UUO remains elusive. The present study found that HDAC inhibition by TSA significantly alleviated renal inflammation and fibrosis. We also found that TSA inhibited the infiltration of M1 and M2a macrophages, enhanced the infiltration of M2c macrophages and directed an M1-to-M2c switch. The TSA-induced upregulation of M2c macrophages correlated with a reduction of renal interstitial fibrosis, and TSA also enhanced the SLAM expression and suppressed profibrotic and proinflammatory phenotypes in cultured M2c macrophages. These data supported that TSA repressed renal fibrosis through augmenting the expression of antifibrotic M2 macrophages. Although we found that TSA reduced UUO-induced renal fibrosis through modulation of the M2 macrophage subpopulation, our findings may not be extrapolated to renal fibrosis attributed to other insults, such as toxin, diabetes or autoimmune diseases. Clearly, more studies will be required to confirm the immunomodulatory and antifibrotic effects of TSA in other models of kidney diseases. In consistency with our findings, Pang et al. found that TSA can mitigate the extent of renal fibrosis in obstructive nephropathy, but the role of TSA on renal inflammation is undefined in their study [25]. A later study by Marumo et al. also found that TSA suppressed tubulointerstitial fibrosis in obstructed kidneys and further showed that TSA reduced renal inflammation in terms of the downregulation of EMR1 and MCP1 expressions, as well as decreased the number of infiltrated macrophages [22]. However, the effect of HDAC inhibition on the phenotypic transition of macrophages was not examined [22]. Taken together, our study provided novel evidence that TSA attenuated renal fibrosis through suppressing the profibrotic M2a macrophage and promoting anti-inflammatory, antifibrotic M2c macrophages. In conclusion, our study showed that HDAC inhibition by TSA significantly attenuated renal fibrosis through promoting an M1-to-M2c macrophage transition in obstructed kidneys. Our study not only added to the knowledge of antifibrotic M2 macrophages but, also, provided the bench evidence that pharmacological HDAC inhibitors can be applied to clinical treatments of renal fibrosis in the future.

4. Materials and Methods

4.1. Animals

Male 6-to-8-week-old C57BL/6J mice weighing 20-25 g were purchased from the National Laboratory Animal Center (Taipei, Taiwan) and housed at the Laboratory Animal Center of the National Yang-Ming University (Taipei, Taiwan). The mice were raised in a sound-attenuated, temperature-controlled (22 ± 1 °C) room with a 12-h light/dark cycle. Standard rodent chow and drinking water were supplied ad libitum. All experimental procedures conformed to the Guide for the Care and Use of Laboratory Animals published by the National Institutes of Health. The study was approved by the Institutional Animal Care and Use Committee of the National Yang-Ming University under the license number 1041244.

4.2. Cell Culture and Treatment

Mouse J774A.1 macrophages (Bioresource Collection and Research Center, Hsin-Chu, Taiwan) were cultured in Dulbecco's modified Eagle's medium (10-013-CM, Corning Inc., Corning, NY, USA) supplemented with 10% fetal bovine serum (Gibco, Grand Island, NY, USA) in a 5% CO_2, 37 °C humidified incubator. To examine the effect of TSA on the macrophage subpopulation, J774A.1 macrophages were first seeded in 6-well dishes (5×10^6 cells/well). Afterwards, J774A.1 macrophages were polarized into the M2a phenotype by stimulation with IL-4 (20 ng/mL, PeproTech, Rocky Hill, NJ, USA) and IL-13 (20 ng/mL, PeproTech) or into the M2c phenotype by stimulation with IL-10 (20 ng/mL, PeproTech) and TGF-b1 (20 ng/mL, PeproTech) for 24 h in the presence or absence of TSA (200 nM and 500 nM, T8552, Sigma-Aldrich, St. Louis, MO, USA) at different concentrations.

Normal rat renal tubular NRK-52E cells (Bioresource Collection and Research Center) were cultured in the low-glucose Dulbecco's modified Eagle's medium (10-014-CV, Corning Inc.) supplemented with 5% fetal bovine serum (Gibco). To determine the effect of TSA on renal myofibroblasts, NRK-52E were stimulated with TGF-β1 (20 ng/mL, PeproTech) for 1, 2 and 4 days in the presence or absence of TSA (500 nM, Sigma-Aldrich).

4.3. Experimental UUO Model

After anesthesia, the UUO model was performed in mice by ligation of the left ureter with 5-O silk through a flank incision, as previously described [26]. After the surgery, the mice were recovered under a warming lamp. For HDAC inhibition experiments, TSA (1 mg/kg, Sigma-Aldrich) or the vehicle were injected intraperitoneally daily. The animals were euthanized, and the obstructed kidneys were harvested 7 and 14 days after UUO for further analyses.

4.4. Histological Analysis of the Kidneys

The kidney tissue was fixed with 4% phosphate-buffered formalin solution (Macron Chemicals, Center Valley, PA, USA), embedded in paraffin block and cut into 4-μm sections. For histological analysis, after deparaffinization and rehydration by xylene and graded alcohols, the sections were subjected to Masson trichrome staining according to the manufacturer's instructions (Accustain, Sigma-Aldrich). Twenty randomly selected nonoverlapping high-power fields (40× objective) were evaluated for each mouse, and the average for each group was then analyzed. The fibrotic area was quantified by ImageJ software (1.52a, US National Institutes of Health, Bethesda, MD, USA).

4.5. Immunohistochemical Staining

Immunohistochemical staining was performed on formalin-fixed paraffin-embedded sections of obstructed kidneys, as previously described [27]. Briefly, after deparaffinization by xylene and rehydration by graded alcohols, consecutive 4-μm sections of kidneys were subjected to heat antigen retrieval in a microwave oven (650W, 12 min) in a 10-mM sodium citrate buffer (pH 6.0). Afterwards, endogenous peroxidase activity was quenched by 3% hydrogen peroxide (Sigma-Aldrich) for 10 min. Thereafter, tissue sections were incubated with the primary antibodies at 4 °C overnight and then with the secondary antibody (Envision$^+$Dual Link System-HRP, Dako, Glostrup, Denmark) for 30 min at room temperature. Signals were developed with diaminobenzidine substrate-chromogen (DAB, Dako), which resulted in a brown-colored precipitate at the antigen site. Finally, sections were counterstained with a Gill's hematoxylin (Merck, Darmstadt, Germany). Primary antibodies included F4/80 (1:100, Cat#sc-25830, Santa Cruz Biotechnology, Santa Cruz, CA, USA), iNOS (1:200, Cat#sc-651, Santa Cruz Biotechnology), Arg1 (1:200, Cat#sc-20150, Santa Cruz Biotechnology), α-SMA (1:200, Cat#ab5694, Abcam, Cambridge, UK), CLEC7A (1:50, Cat#TA322197, OriGene Technologies, Rockville, MD, USA) and SLAM (1:100, Cat#ab156288, Abcam). Twenty randomly selected nonoverlapping high-power fields (40× objective) at the renal cortex were evaluated for each mouse. Analysis of the

DAB-positive area was carried out using Image J with the "Threshold Colour" plug-in (version 1.16, https://imagejdocu.tudor.lu/plugin/color/threshold_colour/start#threshold_colour).

4.6. Western Blotting

Western blotting analysis was performed as previously described [28]. Briefly, protein from the obstructed kidney tissue or cells was extracted in a radioimmunoprecipitation assay buffer containing a protease inhibitor cocktail (cOmplete-Mini, Roche, Indianapolis, IN, USA). The protein concentration was determined by a Bradford assay (Bio-Rad Laboratories, Montreal, Quebec, Canada), separated by sodium dodecyl sulfate-polyacrylamide gel electrophoresis and, subsequently, transferred to polyvinylidene fluoride membranes. The membranes were then probed with primary antibodies against fibronectin (1:1000, Cat#15613-1-AP, Proteintech Group, Chicago, IL, USA), α-SMA (1:5000, Cat#14395-1-AP, Proteintech Group), iNOS (1:1000, Cat#ab3523, Abcam), Arg1 (1:1000, Cat#93668S, Cell Signaling Technology, Boston, MA, USA), CLEC7A (1:500, Cat#TA322197, OriGene Technologies), SLAM (1:1000, Cat#ab156288, Abcam), TNF-α (1:1000, Cat#ab66579, Abcam) and β-actin (1:5000, Cat#60008, Proteintech Group) at 4 °C overnight. Afterwards, the membranes were incubated with horseradish peroxidase-conjugated secondary antibodies (Jackson ImmunoResearch, West Grove, PA, USA) at room temperature for 1.5 h, and the signals were developed using a West Femto Chemiluminescent Substrate kit (Thermo Fisher Scientific, Hudson, NH, USA). Bands were visualized and quantified using a ChemiDoc-It Imaging system (UVP, Cambridge, UK). Data were normalized to the β-actin expression.

4.7. Immunofluorescence

For in vivo experiments, paraffin-embedded 4-μm sections of obstructed kidneys were deparaffinized with xylene, rehydrated with graded alcohols and boiled in a 10-mM citrate buffer. Thereafter, the sections were blocked with hydrogen peroxide and then reacted with primary antibodies against F4/80 (1:100, Cat#MCA497R, Abd Serotec, Oxford, UK), CD206 (1:100, Cat#60143-1-Ig, Proteintech Group), CLEC7A (1:50, Cat#MBS9414183, MyBiosource, San Diego, CA, USA) or SLAM (1:100, Cat#ab156288, Abcam) at 4 °C overnight. Fluorescein isothiocyanate-conjugated goat anti-rat immunoglobulin G (IgG, 1:250, Cat#112-095-003, Jackson ImmunoResearch) and Alexa Fluor 647-conjugated donkey anti-mouse IgG (1:250, Cat# 715-605-151, Jackson ImmunoResearch) were used to visualize the location of F4/80 and CD206, respectively. Alexa Fluor 568-conjugated goat anti-rabbit IgG (1:250, Cat#A11011, Thermo Fisher Scientific) was used to visualize the location of CLEC7A and SLAM. Slides were then mounted with Fluoroshield Mounting Medium with DAPI (ab104139, Abcam).

For in vitro experiments, TGF-β1-stimulated NRK-52E cells were plated in chamber slides (μ-Slide 8-Well, Ibidi, Munich, Germany) for 1, 2 and 4 days in the presence or absence of trichostatin. Afterwards, the chamber slides were fixed with 4% paraformaldehyde for 10 min and blocked with 1% bovine serum albumin for 30 min. Thereafter, slides were incubated with primary antibodies against α-SMA (1:200, ab5694, Abcam) or fibronectin (1:200, 15613-1-AP, Proteintech) at 4 °C overnight, reacted with Alexa Fluor 568-conjugated goat anti-rabbit secondary antibody (1:200, Cat#A11011, Thermo Fisher Scientific) and then counterstained with DAPI (ab104139, Abcam).

4.8. Statistical Analysis

All values are expressed as mean ± SEM. Between-group comparisons were determined by the unpaired Student's *t*-tests or ANOVA, followed by Tukey's post hoc multiple comparison test. Statistical analysis was performed using the Statistical Analysis System (SAS, Version 9.4, SAS Institute, Cary, NC, USA). A value of two-sided $p < 0.05$ was considered statistically significant.

Author Contributions: Conceptualization, W.-C.T.; data curation, M.-T.T.; formal analysis, W.-C.T. and M.-T.T.; funding acquisition, W.-C.T. and D.-C.T.; investigation, W.-C.T.; methodology, W.-C.T.; project administration, D.-C.T.; resources, D.-C.T.; supervision, N.-J.C. and D.-C.T.; validation, M.-T.T.; writing—original draft, W.-C.T. and writing—review and editing, M.-T.T., N.-J.C. and D.-C.T. All authors have read and agreed to the published version of the manuscript.

Acknowledgments: The authors thank the Division of Experimental Surgery, Department of Surgery and Department of Pathology, Taipei Veterans General Hospital for technical assistance. They also thank the Clinical Research Core Laboratory and the Medical Science & Technology Building of Taipei Veterans General Hospital for providing experimental space and facilities.

References

1. Wen, C.P.; Cheng, T.Y.; Tsai, M.K.; Chang, Y.C.; Chan, H.T.; Tsai, S.P.; Chiang, P.H.; Hsu, C.C.; Sung, P.K.; Hsu, Y.H.; et al. All-cause mortality attributable to chronic kidney disease: A prospective cohort study based on 462 293 adults in Taiwan. *Lancet* **2008**, *371*, 2173–2182. [CrossRef]
2. Zeisberg, M.; Neilson, E.G. Mechanisms of tubulointerstitial fibrosis. *J. Am. Soc. Nephrol.* **2010**, *21*, 1819–1834. [CrossRef] [PubMed]
3. Go, A.S.; Chertow, G.M.; Fan, D.; McCulloch, C.E.; Hsu, C.Y. Chronic kidney disease and the risks of death, cardiovascular events, and hospitalization. *N. Engl. J. Med.* **2004**, *351*, 1296–1305. [CrossRef] [PubMed]
4. Sud, M.; Tangri, N.; Pintilie, M.; Levey, A.S.; Naimark, D. Risk of end-stage renal disease and death after cardiovascular events in chronic kidney disease. *Circulation* **2014**, *130*, 458–465. [CrossRef] [PubMed]
5. Braun, L.; Sood, V.; Hogue, S.; Lieberman, B.; Copley-Merriman, C. High burden and unmet patient needs in chronic kidney disease. *Int. J. Nephrol. Renovasc. Dis.* **2012**, *5*, 151–163. [PubMed]
6. Ricardo, S.D.; van Goor, H.; Eddy, A.A. Macrophage diversity in renal injury and repair. *J. Clin. Investig.* **2008**, *118*, 3522–3530. [CrossRef]
7. Anders, H.J.; Ryu, M. Renal microenvironments and macrophage phenotypes determine progression or resolution of renal inflammation and fibrosis. *Kidney Int.* **2011**, *80*, 915–925. [CrossRef]
8. Wermuth, P.J.; Jimenez, S.A. The significance of macrophage polarization subtypes for animal models of tissue fibrosis and human fibrotic diseases. *Clin. Transl. Med.* **2015**, *4*, 2. [CrossRef]
9. Braga, T.T.; Agudelo, J.S.; Camara, N.O. Macrophages during the Fibrotic Process: M2 as Friend and Foe. *Front. Immunol.* **2015**, *6*, 602. [CrossRef]
10. Nikolic-Paterson, D.J.; Wang, S.; Lan, H.Y. Macrophages promote renal fibrosis through direct and indirect mechanisms. *Kidney Int. Suppl.* **2014**, *4*, 34–38. [CrossRef]
11. Ma, F.Y.; Liu, J.; Kitching, A.R.; Manthey, C.L.; Nikolic-Paterson, D.J. Targeting renal macrophage accumulation via c-fms kinase reduces tubular apoptosis but fails to modify progressive fibrosis in the obstructed rat kidney. *Am. J. Physiol. Renal Physiol.* **2009**, *296*, F177–F185. [CrossRef] [PubMed]
12. Lu, J.; Cao, Q.; Zheng, D.; Sun, Y.; Wang, C.; Yu, X.; Wang, Y.; Lee, V.W.; Zheng, G.; Tan, T.K.; et al. Discrete functions of M2a and M2c macrophage subsets determine their relative efficacy in treating chronic kidney disease. *Kidney Int.* **2013**, *84*, 745–755. [CrossRef] [PubMed]
13. Duan, J.; Liu, X.; Wang, H.; Guo, S.W. The M2a macrophage subset may be critically involved in the fibrogenesis of endometriosis in mice. *Reprod. Biomed. Online* **2018**, *37*, 254–268. [CrossRef] [PubMed]
14. Wang, Y.; Wehling-Henricks, M.; Samengo, G.; Tidball, J.G. Increases of M2a macrophages and fibrosis in aging muscle are influenced by bone marrow aging and negatively regulated by muscle-derived nitric oxide. *Aging Cell* **2015**, *14*, 678–688. [CrossRef] [PubMed]
15. Ivashkiv, L.B. Epigenetic regulation of macrophage polarization and function. *Trends Immunol.* **2013**, *34*, 216–223. [CrossRef] [PubMed]
16. Wanner, N.; Bechtel-Walz, W. Epigenetics of kidney disease. *Cell Tissue Res.* **2017**, *369*, 75–92. [CrossRef]
17. Tampe, B.; Zeisberg, M. Evidence for the involvement of epigenetics in the progression of renal fibrogenesis. *Nephrol. Dial. Transplant.* **2014**, *29* (Suppl. 1), i1–i8. [CrossRef]
18. Beckerman, P.; Ko, Y.A.; Susztak, K. Epigenetics: A new way to look at kidney diseases. *Nephrol. Dial. Transplant.* **2014**, *29*, 1821–1827. [CrossRef]
19. Cianciolo Cosentino, C.; Skrypnyk, N.I.; Brilli, L.L.; Chiba, T.; Novitskaya, T.; Woods, C.; West, J.;

Korotchenko, V.N.; McDermott, L.; Day, B.W.; et al. Histone deacetylase inhibitor enhances recovery after AKI. *J. Am. Soc. Nephrol.* **2013**, *24*, 943–953. [CrossRef]
20. Gilbert, R.E.; Huang, Q.; Thai, K.; Advani, S.L.; Lee, K.; Yuen, D.A.; Connelly, K.A.; Advani, A. Histone deacetylase inhibition attenuates diabetes-associated kidney growth: Potential role for epigenetic modification of the epidermal growth factor receptor. *Kidney Int.* **2011**, *79*, 1312–1321. [CrossRef]
21. Van Beneden, K.; Geers, C.; Pauwels, M.; Mannaerts, I.; Verbeelen, D.; van Grunsven, L.A.; Van den Branden, C. Valproic acid attenuates proteinuria and kidney injury. *J. Am. Soc. Nephrol.* **2011**, *22*, 1863–1875. [CrossRef] [PubMed]
22. Marumo, T.; Hishikawa, K.; Yoshikawa, M.; Hirahashi, J.; Kawachi, S.; Fujita, T. Histone deacetylase modulates the proinflammatory and -fibrotic changes in tubulointerstitial injury. *Am. J. Physiol. Renal Physiol.* **2010**, *298*, F133–F141. [CrossRef] [PubMed]
23. Chevalier, R.L.; Forbes, M.S.; Thornhill, B.A. Ureteral obstruction as a model of renal interstitial fibrosis and obstructive nephropathy. *Kidney Int.* **2009**, *75*, 1145–1152. [CrossRef] [PubMed]
24. Huen, S.C.; Cantley, L.G. Macrophages in Renal Injury and Repair. *Annu. Rev. Physiol.* **2017**, *79*, 449–469. [CrossRef] [PubMed]
25. Pang, M.; Kothapally, J.; Mao, H.; Tolbert, E.; Ponnusamy, M.; Chin, Y.E.; Zhuang, S. Inhibition of histone deacetylase activity attenuates renal fibroblast activation and interstitial fibrosis in obstructive nephropathy. *Am. J. Physiol. Renal Physiol.* **2009**, *297*, F996–F1005. [CrossRef] [PubMed]
26. Lo, T.H.; Tseng, K.Y.; Tsao, W.S.; Yang, C.Y.; Hsieh, S.L.; Chiu, A.W.; Takai, T.; Mak, T.W.; Tarng, D.C.; Chen, N.J. TREM-1 regulates macrophage polarization in ureteral obstruction. *Kidney Int.* **2014**, *86*, 1174–1186. [CrossRef]
27. Tseng, W.C.; Yang, W.C.; Yang, A.H.; Hsieh, S.L.; Tarng, D.C. Expression of TNFRSF6B in kidneys is a novel predictor for progression of chronic kidney disease. *Mod. Pathol.* **2013**, *26*, 984–994. [CrossRef]
28. Tseng, W.C.; Chuang, C.W.; Yang, M.H.; Pan, C.C.; Tarng, D.C. Kruppel-like factor 4 is a novel prognostic predictor for urothelial carcinoma of bladder and it regulates TWIST1-mediated epithelial-mesenchymal transition. *Urol. Oncol.* **2016**, *34*, 485.e15–485.e24. [CrossRef]

6

Aminopeptidases in Cardiovascular and Renal Function: Role as Predictive Renal Injury Biomarkers

Félix Vargas [1], Rosemary Wangesteen [2], Isabel Rodríguez-Gómez [1] and Joaquín García-Estañ [3,*]

[1] Depto. Fisiologia, Fac. Medicina, Universidad de Granada, 18071 Granada, Spain; fvargas@ugr.es (F.V.); isabelrg@ugr.es (I.R.-G.)
[2] Depto. Ciencias de la salud, Universidad de Jaén, 23071 Jaén, Spain; rwanges@ujaen.es
[3] Depto. Fisiologia, Fac. Medicina, IMIB, Universidad de Murcia, 30120 Murcia, Spain
* Correspondence: jgestan@um.es

Abstract: Aminopeptidases (APs) are metalloenzymes that hydrolyze peptides and polypeptides by scission of the N-terminus amino acid and that also participate in the intracellular final digestion of proteins. APs play an important role in protein maturation, signal transduction, and cell-cycle control, among other processes. These enzymes are especially relevant in the control of cardiovascular and renal functions. APs participate in the regulation of the systemic and local renin–angiotensin system and also modulate the activity of neuropeptides, kinins, immunomodulatory peptides, and cytokines, even contributing to cholesterol uptake and angiogenesis. This review focuses on the role of four key APs, aspartyl-, alanyl-, glutamyl-, and leucyl-cystinyl-aminopeptidases, in the control of blood pressure (BP) and renal function and on their association with different cardiovascular and renal diseases. In this context, the effects of AP inhibitors are analyzed as therapeutic tools for BP control and renal diseases. Their role as urinary biomarkers of renal injury is also explored. The enzymatic activities of urinary APs, which act as hydrolyzing peptides on the luminal surface of the renal tubule, have emerged as early predictive renal injury biomarkers in both acute and chronic renal nephropathies, including those induced by nephrotoxic agents, obesity, hypertension, or diabetes. Hence, the analysis of urinary AP appears to be a promising diagnostic and prognostic approach to renal disease in both research and clinical settings.

Keywords: urinary aminopeptidases; biomarkers; arterial hypertension; renal function

---

1. Aminopeptidases in the Renin–Angiotensin System

The renin–angiotensin system (RAS) plays an essential role in blood pressure (BP) control, via vascular, renal, brain, and other mechanisms. Abnormalities in RAS activity may lead to the development of arterial hypertension and other cardiovascular and renal diseases. Blockade of this system is an effective therapeutic measure against numerous diseases, and RAS compounds have been found in the kidney, brain, and other tissues. Over recent years, our knowledge of the components of the RAS has increased, including numerous angiotensin peptides with diverse biological activities mediated by different receptor subtypes [1,2].

The enzymatic cascade of the RAS is depicted in Figure 1. It is initiated by angiotensinogen, an alfa 2 globulin of hepatic origin, which generates angiotensin I (AngI) through the enzymatic action of renin on the extreme amino-terminus. The decapeptide AngI is a substrate for angiotensin-converting enzyme (ACE), which splits the dipeptide His-Leu from the extreme carboxy-terminus to generate the octapeptide AngII [1], the major effector peptide of the RAS, which bind to two major receptors, AT1 and AT2, that generally oppose each other.

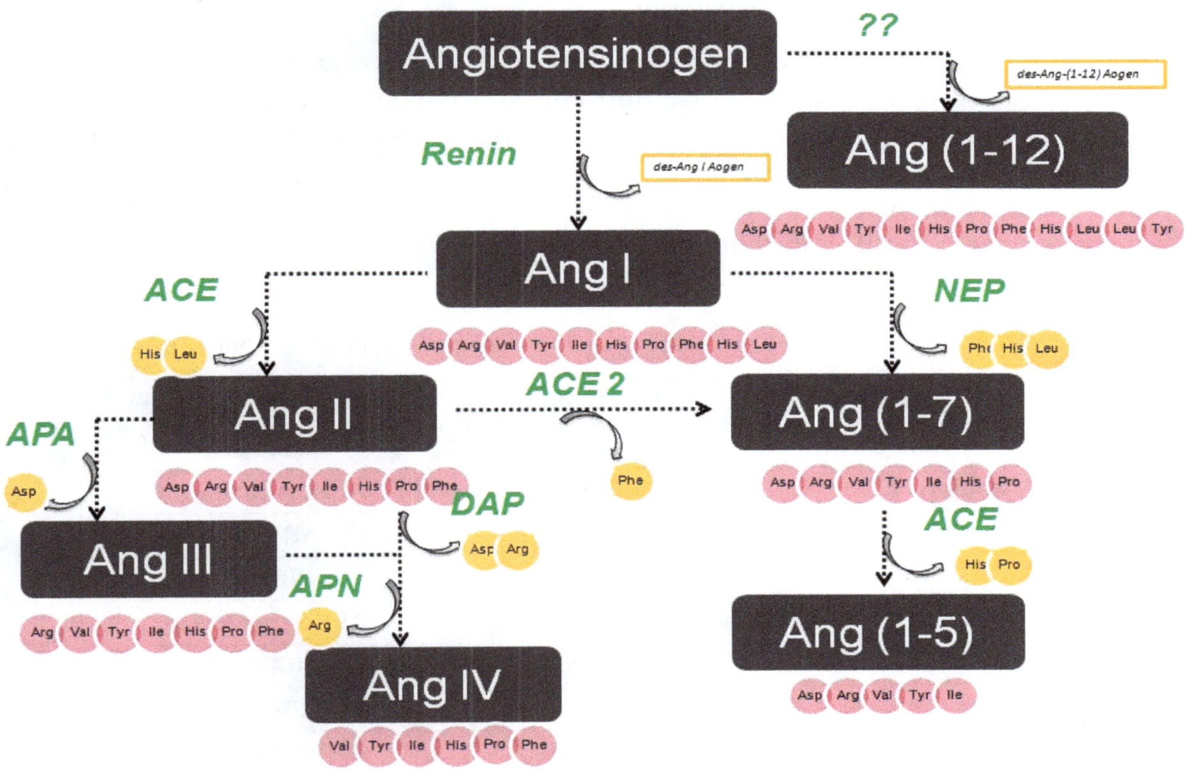

Figure 1. The renin–angiotensin system.

Action of glutamyl aminopeptidase (APA) on AngII removes the Asp residue N-terminus to generate the heptapeptide AngIII. AngIII can also be generated by an AngII-independent pathway via the nonapeptide [des-Asp1]AngI, produced from AngI by AspAP, which is converted to AngIII via ACE. APA also participates in the formation of Ang(1-7), which can also be transformed into Ang(2-7) through cleaving of the Asp-Arg bond.

In the extreme N-terminus, membrane alanyl aminopeptidase N (APN) removes Arg to give hexapeptide angiotensin IV (AngIV). AngIV is also transformed into Ang(3-7) by carboxypeptidase P (Carb-P) and propyl oligopeptidase through scission of the Pro-Phe carboxy-terminus.

ACE2 can also transform AngII into Ang(1-7) through hydrolysis of Phe by Carb-P or through scission of the dipeptide Phe-His from Ang(1-9) [1–4].

Aminopeptidase B (APB), also known as arginine aminopeptidase (Arg-AP), cleaves basic amino acids at the N-terminus. It participates in the conversion of AngIII to AngIV.

Although not part of the RAS, both neuropeptides oxytocin and vasopressin are cleaved at the N-terminus of cysteine next to tyrosine by cystinyl aminopeptidase (CAP), a rat homolog of insulin-regulated AP (IRAP) [5].

All these enzymes are globally called "angiotensinases" because they are responsible for the generation of systemic and local peptides (angiotensins) related to the regulation of BP and the excretion of sodium and water. These enzymes determine the proportions of bioactive compounds.

AngI is biologically inactive, but AngII and AngIII act as agonists for AT1 and AT2 receptors, thereby mediating pressor and dipsogenic effects [6,7]. AngIV has a low affinity for AT1 and AT2 receptors but high affinity and specificity for the AT4 receptor subtype. Interaction with the AT1 receptor subtype reduces the pressor effect of AngIV. A counterregulatory system to the AngII-AngIII/AT1 receptor system is composed of ACE2 and Ang(1-7), which activate the Mas receptor [6–8]. This system induces vasodilatory, antifibrotic, antihypertrophic, and antiproliferative effects.

2. Aminopeptidases in Arterial Hypertension

A list of the most common aminopeptidases with their enzyme commission (EC) numbers and their main abbreviations is shown in Table 1. As was introduced in the previous paragraph, aminopeptidases (Aps) generate the active compounds of the RAS and play an essential role in BP control and sodium handling [9]. APs can also degrade certain peptidergic hormones or neuropeptides such as vasopressin, cholecystokinin, and enkephalins [10]. For this reason, APs have been analyzed in plasma, kidney, and other tissues related to BP control in several rat models of hypertension.

Table 1. Types of aminopeptidases showing their most common abbreviations.

Enzyme	EC Number	Abbreviations
Leucyl AP	3.4.11.1	LAP
Membrane alanyl AP	3.4.11.2	APN, AlaAP
Cystinyl AP	3.4.11.3	CysAP, CAP
Prolyl AP	3.4.11.5	PIP
Aminopeptidase B	3.4.11.6	APB, ArgAP
Glutamyl AP	3.4.11.7	APA, GluAP, EAP
Aminopeptidase P	3.4.11.9	APP
Cytosol alanyl AP	3.4.11.14	AAP, AlaAP
Methionyl AP	3.4.11.18	eMetAP
Aspartyl AP	3.4.11.21	AspAP, DNPEP
Arginyl AP	3.4.22.16	iRAP, APR

Thus, reduced renal membrane-bound APA, iRAP, and APN activities were observed in a reduced renal mass saline model, and reduced APA activity was detected in a two-kidney one-clip Goldblatt hypertension model [11]. In the low renal mass model, a positive correlation was found in both soluble CAP and APN activities between the neurohypophysis and the adrenal gland, but this was not observed in the normotensive rats [12].

The relationship between APs and arterial hypertension has been explored with greater precision. For instance, it has been proposed that endoplasmic reticulum AP 1 (ERAP1) and ERAP2 regulate BP by inactivation of AngII, and these two APs, which also hydrolyze amino acids from the N-terminus of various human antigens and peptide hormones, are widely expressed in human tissues, including heart, endothelial cells, and kidney [13–15]. In vitro, ERAP1 transforms AngII into AngIII and AngIV [14], while ERAP2 converts AngIII to AngIV [15]. ERAP 1 was initially identified as a placental leucine AP that degrades AngII and III and transforms kallidin into bradykinin in vitro, thus has a role in BP regulation [14].

In this sense, several interesting papers have been published. In an in vivo study, an increase in circulating levels of ERAP1 was found to reduce BP and AngII levels [16]. In a genetic study, an association was detected between variants of the gene encoding Arg528 and the development of essential hypertension in a Japanese population [17]. In an investigation of 45 genetic variants of ERAP1 and ERAP2 in 17,255 Caucasian females from the Women's Genome Health Study, ERAP1 was found to be related to increased BP [18]. The ERAP1 genotype also appears to be involved in the reduction of left ventricular mass produced by some antihypertensive treatments [19]. Thus, all these data indicate a possible role for ERAP1 in BP regulation and ventricular remodeling. Finally, other genetic studies have associated variants of ERAP1 and ERAP2 genes with preeclampsia [20], hemolytic uremia [21], and hypertension [17].

Aminopeptidases after Antihypertensive Therapy

Various systemic antihypertensive treatments can alter the activities of brain and systemic APs associated with effects on BP. Thus, in a rat study by Banegas et al. [22], unilateral brain lesions in the nigrostriatal system produced simultaneous and paralleled changes in BP and in brain and plasma AP activities. Later, the same group [23] examined the participation of APs in the metabolism of some angiotensins, vasopressin, cholecystokinin, and enkephalins in the plasma and hypothalamus of spontaneous hypertensive (SHR) rats under normal conditions and after beta-blocker treatment with propranolol. In this rat strain, AP activity in response to propranolol administration differed between plasma and hypothalamus, thus suggesting an interaction between APs and the autonomic nervous system. Moreover, these authors also reported that treatment with ACE inhibitors captopril, propranolol, or the nitric oxide synthesis inhibitor L-NAME, induced a marked modification of brain patterns of neuropeptidase activity in SHR rats [24].

The BP-lowering effect of a diet enriched in extra virgin olive oil in rats was analyzed by Villarejo et al. [25] who observed that rats receiving this diet showed augmented APN and AspAP activity in the renal cortex, suggesting a greater degradation of AngIII and AngIV and an increased generation of the antihypertensive Ang(2-10). Hence, the glomerular formation of Ang(2-10) might compensate the well-known pressor effects of AngII on the glomerular vasculature in this model of hypertension.

Taken together, the data reported in this section indicate that BP changes induced by antihypertensive or prohypertensive drugs are associated with modifications in AP activity. However, no definitive conclusions can be drawn about the functional role of APs in the pathogenesis of hypertension.

3. Brain APA

Aminopeptidase A (APA) is a 109 kDa homodimeric zinc-metallopeptidase that catalyzes the cleavage of glutamatic and aspartatic amino acid residues from the N-terminus of polypeptides. It is encoded by the ENPEP gene and is also known as glutamyl aminopeptidase, gp160, or CD249.

Numerous studies have demonstrated the major role of brain AngIII and both APA and APN in the control of BP and in arterial hypertension [26]. Thus, the intracerebroventricular (icv) injection of APA to induce the transformation of AngII into AngIII was found to elevate BP in normotensive WKY and SHR animals [27]. In contrast, the icv administration of APN, which hydrolyzes AngIII, reduced the BP in WKY rats and to a greater degree in SHR animals [28]. A study of the icv administration of analogs of AngII and AngIII to SHR rats found that a greater BP increase was induced by AngIII than with AngII [29], thus indicating that a major BP reduction is produced by the inhibition of APA activity and consequent interference in the transformation of AngII to AngIII [30], which suggests a greater contribution of brain AngIII than AngII to the BP increase (Figure 2).

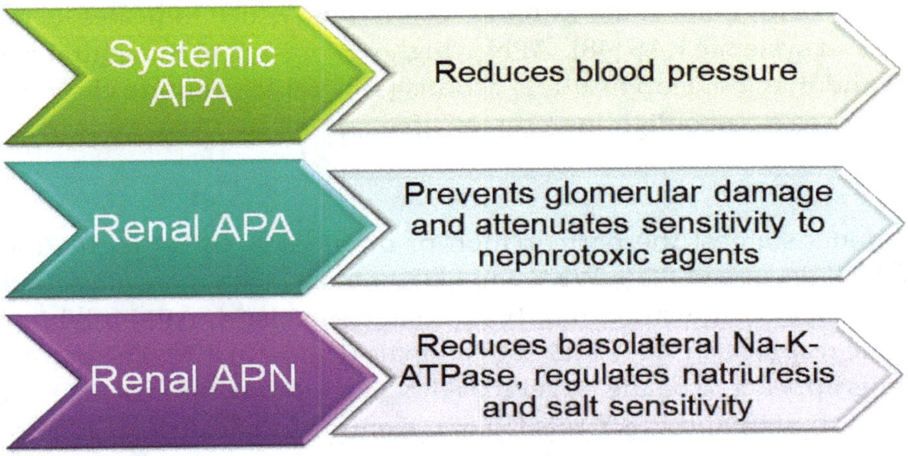

Figure 2. Systemic aminopeptidase A (APA) and aminopeptidase N (APN) in blood pressure control.

Systemic and Renal APA

APA is a membrane-bound enzyme with a major presence in the kidney, in multiple tissues [31], and in a soluble form in the blood, probably due to the cleavage of membrane-bound APA [32]. APA, which thas also been called angiotensinase [33], transforms AngII, the most active systemic peptide, to AngIII, limiting the rate of angiotensin generation [34,35].

The importance of APA in BP control is evidenced by the BP reduction that follows the administration of purified APA [1] and by the BP increase induced by APA inhibitors [36]. In addition, APA-deficient mice are characterized by a high BP and an increased responsiveness to AngII [37]. These data support a role for APA in the regulation of BP under physiological conditions and in hypertensive humans and experimental models.

A study of SHR rats found that a decrease in kidney APA was related to an increase in RAS activity, whereas the administration of APA produced a dose-related reduction in systolic BP [38], showing a 2300-fold increase in activity in comparison to the AT1 blocker candesartan [39]. APA abnormalities have also been observed in the Goldblatt hypertension model [40]. Thus, Prieto et al. [41] reported decreased APA levels in the renal cortex of clipped and non-clipped kidneys in this model, suggesting the involvement of APA in augmenting the AngII-induced reabsorption of sodium and water. Renal RAS is also increased in Dahl salt-sensitive (DSS) rats [42]; in this model, age-related glomerular injury is associated with an increasing elevation of AngII levels because sclerotic glomeruli are less active in synthesizing APA [43]. In human subjects, serum APA activity increases in an age-dependent manner in both men and women [44], and this may be in relation to the metabolic clearance of AngII [45].

At the renal level, Velez et al. [46] observed an increased sensitivity to glomerular damage in APA-deficient BALB/c mice. The authors injected the APA-knockout (KO) mice with a nephrotoxic serum and observed glomerular hyalinosis and albuminuria at 96 h post-administration, whereas no renal injury was observed in the wild-type controls. Likewise, the 4-week infusion of AngII reduced podocyte nephrin levels in APA-KO mice but not in wild-type controls. These data indicate that the degradation of AngII induced by APA plays a protective role in glomerular injury.

Taken together, the above data indicate that an increase in systemic APA protects against hypertension. Conversely, a reduction in the activity of this enzyme maintains high levels of AngII and therefore promotes hypertension (Figure 2). As a conclusion, increased APA activity in the brain raises BP through an increased generation of AngIII, which is the main AT1 receptor agonist in the brain, whereas increased APA activity in the peripheral circulation lowers BP through the degradation of AngII (Figure 2).

4. APN

Aminopeptidase N (APN), also called leucine aminopeptidase and alanyl aminopeptidase, is a homodimeric, membrane-bound, zinc-dependent aminopeptidase [47]. APN cleaves AngIII to AngIV via the scission of arginine at the extreme N-terminus, which indicates its participation in the regulation of tissue and systemic RAS [48]. APN is highly expressed in the central nervous system and kidneys [47,49,50] and may develop multiple actions [47] besides peptide cleavage [51,52]. For this reason, APN is known as a "moonlighting protein" [53].

4.1. Brain APN in BP Regulation

Studies in rodents suggest the participation of brain APN in BP regulation [54]. Thus, icv administration of APN decreased BP in WKY and SHR animals, with more effect in the hypersensitive rats [55]. Conversely, icv administration of bestatin and amistatin, APN inhibitors, raised BP and induced a dipsogenic response in WKY and SHR animals (Figure 3) [55]. The paraventricular nucleus of the hypothalamus appears to be the target for APN in the brain, because its microinfusion at this site reduced BP in both SHR and WKY rats [56,57]. Central APN exerts its effects by transforming the pressor AngIII in the brain into AngIV. In this way, the pressor response induced by icv AngIII is potentiated by the APN antagonists bestatin and amistatin [38,58]. In line with these observations, administration of an angiotensin antagonist was found to inhibit the increase in BP produced by the icv administration of APN inhibitors [30,57].

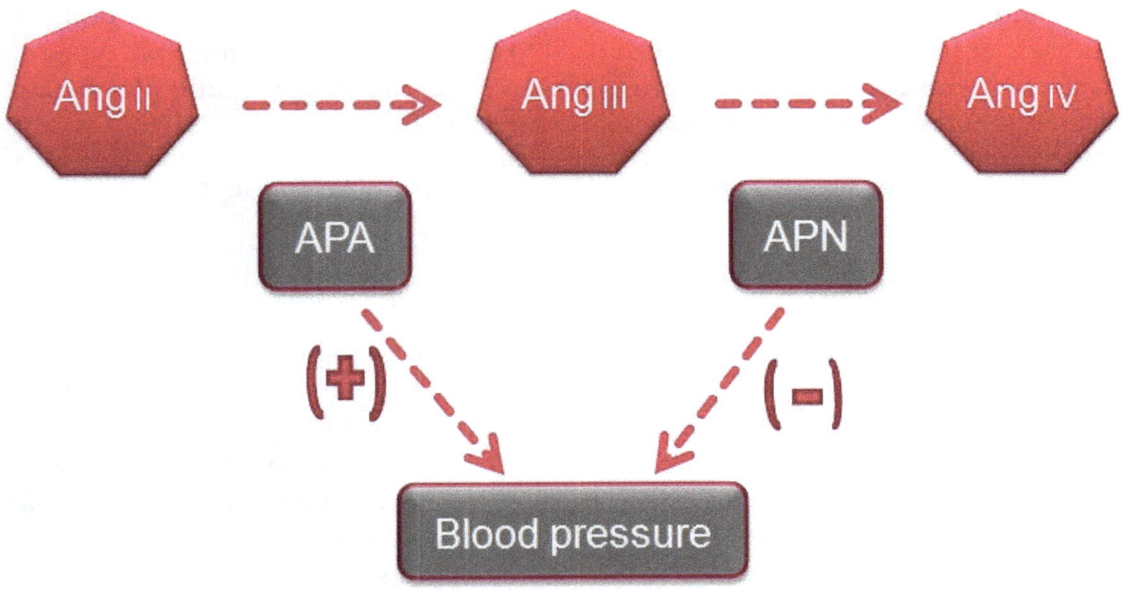

Figure 3. Systemic and renal APA and APN in the control of blood pressure and renal function.

4.2. *Renal APN in BP Control*

APN is widely distributed in the kidney and has been detected in glomeruli, mesangial cells, and on the luminal surface of tubules [47,58]. Renal APN generates AngIV [59,60], and infusion of AngIV in the renal artery increased sodium excretion [61–63], an effect related to the reduced activity of basolateral tubular Na-K-ATPase [64]. This mechanism may also participate in the adaptative response to increased salt intake, thus protecting against hypertension. Moreover, abnormalities in renal APN have also been observed in several models of experimental hypertension. Thus, the Goldblatt model showed increased APN activity in the renal cortex of the non-clipped kidney [41] and APN protein abundance and activity in the kidney were increased in Dahl salt-resistant versus Dahl salt-sensitive animals (64). APN has also been associated with essential hypertension in humans [65].

APN as a Regulator of Salt Sensitivity

Renal APN regulates mechanisms that facilitate renal sodium excretion after increased saline intake, producing a coordinated decrease in Na-K-ATPase abundance on the basal side of the tubule (by endocytosis) and a reduction in sodium transporters (by internalization) [66–68].

APN abundance is higher in Dahl salt-resistant rats. In these animals, APN may reduce basolateral Na^+-K^+-ATPase as a protective mechanism in response to the increased saline intake [64]. Reduced tissue and plasma APN levels have also been reported in the L-NAME model but not in the controls [68]. In conclusion, renal tubule levels of APN can regulate sodium excretion and, therefore, salt sensitivity and BP.

4.3. *Other Actions of APN Related to the Cardiovascular System*

APN activation has been reported in diabetic nephropathy, renal damage, connective vascular disease, and cerebral ischemia [69]. In mice, APN is also essential for inflammatory trafficking after coronary artery occlusion and for sustaining the reparative response [70]. Hence, APN blockade of APN is a therapeutic approach to these vascular abnormalities.

Stimulation of AT4 receptors by APN-generated AngIV exerts proangiogenic action. Thus, APN is augmented in pathologic angiogenesis, especially in tumor vasculature [71], and APN blockade reduces angiogenesis in vivo [72]. In APN-null mice, angiogenesis alterations are manifested in pathological situations but not under physiological conditions [73]. According to these observations, APN activity promotes angiogenesis in various conditions and its blockade prevents new blood vessel growth. Indeed, molecular imaging of APN has been used to detect and monitor multiple types of cancer and the surface of vasculature undergoing angiogenesis in cardiac regeneration [74]. Hence, APN is a potential biomarker of angiogenesis and therapeutic tool.

5. Therapeutic Strategies to Treat Arterial Hypertension with Aminopeptidases

The vast majority of studies on the control of BP and treatment of hypertension have addressed the blockade of AngII or its receptors, and there has been less research on the regulation of other angiotensin peptides. Thus, blockade of the brain RAS has been found to simultaneously decrease sympathetic tone, vasopressin release, and baroreflex activity, thereby reducing cardiac output and peripheral resistance [75].

An action on central or peripheral APs represents a new approach to the treatment of hypertension. Thus, new antihypertensive treatments have been developed based on potent orally-active inhibitors of APA or activators of aspartyl-aminopeptidase (DNPEP), since brain aspartyl aminopeptidase exerts BP-lowering effects by transforming AngI into angiotensin 2-10. Currently, the search for new antihypertensive compounds that affect the RAS multi-enzyme cascade is an important line of research.

5.1. *Inhibition of APA*

The icv administration of EC33, a specific APA inhibitor, prevented the BP increase produced by the icv administration of AngII in SHR animals, indicating that the central response to AngII requires its transformation into AngIII by APA. A marked BP decrease has also been observed in conscious SHR and DOCA-salt hypertensive rats after the icv infusion of EC33 [76,77]. In contrast, the peripheral iv infusion of EC33 did not reduce BP, indicating that EC33 does not cross the blood–brain barrier and/or is inactive in systemic circulation.

The BP of SHR rats increased after the central icv administration of APA [78], probably due to an increased endogenous generation of AngIII, whereas APA blockade with an antiserum attenuated the pressor response to AngII by around 60% [78]. It is interesting to note that a selective APA inhibitor (RB150) with antihypertensive properties can be given either intravenously [77] or orally [79] because it can cross the blood–brain barrier.

The peripheral activity of the AT1 receptor depends on the transformation of AngII into AngIII by APA [80]. Thus, antihypertensive effects were observed in SHR rats after the systemic administration of recombinant APA [81] at a dose that was one-tenth of the usual candesartan dose [82]; the joint i.v. administration of APA and APN attenuated the pressor effect of AngII in normal rats and treatment with APA reduced the BP of SHR rats to normal levels [83].

Considered together, these data clearly demonstrate that APA reduces BP, while abnormalities in APA activity promote hypertension, as supported by the lower renal APA activity in SHR versus WKY rats [84]. The administration of APA has therefore been proposed for the treatment of acute heart failure, acute hypertensive crisis, preeclampsia, and hypertensive encephalopathy, among other hypertensive emergencies [85,86].

5.2. *APN Blockade in the Treatment of Hypertension*

The administration of PC18, an inhibitor of APN, generates a pressor response through the accumulation of endogenous AngIII, which is mediated via the AT1 receptor. In this way, pretreatment with the AT1 blocker losartan can suppress the pressor response, while the AT2 antagonist PD123319 is unable to prevent the BP increase [87]. The enhanced proximal tubular sodium reabsorption of SHR rats is prevented by the intrarenal infusion of PC18 [88]. This finding indicates that the blockade of

AngIII degradation achieved by APN inhibition improved sodium excretion in the proximal tubule of these rats when it was administered in the renal interstitium [89]. Hence, the transformation of AngII into AngIII is required for this natriuretic response, which is not affected by the AT1 blocker candesartan. Research on the usefulness of APN inhibitors to treat hypertensive patients is at an early stage, and further studies are required.

6. APs as Urinary Biomarkers of Renal Injury

Serum creatinine and blood urea nitrogen (BUN) are widely used markers of renal disease, but their sensitivity and specificity are limited, and they are not useful in distinguishing the stages of acute kidney injury (AKI) [90]. They lack sensitivity because they increase only when the renal lesion is evident. Thus, serum creatinine levels rise gradually, and the kidneys have already lost half of their functionality by the time normal levels are doubled [91,92]. Besides, normal levels of these markers can be affected by protein-rich diets, intestinal bleeding, muscle disease, and dehydration, generating false positives in the diagnosis of renal disease. There is a need for biomarkers to allow an earlier diagnosis of AKI, a better prediction of renal disease severity, and an improved assessment of adverse effects in drug development [90].

Various urinary biomarkers for the early detection of AKI have emerged over recent years [91,92], including tubular enzymes that are increased in urine after damage to the tubular epithelium [92], which can precede or even trigger renal dysfunction. Major advantages of urinary markers include the non-invasiveness of the sampling and their usefulness to elucidate the size and localization of tubular cell lesions and to detect the presence of necrosis or other alterations that evoke renal dysfunction [93]. The measurement of urinary enzymes and other urinary biomarkers may therefore be a valuable tool to obtain an early diagnosis during initial stages of renal disease and to follow its progression or regression, facilitating prediction of the prognosis. Urinary APs are considered promising and useful biomarkers of renal disease of different pathophysiological origin, and an automated photometric assay has been developed for their measurement [94].

APA, APN, and CAP are present in the brush border membrane of renal tubular cells [95], have molecular weights above 140 kDa, and are highly organ-specific. These conditions ensure the tubular origin of these urinary enzymes, which cannot pass easily into the urine through the glomerular barrier (Figure 4).

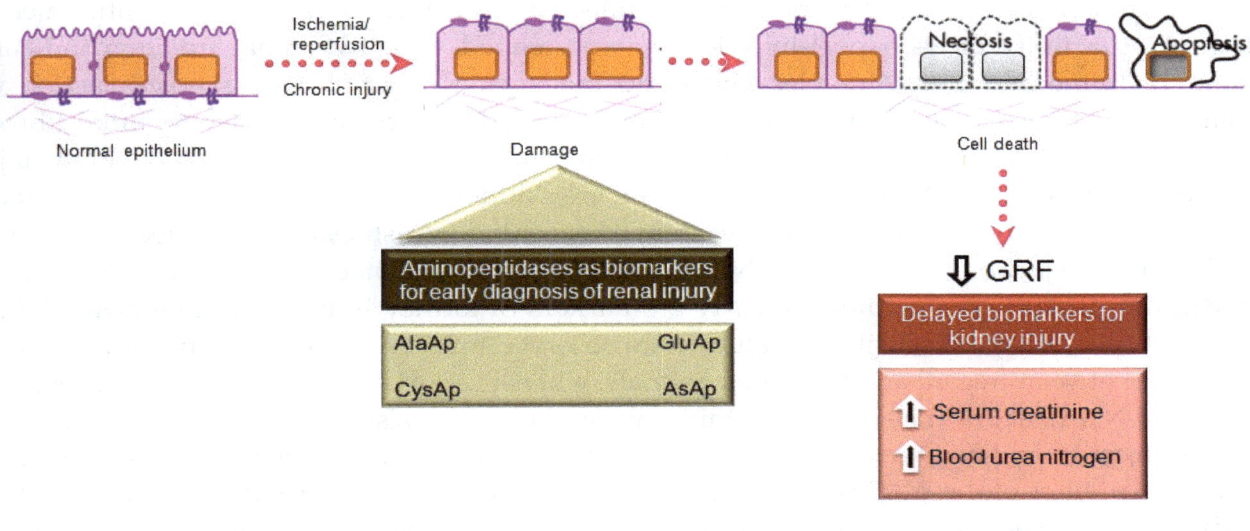

Figure 4. Main aminopeptidases studied as biomarkers of acute and chronic kidney injury.

APs participate in AngII metabolism, forming part of the renal renin–angiotensin–aldosterone system (RAAS) [96], which is elevated in renal diseases. One of these enzymes, alanine aminopeptidase (APN), is a brush border enzyme that was proposed in the early 1970s as a urinary marker of renal disease [97]. Later, Marchewka et al. [98] demonstrated that the measurement of APN and its isoforms was of diagnostic relevance in nephrolithiasis. They also observed significantly higher APN excretion in patients with glomerulonephritis than in controls and a positive correlation between urinary protein concentrations and APN activity [99]. Their findings supported the association between proteinuria and elevated activity of renal tubular brush border enzymes reported in other studies of chronic glomerulonephritis [100]. As an explanation of this association, these authors [99] proposed that the protein present in the ultrafiltrate produces a release of APN from the external membrane of renal tubule microvilli. Because of its external localization, its release into the urine can be caused by a weak destructive action and is not necessarily linked to disruption of the integrity of kidney tubule cells [101].

Jung et al. [102] reported that the urinary excretion of APN, alkaline phosphatase, γ-glutamyltransferase, and N-acetyl-β-D-glucosaminidase is age-dependent in humans. These enzymes were determined in random morning urine samples from 442 individuals aged from 5 days to 58 years, and their creatinine-normalized activity significantly decreased with increasing age. APN activity has also been proposed as a biomarker of the nephrotoxicity induced by vancomycin [101] or amphotericin B [103] in experimental models and in several human diseases, such as glomerulopathy [104], IgA nephropathy [105], and diabetes [106]. However, conflicting results have been published on its usefulness as a biomarker of renal function in kidney transplantation patients [107,108].

Acute Kidney Injury

AKI is defined by an abrupt increase in serum creatinine during the 48 h period after an insult responsible for functional or structural changes in the kidney, and it is mainly caused by the acute apoptosis or necrosis of renal tubular cells [109]. The early detection of AKI is a current preclinical and clinical research priority. The administration of nephrotoxic drugs that alter tubular function is the most common experimental model to relate the excretion of different biomarkers to renal dysfunction. Cisplatin is an antineoplastic drug with a potent nephrotoxic effect, mainly due to its action on the proximal tubule, causing AKI in experimental animal models and patients [110,111]. Its administration induces tubular and glomerular disturbances that lead to the development of interstitial fibrosis [112].

Our group investigated whether urinary activities of APN, APA, and CAP could serve as biomarkers of renal dysfunction by using a rat model of cisplatin-induced nephrotoxicity [113]. Their activity was determined in urine samples collected at 24, 48, and 72 h after cisplatin injection. Their urinary activity at 24 h post-injection was correlated with two renal function indicators (plasma creatinine and creatinine clearance) and their activity at two weeks post-injection was correlated with two indicators of structural damage (renal hypertrophy and interstitial fibrosis). A comparative analysis was also performed with other proposed urinary biomarkers of kidney injury, i.e., albumin, proteinuria, NAG, and NGAL. The area under the curve (AUC) was calculated to quantify the sensitivity and specificity of each marker to distinguish cisplatin-treated from control rats at 24 h post-injection (Figure 5). APN, APA, CAP, and DNPEP had an AUC value greater than 0.5, indicating that these enzymes are early biomarkers of kidney injury in cisplatin-treated rats. The greatest specificity and sensitivity values were observed for APN, which was the best variable to discriminate between treated and untreated animals, whereas an AUC value below 0.5 was observed for NAG and NGAL at this time point. A significant correlation was also found between AP activities at day 1 post-injection and functional and structural variables at day 14. It can therefore be concluded that the urinary activities of these APs may serve as early and predictive biomarkers of cisplatin-induced renal dysfunction. The measurement of urinary AP activities can be useful in preclinical research for the early detection and follow-up of renal damage and for the evaluation of drug nephrotoxicity, and it may offer a useful prognostic and diagnostic tool for renal diseases in the clinical setting.

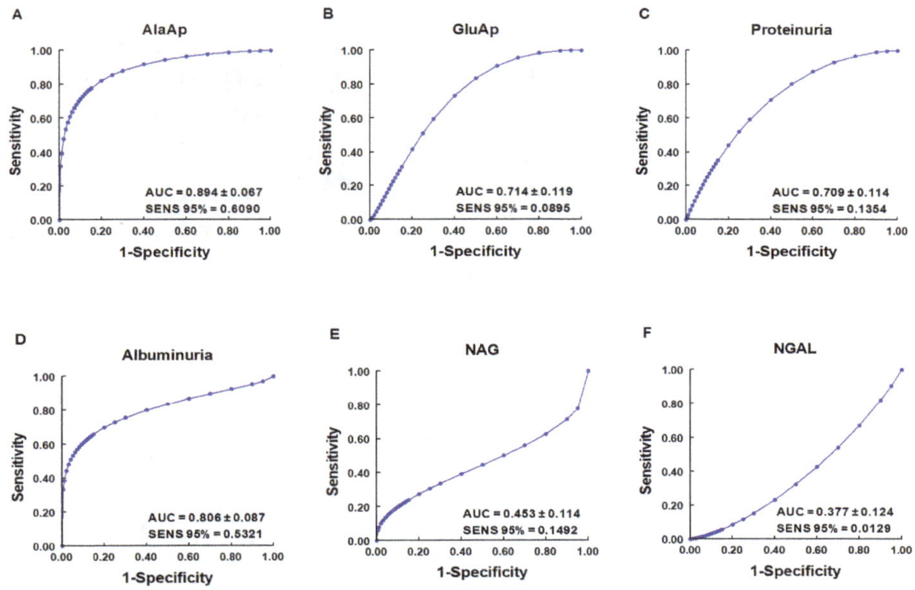

Figure 5. ROC curves showing specificity and sensitivity for APN (AlaAp) (**A**), APA (GluAp) (**B**), proteinuria (**C**), albuminuria (**D**), N-acetyl-β-D-glucosaminidase (NAG) (**E**), and neutrophil gelatinase-associated lipocalin (NGAL) (**F**) to differentiate cisplatin-treated rats from control rats 24 h after injection of saline, 3.5 or 7 mg/kg of cisplatin (n = 8 each group). All cisplatin-treated rats displayed tubular dysplasia and interstitial fibrosis 14 days after injection. Urinary markers were expressed in daily total activity or excretion per 100 g of body weight. AUC = area under the curve. SENS 95 % = calculated sensitivity at 95 % of specificity.

7. Quantification of Urinary APs

APs activities can be readily quantified in biological samples by kinetic methods using photometric [94] or fluorometric [113] assays. Widely applied immunological techniques such as immunoblotting or ELISA can be used to analyze the amount/expression of these proteins in biological samples. Our group used ELISA and Western blot to measure the amount of APN excreted in the urine of cisplatin-treated rats and correlated its excretion 24 h post-injection with increased serum creatinine and decreased body weight at two weeks [114]. In addition, the quantification of APN by ELISA showed a very high correlation with urinary APA activity. The above findings confirm that the immunological determination of this enzyme can also serve as an early marker of renal damage. Further studies are warranted to compare the sensitivity and specificity of kinetic and fluorometric methods in other experimental models and in human diseases that involve renal dysfunction.

7.1. Aminopeptidases in Urinary Vesicles and Exosomes

Extracellular vesicles (EVs) released by the renal epithelium into the tubular fluid are excreted and may be detected in urine samples [115,116]; they include microvesicles and exosomes. Exosomes are nanovesicles (30–120 nm) released by epithelial cells throughout the urinary tract [117,118]. Thus, the exosomic fraction of urine contains potential biomarkers of various renal diseases. Since exosomes secrete mRNAs, miRNAs, and proteins that affect the function of recipient cells [119], it has been proposed that the biological role of exosomes in the kidney is to regulate the co-functionality of different sections of the nephron.

However, the content of biomarkers in urinary microvesicles has not been fully elucidated. The release of microvesicles into the urine has been studied in some renal diseases [120], and their content can also transmit biological signals within the kidney [121–124].

Our group therefore investigated whether the microvesicular and exosomic content of APA in urine was related to cisplatin-induced renal dysfunction in rats [125]. An increased APA content was observed in microvesicular and exosomic fractions at the peak of toxicity, 3 days post-cisplatin injection, and it showed a significant predictive correlation with serum creatinine, regardless of the method of normalization used for APA values (Figure 6). It was concluded that APA content and activity in urinary microvesicles and exosomes may serve as renal dysfunction biomarkers in this nephrotoxicity model.

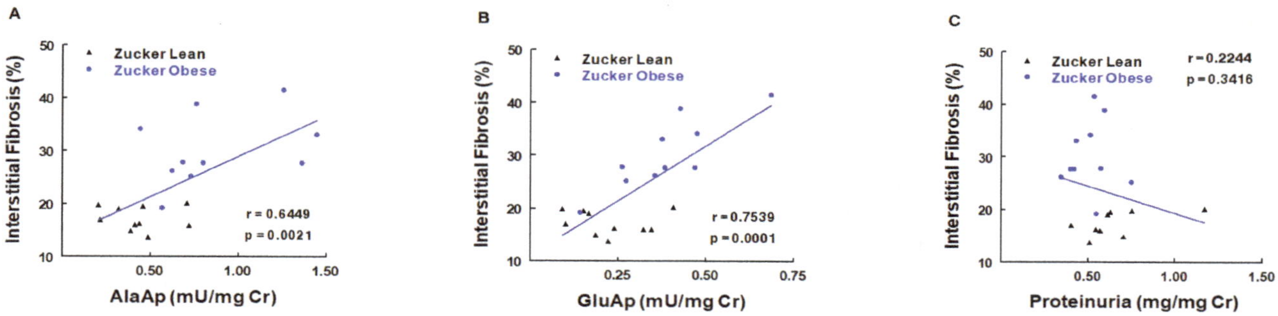

Figure 6. Correlations of urinary activities of APN (AlaAp) (**A**), APA (GluAp) (**B**), and proteinuria (**C**) with percentage of renal interstitial fibrosis in urine samples of Zucker lean and obese rats (n = 10 each group). Cr = creatinine (adapted from reference [126]).

Thus, the determination of GluAp in microvesicular and exosomic fractions can be useful to study proximal tubular lesions independently of the glomerular filtration rate. From a technical viewpoint, it is interesting to note that the microvesicular fraction can be obtained more rapidly than can the exosomic fraction. In addition, the analysis of these fractions can avoid interference due to urea content, ionic strength, or other components of urine, because the samples are centrifuged and dissolved in a buffer. According to these observations, examination of the content of the microvesicular fraction can also be a relevant diagnostic tool in nephropathies.

7.2. AKI Induced by Surgical Procedures

Patients undergoing a cardiopulmonary bypass (CPB) can develop AKI as a post-surgical complication. The diagnosis of AKI in these patients is based on an increase in serum creatinine (SCr) concentration over baseline values during the 48 h postoperative period; however, the slow progressive rise of SCr can delay the detection of renal dysfunction. Kim et al. [127] analyzed the serum and urinary enzymatic activity of vasopressinase and SCr in 31 patients at different time points after CPB surgery. Results showed maximum serum and urine activity of vasopressinase at intensive care unit (ICU) admission in patients developing AKI as a complication of CPB earlier than the peak of SCr activity, which is usually observed at 48 h post-surgery. The authors therefore proposed vasopressinase (cystil AP, CAP) activity as an early biomarker for AKI. Animal models of renal ischemia also showed that AKI was related to vasopressinase activity [128].

In a similar study of 103 patients, our group observed a significant increase in urinary APA activity at ICU admission in patients who developed persistent AKI in comparison to those who did not experience AKI or developed only transient AKI. Urinary APA activity showed a higher sensitivity than SCr at this time point, obtaining a higher total number of correctly diagnosed cases in comparison to the application of criteria published by the Acute Kidney Injury Network [129]. These observations also indicate that tubular injury increases the risk of post-surgery AKI.

7.3. Urinary Aminopeptidases as Biomarkers of Renal Dysfunction in Chronic Diseases

7.3.1. Obesity

Obesity and hypertension are chronic diseases that can ultimately lead to renal failure. Experimental models of these diseases have been used for long-term evaluation of the usefulness of urinary APs as renal injury biomarkers.

The obese Zucker rat is an animal model of human type II diabetes [130] characterized by obesity, dyslipidemia, insulin resistance, and kidney damage. Male obese (ZO) and lean (ZL) Zucker rats were studied for 6 months (age of 2–8 months) [131]. At the age of 8 months, ZO rats exhibited various renal lesions, including mild focal and segmental glomerulosclerosis and moderate tubulointerstitial damage. Urinary GluAp (APA) and AlaAp (APN) activities were measured monthly and were increased in ZO rats. Both APA and APN activities correlated with renal lesions and can be considered early diagnostic biomarkers of these lesions (Figure 6). AP activities also showed predictive correlations with the level of interstitial fibrosis in the kidney and with the amount of hydroxyproline accumulated in renal tissue at the age of 8 months. Hence, the early excretion of these markers also serves to evaluate the development of fibrosis in this experimental model.

7.3.2. Hypertension

The SHR model of essential hypertension in humans is widely used [132,133] and is characterized by an increase in BP and development of renal injury as age advances [126,133]. This model has been used to analyze the urinary enzymatic activities of APA, APN, and dipeptidyl peptidase-4 (DPP4) as biomarkers of renal injury in hypertension. These activities were measured in male SHR and WKY rats from the age of 2 to 8 months [134]. The SHR animals did not develop relevant signs of histopathological kidney alterations at the end of the study, but they showed increased glomerular area and cellularity. These activities were increased in monthly-collected urine samples from SHR rats and were correlated with systolic blood pressure throughout the study. Their increased activity in SHR animals indicate that a certain degree of tubular injury can be detected before the appearance of all histopathological manifestations of renal disease. These markers can therefore be used for the diagnosis of renal disease in early stages of hypertension and offer a non-invasive method to follow the progression of renal dysfunction in hypertension and other diseases.

7.3.3. Hyperthyroidism

In rats, hyperthyroidism is an endocrine disease associated with hypertension and renal abnormalities, accelerating the course of experimental hypertension, whereas hypothyroidism is associated with hypotension, preventing the development of hypertension and protecting against renal injury [135]. Ethanol-binding protein and N-acetyl-β-D-glycosaminidase, urinary biomarkers of tubular damage, are increased in hyperthyroid humans [136] and cats [137].

Our group studied the urinary excretion of APN, APA, CAP, and AspAp in control, hyperthyroid, and hypothyroid rats receiving a normal- or high-sodium diet. All APs were augmented in hyperthyroid rats, whereas their levels were similar between hypothyroid and control rats [138]. Hyperthyroid rats receiving a high sodium diet showed increased hypertension, cardiac/renal hypertrophy, albuminuria, and oxidative stress and a marked rise in urinary AP activities. AP activity was modestly elevated in the controls on a high-sodium diet but did not differ between hypothyroid rats on a high- versus normal-sodium diet. According to these results, the combination of T4 treatment and salt exert additive effects on the production of tubular damage, whereas hypothyroidism confers resistance to the effects of high salt intake on urinary AP activities. These findings support previous descriptions of hypothyroid status as beneficial in chronic kidney diseases [139]. It can be concluded that urinary AP activities are diagnostic biomarkers of renal injury in this experimental model. Our group [140] also determined APA activities in renal tissue and plasma samples from adult male euthyroid, hyperthyroid, and hypothyroid rats, and found a significantly higher expression of renal APA in hyperthyroid versus control or hypothyroid rats. However, plasma APA activity was lower in hyperthyroid versus control rats, indicating that the increased APA in these animals is focalized in renal tissue.

7.3.4. Diabetes Mellitus

In a study of urinary levels of enzymes and low-molecular-mass proteins as indicators of diabetes nephropathy, Jung et al. [141] observed an increase in urinary alanine aminopeptidase in diabetic patients and an even greater increase in diabetic patients with proteinuria. However, a study by Lazarevic et al. [106] on the impact of aerobic exercise on microalbuminuria and enzymuria in type II diabetic patients found no significant difference in urinary or plasma APN activities over the study period between patients with and without diabetes or within the diabetes group. Numerous factors may be implicated in these discrepancies between studies.

7.3.5. Urinary APs in Other Chronic Diseases

Sorokman et al. [142] measured urinary levels of renal-specific enzymes (neutral α-glucosidase, L-alanine aminopeptidase, and γ-glutamyltranspeptidase) as markers of proximal tubule damage in children with pyelonephritis, the most common cause of fever in patients with urinary system disorders. They observed an increase in urinary levels of these enzymes during the active phase of pyelonephritis, which correlated with leukocyturia and C-Reactive Protein levels. Finally, Spasovski et al. [143] studied urinary levels of brush border enzymes of the proximal renal tubules (e.g., APN, gamma-glutamyl transferase, and beta2 microglobulin) in patients with untreated rheumatoid arthritis to explore the possible relationship between this disease and dysfunction of the brush border of proximal tubules. They found that urinary APN activity was a superior indicator of asymptomatic renal lesions in untreated rheumatoid arthritis patients compared with measurements of gamma-GT or beta2m.

Author Contributions: All authors have contributed to the review and have read and agreed to the published version of the manuscript.

Abbreviations

ACE	Angiotensin converting enzyme
AKI	Acute kidney injury
AngI	Angiotensin I
AngII	Angiotensin II
AngIII	Angiotensin III
AngIV	Angiotensin IV
APs	Aminopeptidases
APA	Aminopeptidase A
APN	Aminopeptidase N
AT1	Angiotensin receptor type 1
AT2	Angiotensin receptor type 2
BP	Blood pressure
CAP	Cystinil AP
DOCA	Deoxycorticosterone
L-NAME	N(ω)-nitro-L-arginine methyl ester
RAS	Renin–angiotensin system
SHR	Spontaneous hypertensive rat
WKY	Wistar Kyoto rat
ZO	Zucker obese rats

References

1. Johnston, C.I. Biochemistry and pharmacology of the renin-angiotensin system. *Drugs* **1990**, *39*, 21–31. [CrossRef] [PubMed]
2. Reudelhuber, T.L. The renin-angiotensin system: Peptides and enzymes beyond angiotensin II. *Curr. Opin. Nephrol. Hypertens.* **2005**, *14*, 155–159. [CrossRef] [PubMed]
3. Ferrario, C.M.; Chappell, M.C. Novel Angiotensin peptides. *Cell. Mol. Life. Sci.* **2004**, *61*, 2720–2727. [CrossRef]
4. Vauquelin, G.; Michotte Smolders, Y.I.; Sarre, S.; Ebinger, G.; Dupont, A.; Vanderheyden, P. Cellular targets for angiotensin II fragments: Pharmacological and molecular evidence. *J. Renin Angiotensin Aldosterone Syst.* **2002**, *3*, 195–204. [CrossRef] [PubMed]
5. Enzyme Nomenclature. Recommendations of the Nomenclature Committee of the International Union of Biochemistry and Molecular Biology on the Nomenclature and Classification of Enzymes by the Reactions they Catalyse. Available online: https://www.qmul.ac.uk/sbcs/iubmb/enzyme/ (accessed on 18 June 2020).
6. De Gasparo, M.; Catt, K.J.; Inagami, T.; Wright, J.W.; Unger, T. International union of pharmacology. XXIII. The angiotensin II receptors. *Pharmacol. Rev.* **2000**, *52*, 415–472. [PubMed]
7. Dinh, D.T.; Frauman, A.G.; Johnston, C.I.; Fabiani, M.E. Angiotensin receptors: Distribution, signalling and function. *Clin. Sci.* **2001**, *100*, 481–492. [CrossRef]
8. Chappell, M.C. Nonclassical renin-angiotensin system and renal function. *Compr. Physiol.* **2012**, *2*, 2733–2735. [PubMed]
9. Prieto, I.; Villarejo, A.B.; Segarra, A.B.; Banegas, I.; Wangensteen, R.; Martinez-Cañamero, M.; de Gasparo, M.; Vives, F.; Ramírez-Sánchez, M. Brain, heart and kidney correlate for the control of blood pressure and water balance: Role of angiotensinases. *Neuroendocrinology* **2014**, *100*, 198–208. [CrossRef]
10. Ramírez, M.; Prieto, I.; Alba, F.; Vives, F.; Banegas, I.; de Gasparo, M. Role of central and peripheral aminopeptidase activities in the control of blood pressure: A working hypothesis. *Heart Fail. Rev.* **2008**, *13*, 339–353. [CrossRef]
11. Ramírez, M.; Prieto, I.; Martinez, J.M.; Vargas, F.; Alba, F. Renal aminopeptidase activities in animal models of hypertension. *Regul. Pept.* **1997**, *72*, 155–159. [CrossRef]
12. Prieto, I.; Martinez, A.; Martinez, J.M.; Ramírez, M.J.; Vargas, F.; Alba, F.; Ramírez, M. Activities of aminopeptidases in a rat saline model of volume hypertension. *Horm. Metab. Res.* **1998**, *30*, 246–248. [CrossRef] [PubMed]
13. Tsujimoto, M.; Goto, Y.; Maruyama, M.; Hattori, A. Biochemical and enzymatic properties of the m1 family of aminopeptidases involved in the regulation of blood pressure. *Heart Fail. Rev.* **2008**, *13*, 285–291. [CrossRef] [PubMed]
14. Hattori, A.; Kitatani, K.; Matsumoto, H.; Miyazawa, S.; Rogi, T.; Tsuruoka, N.; Mizutani, S.; Natori, Y.; Tsujimoto, M. Characterization of recombinant human adipocyte-derived leucine aminopeptidase expressed in Chinese hamster ovary cells. *J. Biochem.* **2000**, *128*, 755–762. [CrossRef] [PubMed]
15. Tanioka, T.; Hattori, A.; Masuda, S.; Nomura, Y.; Nakayama, H.; Mizutani, S.; Tsujimoto, M. Human leukocytederived arginine aminopeptidase. The third member of the oxytocinase subfamily of aminopeptidases. *J. Biol. Chem.* **2003**, *278*, 32275–32283. [CrossRef] [PubMed]
16. Hisatsune, C.; Ebisui, E.; Usui, M.; Ogawa, N.; Suzuki, A.; Mataga, N.; Hiromi Takahashi-Iwanaga, H.; Katsuhiko Mikoshiba, K. ERp44 exerts redox dependent control of blood pressure at the ER. *Mol. Cell* **2015**, *58*, 1015–1027. [CrossRef] [PubMed]
17. Yamamoto, N.; Nakayama, J.; Yamakawa-Kobayashi, K.; Hamaguchi, H.; Miyazaki, R.; Arinami, T. Identification of 33 polymorphisms in the adipocyte-derived leucine aminopeptidase (ALAP) gene and possible association with hypertension. *Hum. Mutat.* **2002**, *19*, 251–257. [CrossRef]
18. Robert, Y.; Zee, L.; Rivera, A.; Inostroza, Y.; Ridker, P.M.; Daniel, I.; Chasman, D.I.; Romero, J.R. Gene variation of endoplasmic reticulum aminopeptidases 1 and 2, and risk of blood pressure progression and incident hypertension among 17,255 initially healthy women. *Int. J. Genom.* **2018**, *2018*, 2308585.
19. Hallberg, P.; Lind, L.; Michaelsson, K.; Kurland, L.; Kahan, T.; Malmqvist, K.; Ohman, K.P.; Nystrom, F.; Liljedahl, U.; Syvanen, A.C.; et al. Adipocyte-derived leucine aminopeptidase genotype and response to antihypertensive therapy. *BMC Cardiovasc. Disord.* **2003**, *3*, 11. [CrossRef]

20. Johnson, M.P.; Roten, L.T.; Dyer, T.D.; East, C.E.; Forsmo, S.; Blangero, J.; Brennecke, S.P.; Austgulen, R.; Moses, E.K. The ERAP2 gene is associated with preeclampsia in Australian and Norwegian populations. *Hum. Genet.* **2009**, *126*, 655–666. [CrossRef]
21. Taranta, A.; Gianviti, A.; Palma, A.; De Luca, V.; Mannucci, L.; Procaccino, M.A.; Ghiggeri, G.M.; Caridi, G.; Fruci, D.; Ferracuti, S.; et al. Genetic risk factors in typical haemolytic uraemic syndrome. *Nephrol. Dial. Transplant.* **2009**, *24*, 1851–1857. [CrossRef]
22. Banegas, I.; Ramírez, M.; Vives, F.; Alba, F.; Segarra, A.B.; Duran, R.; De Gasparo, M.; Prieto, I. Aminopeptidase activity in the nigrostriatal system and prefrontal cortex of rats with experimental hemiparkinsonism. *Horm. Metab. Res.* **2005**, *37*, 53–55. [CrossRef] [PubMed]
23. Prieto, I.; Segarra, A.B.; de Gasparo, M.; Martínez-Cañamero, M.; Ramírez-Sánchez, M. Divergent profile between hypothalamic and plasmatic aminopeptidase activities in WKY and SHR. Influence of beta-adrenergic blockade. *Life Sci.* **2018**, *192*, 9–17. [CrossRef] [PubMed]
24. Prieto, I.; Segarra, A.B.; Villarejo, A.B.; de Gasparo, M.; Martínez-Cañamero, M.M.; Ramírez-Sánchez, M. Neuropeptidase activity in the frontal cortex of Wistar-Kyoto and spontaneously hypertensive rats treated with vasoactive drugs: A bilateral study. *J. Hypertens.* **2019**, *37*, 612–628. [CrossRef] [PubMed]
25. Villarejo, A.B.; Ramírez-Sánchez, M.; Segarra, A.B.; Martínez-Cañamero, M.; Prieto, I. Influence of extra virgin olive oil on blood pressure and kidney angiotensinase activities in spontaneously hypertensive rats. *Planta Med.* **2015**, *81*, 664–669. [CrossRef]
26. Wright, J.W.; Mizutani, S.; Harding, J.W. Focus on Brain Angiotensin III and Aminopeptidase A in the Control of Hypertension. *Int. J. Hypertens.* **2012**, *2012*, 124758. [CrossRef]
27. Wright, J.W.; Mizutani, S.; Murray, C.E.; Amir, H.Z.; Harding, J.W. Aminopeptidase-induced elevations and reductions in blood pressure in the spontaneously hypertensive rat. *J. Hypertens.* **1990**, *8*, 969–974. [CrossRef]
28. Jensen, L.L.; Harding, J.W.; Wright, J.W. Increased blood pressure induced by central application of aminopeptidase inhibitors is angiotensinergic-dependent in normotensive and hypertensive rat strains. *Brain Res.* **1989**, *490*, 48–55. [CrossRef]
29. Wright, J.W.; Roberts, K.A.; Cook, V.I.; Murray, C.E.; Sardinia, M.F.; Harding, J.W. Intracerebroventricularly infused [D-Arg1]angiotensin III, is superior to [D-Asp1]angiotensin II, as a pressor agent in rats. *Brain Res.* **1990**, *514*, 5–10. [CrossRef]
30. Wright, J.W.; Tamura-Myers, E.; Wilson, W.L.; Roques, B.P.; Llorens-Cortes, C.; Speth, R.C.; Harding, J.W. Conversion of brain angiotensin II to angiotensin III is critical for pressor response in rats. *Am. J. Physiol. Regul. Integr. Comp. Physiol.* **2003**, *284*, R725–R733. [CrossRef]
31. Lodja, Z.; Gossrau, R. Study on aminopeptidase A. *Histochemistry* **1980**, *67*, 237–290.
32. Wright, J.W.; Harding, J.W. Brain angiotensin receptor subtypes AT1, AT2 and AT4 and their functions. *Regul. Pept.* **1995**, *59*, 269–295. [CrossRef]
33. Speth, R.C.; Thompson, S.M.; Johns, S.J. Angiotensin II receptors: Structural and functional considerations. *Adv. Exp. Med. Biol.* **1995**, *377*, 169–192. [PubMed]
34. Mizutani, S.; Akiyama, H.; Kurauchi, O.; Taira, H.; Narita, O.; Tomoda, Y. In vitro degradation of angiotensin II (A-II) by human placental subcellular fractions, pregnancy sera and purified placental aminopeptidases. *Acta Endocrinol.* **1985**, *110*, 135–139. [CrossRef]
35. Yamada, R.; Mizutani, S.; Kurauchi, O.; Okano, K.; Imaizumi, H.; Narita, O.; Tomoda, Y. Purification and characterization of human placental aminopeptidase A. *Enzyme* **1988**, *40*, 223–230. [CrossRef]
36. Chauvel, E.N.; Llorens-Cortes, C.; Coric, P.; Wilk, S.; Roques, B.P.; Fournie-Zaluski, M.C. Differential inhibition of aminopeptidase A and aminopeptidase N by new-amino thiols. *J. Med. Chem.* **1994**, *37*, 2950–2957. [CrossRef] [PubMed]
37. Mitsui, T.; Nomura, S.; Okada, M.; Ohno, Y.; Kobayashi, H.; Nakashima, Y.; Murata, Y.; Takeuchi, M.; Kuno, N.; Nagasaka, T.; et al. Hypertension and Angiotensin II hypersensitivity in aminopeptidase A-deficient mice. *Mol. Med.* **2003**, *9*, 57–62. [CrossRef]
38. Mizutani, S.; Furuhashi, M.; Imaizumi, H.; Ito, Y.; Kurauchi, O.; Tomoda, Y. Effects of human placental aminopeptidases in spontaneously hypertensive rats. *Med. Sci. Res.* **1987**, *15*, 1203–1204.
39. Goto, Y.; Hattori, A.; Ishii, Y.; Mizutani, S.; Tsujimoto, M. Enzymatic properties of aminopeptidase A: Regulation of its enzymatic activity by calcium and angiotensin IV. *J. Biol. Chem.* **2006**, *281*, 23503–23513. [CrossRef]

40. Bivol, L.M.; Vagnes, O.B.; Iversen, B.M. The renal vascular response to ANG II injection is reduced in the nonclipped kidney of two-kidney, one-clip hypertension. *Am. J. Physiol. Ren. Physiol.* **2005**, *289*, F393–F400. [CrossRef]
41. Prieto, I.; Hermoso, F.; Gaspara, M.; Vargas, F.; Alba, F.; Segarra, A.B.; Banegas, I.; Ramirez, M. Angiotensinase activities in the kidney of renovascular hypertensive rats. *Peptides* **2003**, *24*, 755–760. [CrossRef]
42. Kobori, H.; Nishiyama, A.; Abe, Y.; Navar, G. Enhancement of intrarenal angiotensinogen in Dahl salt-sensitive rats on high salt diet. *Hypertension* **2003**, *41*, 592–597. [CrossRef] [PubMed]
43. Nomura, M.; Nomura, S.; Mitsui, T.; Suzuki, M.; Kobayashi, H.; Ito, T.; Itakura, A.; Kikkawa, F.; Mizutani, S. (2005) Possible involvement of aminopeptidase A in hypertension and renal damage in Dahl saltsensitive rats. *Am. J. Hypertens.* **2005**, *18*, 538–543. [CrossRef] [PubMed]
44. Martinez, J.M.; Prieto, I.; Ramirez, M.J.; de Gasparo, M.; Hermoso, F.; Arias, J.M.; Alba, F.; Ramirez, M. Sex differences and agerelated changes in human serum aminopeptidase A activity. *Clin. Chim. Acta* **1998**, *274*, 53–61. [CrossRef]
45. Baylis, C.; Engels, K.; Hymel, A.; Navar, L.G. Plasma rennin activity and metabolic rate of angiotensin II in the unstressed aging rat. *Mech. Aging Dev.* **1997**, *97*, 163–172. [CrossRef]
46. Velez, J.C.; Arif, E.; Rodgers, J.; Hicks, M.P.; Arthur, J.M.; Nihalani, D.; Bruner, E.T.; Budisavljevic, M.N.; Atkinson, C.; Fitzgibbon, W.R.; et al. Deficiency of the Angiotensinase Aminopeptidase A Increases Susceptibility to Glomerular Injury. *J. Am. Soc. Nephrol.* **2017**, *28*, 2119–2132. [CrossRef] [PubMed]
47. Sjostrom, H.; Noren, O.; Olsen, J. Structure and function of aminopeptidase N. *Adv. Exp. Med. Biol.* **2000**, *477*, 25–34.
48. Paul, M.; Poyan, M.A.; Kreutz, R. Physiology of local renin-angiotensin systems. *Physiol. Rev.* **2006**, *86*, 747–803. [CrossRef]
49. Robert, S.D. Aminopeptidase N in arterial hypertension. *Heart Fail. Rev.* **2008**, *13*, 293–298.
50. Amin, S.A.; Adhikari, N.; Jha, T. Design of aminopeptidase N inhibitors as anti-cancer agents. *J. Med. Chem.* **2018**, *61*, 6468–6490.
51. Dan, H.; Tani, K.; Hase, K.; Shimizu, T.; Tamiya, H.; Biraa, Y.; Huang, L.; Yanagawa, H.; Sone, S. CD13/aminopeptidase N in collagen vascular diseases. *Rheumatol. Int.* **2003**, *23*, 271–276. [CrossRef]
52. Khatun, A.; Kang, K.H.; Ryu, D.Y.; Rahman, M.S.; Kwon, W.S.; Pang, M.G. Effect of Aminopeptidase N on functions and fertility of mouse spermatozoa in vitro. *Theriogenology* **2018**, *118*, 182–189. [CrossRef] [PubMed]
53. Mina-Osorio, P. The moonlighting enzyme CD13: Old and new functions to target. *Trends Mol. Med.* **2008**, *14*, 361–371. [CrossRef]
54. Banegas, I.; Prieto, I.; Vives, F.; Alba, F.; de Gasparo, M.; Segarra, A.B.; Hermoso, F.; Durán, R.; Ramírez, M. Brain aminopeptidases and hypertension. *J. Renin Angiotensin Aldosterone Syst.* **2006**, *7*, 129–134. [CrossRef] [PubMed]
55. Wright, J.W.; Jensen, L.L.; Cushing, L.L.; Harding, J.W. Leucine aminopeptidase M-induced reductions in blood pressure in spontaneously hypertensive rats. *Hypertension* **1989**, *13*, 910–915. [CrossRef] [PubMed]
56. Batt, C.M.; Jensen, L.L.; Harding, J.W.; Wright, J.W. Microinfusion of aminopeptidase M into the paraventricular nucleus of the hypothalamus in normotensive and hypertensive rats. *Brain Res. Bull.* **1996**, *39*, 235–240. [CrossRef]
57. Abhold, R.H.; Sullivan, M.J.; Wright, J.W.; Harding, J.W. Binding, degradation and pressor activity of angiotensins II and III after aminopeptidase inhibition with amastatin and bestatin. *J. Pharmacol. Exp. Ther.* **1987**, *242*, 957–962.
58. Kenny, A.J.; Maroux, S. Topology of microvillar membrance hydrolases of kidney and intestine. *Physiol. Rev.* **1982**, *62*, 91–128. [CrossRef]
59. Albiston, A.L.; McDowall, S.G.; Matsacos, D.; Sim, P.; Clune, E.; Mustafa, T.; Lee, J.; Mendelsohn, F.A.; Simpson, R.J.; Connolly, L.M.; et al. Evidence that the angiotensin IV [AT(4)] receptor is the enzyme insulin-regulated aminopeptidase. *J. Biol. Chem.* **2001**, *276*, 48623–48626. [CrossRef]
60. Chai, S.Y.; Fernando, R.; Peck, G.; Ye, S.Y.; Mendelsohn, F.A.; Jenkins, T.A.; Albiston, A.L. The angiotensin IV/AT4 receptor. *Cell. Mol. Life Sci.* **2004**, *61*, 2728–2737. [CrossRef]
61. Hamilton, T.A.; Handa, R.K.; Harding, J.W.; Wright, J.W. A role for the angiotensin IV/AT4 system in mediating natriuresis in the rat. *Peptides* **2001**, *22*, 935–944. [CrossRef]
62. Handa, R.K.; Krebs, L.T.; Harding, J.W.; Handa, S.E. Angiotensin IV AT4-receptor system in the rat kidney. *Am. J. Physiol. Ren. Physiol.* **1998**, *274*, F290–F299. [CrossRef] [PubMed]

63. Kotlo, K.; Shukla, S.; Tawar, U.; Skidgel, R.A.; Danziger, R.S. Aminopeptidase N reduces basolateral Na_-K_-ATPase in proximal tubule cells. *Am. J. Physiol. Ren. Physiol.* **2007**, *293*, F1047–F1053. [CrossRef] [PubMed]
64. Farjah, M.; Roxas, B.; Danziger, R.S. Dietary NaCl regulates in renal APN transcript/protein abundance and activity: Relevance to hypertension in the Dahl rat. *Hypertension* **2004**, *43*, 282–285. [CrossRef]
65. Williams, J.S.; Raji, A.; Williams, G.H.; Conlin, P.R. Nonmodulating hypertension is associated with insulin resistance and the Lys528Arg variant human adipocyte-derived leucine aminopeptidase. *Hypertension* **2006**, *48*, 331–336.
66. Ogimoto, G.; Yudowski, G.A.; Barker, C.J.; Kohler, M.; Katz, A.I.; Feraille, E.; Pedemonte, C.H.; Berggren, P.O.; Bertorello, A.M. G protein-coupled receptors regulate Na,K-ATPase activity and endocytosis by modulating the recruitment of adaptor protein 2 and clathrin. *Proc. Natl. Acad. Sci. USA* **2000**, *97*, 3242–3247. [CrossRef] [PubMed]
67. Periyasamy, S.M.; Liu, J.; Tanta, F.; Kabak, B.; Wakefield, B.; Malhotra, D.; Kennedy, D.J.; Nadoor, A.; Fedorova, O.V.; Gunning, W.; et al. Salt loading induces redistribution of the plasmalemmal Na-K-ATPase in proximal tubule cells. *Kidney Int.* **2005**, *67*, 1868–1877. [CrossRef]
68. Linardi, A.; Panunto, P.C.; Ferro, E.S.; Hyslop, S. Peptidase activities in rats treated chronically with N (omega)-nitro-L-arginine methyl ester (L-NAME). *Biochem. Pharmacol.* **2004**, *68*, 205–214. [CrossRef]
69. Röhnert, P.; Schmidt, W.; Emmerlich, P.; Goihl, A.; Wrenger, S.; Bank, U.; Nordhoff, K.; Täger, M.; Ansorge, S.; Reinhold, D.; et al. Dipeptidyl peptidase IV, aminopeptidase N and DPIV/APN-like proteases in cerebral ischemia. *J. Neuroinflamm.* **2012**, *9*, 44. [CrossRef]
70. Pereira, F.E.; Cronin, C.; Ghosh, M.; Zhou, S.Y.; Agosto, M.; Subramani, J.; Wang, R.; Shen, J.B.; Schacke, W.; Liang, B.; et al. CD13 is essential for inflammatory trafficking and infarct healing following permanent coronary artery occlusion in mice. *Cardiovasc. Res.* **2013**, *100*, 74–83. [CrossRef]
71. Khakoo, A.Y.; Sidman, R.L.; Pasqualini, R.; Arap, W. Does the renin-angiotensin system participate in regulation of human vasculogenesis and angiogenesis? *Cancer Res.* **2008**, *68*, 9112–9115. [CrossRef]
72. Pasqualini, R.; Koivunen, E.; Kain, R.; Lahdenranta, J.; Sakamoto, M.; Stryhn, A.; Ashmun, R.A.; Shapiro, L.H.; Arap, W.; Ruoslahti, E. Aminopeptidase Nis a receptor for tumor-homing peptides and a target for inhibiting angiogenesis. *Cancer Res.* **2000**, *60*, 722–727.
73. Rangel, R.; Sun, Y.; Guzman-Rojas, L.; Ozawa, M.G.; Sun, J.; Giordano, R.J.; Van Pelt, C.S.; Tinkey, P.T.; Behringer, R.R.; Sidman, R.L.; et al. Impaired angiogenesis in aminopeptidase N-null mice. *Proc. Natl. Acad. Sci. USA* **2007**, *104*, 4588–4593. [CrossRef] [PubMed]
74. Schreiber, C.L.; Smith, B.D. Molecular Imaging of Aminopeptidase N in Cancer and Angiogenesis. *Contrast Media Mol. Imaging* **2018**, *2018*, 5315172. [CrossRef] [PubMed]
75. Marc, Y.; Llorens-Cortes, C. The role of the brain renin-angiotensin system in hypertension: Implications for new treatment. *Prog. Neurobiol.* **2011**, *95*, 89–103. [CrossRef] [PubMed]
76. Morton, J.J.; Casals-Stenzel, J.; Lever, A.F. Inhibitors of the renin-angiotensin system in experimental hypertension, with a note on the measurement of angiotensin I, II and III during infusion of converting-enzyme inhibitor. *Br. J. Clin. Pharmacol.* **1979**, *2*, 233S–241S. [CrossRef]
77. Fournie-Zaluski, M.C.; Fassot, C.; Valentin, B.; Djordjijevic, D.; Reaux-Le Goazigo, A.; Corvol, P.; Roques, B.P.; Llorens-Cortes, C. Brain renin-angiotensin system blockade by systemically active aminopeptidase A inhibitors: A potential treatment of salt-dependent hypertension. *Proc. Natl. Acad. Sci. USA* **2004**, *101*, 7775–7780. [CrossRef]
78. Song, L.; Wilk, S.; Healy, D.P. Aminopeptidase A antiserum inhibits intracerebroventricular angiotensin IIinduced dipsogenic and pressor responses. *Brain Res.* **1997**, *744*, 1–6. [CrossRef]
79. Bodineau, L.; Frugière, A.; Marc, Y.; Inguimbert, N.; Fassot, C.; Balavoine, F.; Roques, B.; Llorens-Cortes, C. Orally active aminopeptidase A inhibitors reduce blood pressure: A new strategy for treating hypertension. *Hypertension* **2008**, *51*, 1318–1325. [CrossRef]
80. Wright, J.W.; Harding, J.W. Brain renin-angiotensin-A new look at an old system. *Prog. Neurobiol.* **2011**, *95*, 49–67. [CrossRef]
81. Goto, Y.; Hattori, A.; Ishii, Y.; Tsujimoto, M. Reduced activity of the hypertension-associated Lys528Arg mutant of human adipocyte-derived leucine aminopeptidase (ALAP)/ ER-aminopeptidase-1. *FEBS Lett.* **2006**, *580*, 1833–1838. [CrossRef]

82. Ishii, M.; Hattori, A.; Numaguchi, Y.; Tsujimoto, M.; Ishiura, S.; Kobayashi, H.; Murohara, T.; Wrght, J.W.; Mizutani, S. The effect of recombinant aminopeptidase a on hypertension in spontaneously hypertensive rats: Its effect in comparison with candesartan. *Horm. Metab. Res.* **2008**, *40*, 887–891. [CrossRef] [PubMed]
83. Mizutani, S.; Okano, K.; Hasegawa, E. Human placental leucine aminopeptidase (P-LAP) as a hypotensive agent. *Experientia* **1982**, *38*, 821–822. [CrossRef] [PubMed]
84. Nakashima, Y.; Ohno, Y.; Itakura, A.; Takeuchi, M.; Murata, Y.; Kuno, N.; Mizutani, S. Possible involvement of aminopeptidase A in hypertension in spontaneously hypertensive rats (SHRs) and change of refractoriness in response to angiotensin II in pregnant SHRs. *J. Hypertens.* **2002**, *20*, 2233–2238. [CrossRef] [PubMed]
85. Mizutani, S.; Wright, J.; Kobayashi, H. A new approach regarding the treatment of preeclampsia and preterm labor. *Life Sci.* **2011**, *88*, 17–23. [CrossRef]
86. Kobayashi, H.; Mizutani, S.; Wright, J.W. Placental leucine aminopeptidase- and aminopeptidase A-deficient mice offer insight concerning the mechanisms underlying preterm labor and preeclampsia. *J. Biomed. Biotechnol.* **2011**, *2011*, 286947.
87. Carey, R.M.; Padia, S.H. Role of angiotensin at2 receptors in natriuresis: Intrarenal mechanisms and therapeutic potential. *Clin. Exp. Pharmacol. Physiol.* **2013**, *40*, 527–534. [CrossRef]
88. Padia, S.H.; Howell, N.L.; Kemp, B.A.; Fournie-Zaluski, M.C.; Roques, B.P.; Carey, R.M. Intrarenal aminopeptidase N inhibition restores defective angiontesin II type 2-mediated natriuresis in spontaneously hypertensive rats. *Hypertension* **2010**, *55*, 474–480. [CrossRef]
89. Padia, S.H.; Kemp, B.A.; Howell, N.L.; Gildea, J.J.; Keller, S.R.; Carey, R.M. Intrarenal angiotensin III infusion induces natriuresis and angiotensin type 2 receptor translocation in Wistar-Kyoto but not in spontaneously hypertensive rats. *Hypertension* **2009**, *53*, 338–343. [CrossRef]
90. Vaidya, V.S.; Ferguson, M.A.; Bonventre, J.V. Biomarkers of acute kidney injury. *Annu. Rev. Pharmacol. Toxicol.* **2008**, *48*, 463–493. [CrossRef]
91. Bonventre, J.V.; Vaidya, V.S.; Schmouder, R.; Feig, P.; Dieterle, F. Nextgeneration biomarkers for detecting kidney toxicity. *Nat. Biotechnol.* **2010**, *28*, 436–440. [CrossRef]
92. Devarajan, P. Emerging biomarkers of acute kidney injury. *Contrib. Nephrol.* **2007**, *156*, 203–212. [PubMed]
93. Lisowska-Myjak, B. Serum and urinary biomarker of acute kidney injury. *Blood. Purif.* **2010**, *29*, 357–365. [CrossRef] [PubMed]
94. Holdt, B.; Peters, E.; Nagel, H.R.; Steiner, M. An automated assay of urinary alanine aminopeptidase activity. *Clin. Chem. Lab. Med.* **2008**, *46*, 537–540. [CrossRef] [PubMed]
95. Song, L.; Ye, M.; Troyanovskaya, M.; Wilk, E.; Wilk, S.; Healy, D.P. Rat kidney glutamyl aminopeptidase (aminopeptidase A): Molecular identity and cellular localization. *Am. J. Physiol.* **1994**, *267*, F546–F557. [CrossRef] [PubMed]
96. Segarra, A.B.; Ramírez, M.; Banegas, I.; Hermoso, F.; Vargas, F.; Vives, F.; Alba, F.; de Gasparo, M.; Prieto, I. Influence of thyroid disorders on kidney angiotensinase activity. *Horm. Metab. Res.* **2006**, *38*, 48–52. [CrossRef]
97. Peters, J.E.; Mampel, E.; Schneider, I.; Burchardt, U.; Fukala, E.; Ahrens, I.; Haschen, R.J. Alanine aminopeptidase in urine in renal diseases. *Clin. Chim. Acta* **1972**, *37*, 213–224. [CrossRef]
98. Marchewka, Z.; Długosz, A.; Kúzniar, J. Diagnostic application of AAP isoenzyme separation. *Int. Urol. Nephrol.* **1999**, *31*, 409–416. [CrossRef]
99. Marchewka, Z.; Kúzniar, J.; Długosz, A. Enzymuria and β2-Mikroglobulinuria in the assessment of the influence of proteinuria on the progression of glomerulopathies. *Int. Urol. Nephrol.* **2001**, *33*, 673–676. [CrossRef]
100. Idasiak-Piechocka, I.; Krzymánski, M. The role of tubulointerstitial changes in progression of chronic glomerulonephritis (GN). *Przegl. Lek.* **1996**, *53*, 443–453.
101. Naghibi, B.; Ghafghazi, T.; Hajhashemi, V.; Talebi, A. Vancomycin-induced nephrotoxicity in rats: Is enzyme elevation a consistent finding in tubular injury? *J. Nephrol.* **2007**, *20*, 482–488.
102. Jung, K.; Hempel, A.; Grutzmann, K.D.; Hempel, R.D.; Schreiber, G. Age-dependent excretion of alanine aminopeptydase, alkaline phosphatase, γ -glutamyltransferase and N-acetyl-β-D-glucosaaminidase in human urine. *Enzyme* **1990**, *43*, 10–16. [CrossRef] [PubMed]
103. Inselmann, G.; Balaschke, M.; Heidemann, H.T. Enzymuria following amphotericin B application in the rat. *Mycoses* **2003**, *46*, 169–173. [CrossRef] [PubMed]

104. Mitic, B.; Lazarevic, G.; Vlahovic, P.; Rajic, M.; Stefanovic, V. Diagnostic value of the aminopeptidase N, N-acetyl-beta-D-glucosaminidase and dipeptidylpeptidase IV in evaluating tubular dysfunction in patients with glomerulopathies. *Ren. Fail.* **2008**, *30*, 896–903. [CrossRef] [PubMed]
105. Moon, P.G.; Lee, J.E.; You, S.; Kim, T.K.; Cho, J.H.; Kim, I.S.; Kwon, T.H.; Kim, C.D.; Park, S.H.; Hwang, D.; et al. Proteomic analysis of urinary exosomes from patients of early IgA nephropathy and thin basement membrane nephropathy. *Proteomics* **2011**, *11*, 2459–2475. [CrossRef] [PubMed]
106. Lazarevic, G.; Antic, S.; Vlahovic, P.; Djordjevic, V.; Zvezdanovic, L.; Stefanovic, V. Effects of aerobic exercise on microalbuminuria and enzymuria in type 2 diabetic patients. *Ren. Fail.* **2007**, *29*, 199–205. [CrossRef] [PubMed]
107. Kuzniar, J.; Marchewka, Z.; Krasnowski, R.; Boratynska, M.; Długosz, A.; Klinger, M. Enzymuria and low molecular weight protein excretion as the differentiating marker of complications in the early post kidney transplantation period. *Int. Urol. Nephrol.* **2006**, *38*, 753–758. [CrossRef]
108. Marchewka, Z.; Kuzniar, J.; Zynek-Litwin, M.; Falkiewicz, K.; Szymanska, B.; Roszkowska, A.; Klinger, M. Kidney graft function in long-term cyclosporine and tacrolimus treatment: Comparative study with nephrotoxicity markers. *Transplant. Proc.* **2009**, *41*, 1660–1665. [CrossRef]
109. Molitoris, B.A.; Levin, A.; Warnock, D.G.; Joannidis, M.; Mehta, R.L.; Kellum, J.A.; Ronco, C.; Shah, S. Improving outcomes from acute kidney injury. *J. Am. Soc. Nephrol.* **2007**, *18*, 1992–1994. [CrossRef]
110. Safirstein, R.; Winston, J.; Moel, D.; Dikman, S.; Guttenplan, J. Cisplatin nephrotoxicity-insights into mechanism. *Int. J. Androl.* **1987**, *10*, 325–346. [CrossRef]
111. Winston, J.A.; Safirstein, R. Reduced renal blood-flow in early cisplatin induced acute renal failure in the rat. *Am. J. Physiol.* **1985**, *249*, F490–F496. [CrossRef]
112. Yao, X.; Panichpisal, K.; Kurtzman, N.; Nugent, K. Cisplatin nephrotoxicity: A review. *Am. J. Med. Sci.* **2007**, *334*, 115–124. [CrossRef] [PubMed]
113. Quesada, A.; Vargas, F.; Montoro-Molina, S.; O'Valle, F.; Rodríguez-Martínez, M.D.; Osuna, A.; Prieto, I.; Ramírez, M.; Wangensteen, F. Urinary Aminopeptidase Activities as Early and Predictive Biomarkers of Renal Dysfunction in Cisplatin-Treated Rats. *PLoS ONE* **2012**, *7*, e40402. [CrossRef] [PubMed]
114. Montoro-Molina, S.; Quesada, A.; Zafra-Ruiz, P.V.; O'Valle, F.; Vargas, F.; de Gracia, M.C.; Osuna, A.; Wangensteen, F. Immunological detection of glutamyl aminopeptidase in urine samples from cisplatin-treated rats. *Proteom. Clin. Appl.* **2015**, *9*, 630–635. [CrossRef] [PubMed]
115. Salih, M.; Zietse, R.; Hoorn, E.J. Urinary extracellular vesicles and the kidney: Biomarkers and beyond. *Am. J. Physiol. Ren. Physiol.* **2014**, *306*, 1251–1259. [CrossRef] [PubMed]
116. Gámez-Valero, A.; Lozano-Ramos, S.I.; Bancu, I.; Lauzurica-Valdemoros, R.; Borras, F.E. Urinary extracellular vesicles as source of biomarkers in kidney diseases. *Front. Inmunol.* **2015**, *6*, 6.
117. Pisitkun, T.; Johnstone, R.; Knepper, M.A. Discovery of urinary biomarkers. *Mol. Cell. Proteom.* **2006**, *5*, 1760–1771. [CrossRef]
118. Ohno, S.; Ishikawa, A.; Kuroda, M. Roles of exosomes and microvesicles in disease pathogenesis. *Adv. Drug. Deliv. Rev.* **2013**, *65*, 398–401. [CrossRef]
119. Dimov, I.; Jankovic, V.L.; Stefanovic, V. Urinary exosomes. *Sci. World J.* **2009**, *9*, 1107–1118. [CrossRef]
120. Jayachandran, M.; Lugo, G.; Heiling, H.; Miller, V.M.; Rule, A.D.; Lieske, J.C. Extracellular vesicles in urine of women with but not without kidney stones manifest patterns similar to men: A case control study. *Biol. Sex. Differ.* **2015**, *6*, 2. [CrossRef]
121. Lv, L.L.; Cao, Y.; Liu, D.; Xu, M.; Liu, H.; Tang, R.N.; Ma, K.L.; Liu, B.C. Isolation and quantification of microRNAs from urinary exosomes/microvesicles for biomarker discovery. *Int. J. Biol. Sci.* **2013**, *9*, 1021–1031. [CrossRef]
122. Murakami, T.; Oakes, M.; Ogura, M.; Tovar, V.; Yamamoto, C.; Mitsuhashi, M. Development of glomerulus-, tubule-, and collecting duct-specific mRNA assay in human urinary exosomes and microvesicles. *PLoS ONE* **2014**, *2*, e109074. [CrossRef] [PubMed]
123. Álvarez, S.; Suazo, C.; Boltansky, A.; Ursu, M.; Carvajal, D.; Innocenti, G.; Vukusich, A.; Hurtado, M.; Villanueva, S.; Carreño, J.E. Urinary exosomes as a source of kidney dysfunction biomarker in renal transplantation. *Transplant. Proc.* **2013**, *45*, 3719–3723. [CrossRef] [PubMed]
124. Dear, J.W.; Street, J.M.; Bailey, M.A. Urinary exosomes: A reservoir for biomarker discovery and potential mediators of intrarenal signalling. *Proteomics* **2013**, *13*, 1572–1580. [CrossRef] [PubMed]

125. Quesada, A.; Segarra, A.B.; Montoro-Molina, S.; de Gracia, M.D.C.; Osuna, A.; O'Valle, F.; Gómez-Guzmán, M.; Vargas, F.; Wangensteen, R. Glutamyl aminopeptidase in microvesicular and exosomal fractions of urine is related with renal dysfunction in cisplatin-treated rats. *PLoS ONE* **2017**, *12*, e0175462. [CrossRef]
126. Hultström, M. Development of structural kidney damage in spontaneously hypertensive rats. *J. Hypertens.* **2012**, *30*, 1087–1091. [CrossRef]
127. Kim, N.; Dai, S.Y.; Pang, V.; Mazer, C.D. Vasopressinase Activity: A Potential Early Biomarker for Detecting Cardiopulmonary Bypass-Associated Acute Kidney Injury? *Thorac. Cardiovasc. Surg.* **2016**, *64*, 555–560. [CrossRef]
128. Munshi, R.; Hsu, C.; Himmelfarb, J. Advances in understanding ischemic acute kidney injury. *BMC Med.* **2011**, *9*, 11. [CrossRef]
129. Osuna, A.; de Gracia, M.C.; Quesada, A.; Manzano, F.; Wangensteen, R. Alanil aminopeptidase como marcador temprano del daño renal agudo persistente en pacientes sometidos a cirugía cardíaca. In Proceedings of the XLIX Congreso de la Soc Esp Nefrol, A Coruña, España, 5 October 2019.
130. de Artinano, A.A.; Castro, M.M. Experimental rat models to study the metabolic syndrome. *Br. J. Nutr.* **2009**, *102*, 1246–1253. [CrossRef]
131. Montoro-Molina, S.; López-Carmona, A.; Quesada, A.; O'Valle, F.; Martín-Morales, N.; Osuna, A.; Vargas, F.; Wangensteen, R. Klotho and Aminopeptidases as Early Biomarkers of Renal Injury in Zucker Obese Rats. *Front. Physiol.* **2018**, *9*, 1599. [CrossRef]
132. Llorens, S.; Fernandez, A.P.; Nava, E. Cardiovascular and renal alterations on the nitric oxide path way in spontaneous hypertension and ageing. *Clin. Hemorheol. Microcirc.* **2007**, *37*, 149–156.
133. Sun, Z.J.; Zhang, Z.E. Historic perspectives and recent advances in major animal models of hypertension. *Acta Pharmacol. Sin.* **2005**, *26*, 295–301. [CrossRef] [PubMed]
134. Montoro-Molina, S.; Quesada, A.; O'Valle, F.; Osuna, A.; de Gracia, M.C.; Vargas, F.; Wangensteen, R. Urinary aminopeptidase activities in spontaneously hypertensive rats. In Proceedings of the Physiology 2016, Dublin, Ireland, 39–31 July 2016. PCA320.
135. Vargas, F.; Moreno, J.M.; Rodríguez-Gómez, I.; Wangensteen, R.; Osuna, A.; Alvarez-Guerra, M.; García-Estañ, J. Vascular and renal function in experimental thyroid disorders. *Eur. J. Endocrinol.* **2006**, *154*, 197–212. [CrossRef] [PubMed]
136. Nakamura, S.; Ishiyama, M.; Kosaka, J.; Mutoh, J.; Umemura, N.; Harase, C. Urinary N-acetyl-beta-D-glucosaminidase (NAG) activity in patients with Graves' disease, subacute thyroiditis, and silent thyroiditis: A longitudinal study. *Endocrinol. Jpn.* **1991**, *38*, 303–308. [CrossRef] [PubMed]
137. Van Hoek, I.; Meyer, E.; Duchateau, L.; Peremans, K.; Smets, P.; Daminet, S. Retinol-binding protein in serum and urine of hyperthyroid cats before and after treatment with radioiodine. *J. Vet. Intern. Med.* **2009**, *23*, 1031–1037. [CrossRef]
138. Pérez-Abud, R.; Rodríguez-Gómez, I.; Villarejo, A.B.; Moreno, J.M.; Wangensteen, R.; Tassi, M.; O'Valle, F.; Osuna, A.; Vargas, F. Salt sensitivity in experimental thyroid disorders in rats. *Am. J. Physiol. Endocrinol. Metab.* **2011**, *301*, E281–E287. [CrossRef]
139. Conger, J.D.; Falk, S.A.; Gillum, D.M. The protective mechanism of thyroidectomy in a rat model of chronic renal failure. *Am. J. Kidney Dis.* **1989**, *13*, 217–225. [CrossRef]
140. Wangensteen, R.; Segarra, A.B.; Ramirez-Sanchez, M.; Gasparo, M.D.; Dominguez, G.; Banegas, I.; Vargas, F.; Vives, F.; Prieto, I. Influence of thyroid disorders on the kidney expression and plasma activity of aminopeptidase A. *Endocr. Regul.* **2015**, *49*, 68–72. [CrossRef]
141. Jung, K.; Pergande, M.; Schimie, E.; Ratzmann, K.P.; Illus, A. Urinary enzymes and low-molecular-mass proteins as indicator of diabetes nephropathy. *Clin. Chem.* **1988**, *34*, 544–547. [CrossRef]
142. Sorokman, T.; Sokolnyk, S.; Popelyuk, O.; Makarova, O.; Kopchuk, T. Biomarkers of renal injury risk in children with pyelonephritis. *Georgian Med. News* **2018**, *280–281*, 98–103.
143. Spasovski, D.; Masin-Spasovska, J.; Nada, M.; Calovski, J.; Sandevska, E.; Osmani, B.; Sotirova, T.; Balkanov, S.; Dukovski, D.; Ljatifi, A.; et al. Diagnostic value of brush border enzymes of the proximal renal tubules in rheumatoid arthritis. *Clin. Lab.* **2011**, *57*, 305–314.

7

Proteomics-Based Machine Learning Approach as an Alternative to Conventional Biomarkers for Differential Diagnosis of Chronic Kidney Diseases

Yury E. Glazyrin [1,2,*], Dmitry V. Veprintsev [2], Irina A. Ler [3], Maria L. Rossovskaya [3], Svetlana A. Varygina [3], Sofia L. Glizer [3,4], Tatiana N. Zamay [1], Marina M. Petrova [4], Zoran Minic [5], Maxim V. Berezovski [5] and Anna S. Kichkailo [1,2]

1 Laboratory for Biomolecular and Medical Technologies, Krasnoyarsk State Medical University Named after Prof. V.F. Voyno-Yasenetsky, 660022 Krasnoyarsk, Russia; tzamay@yandex.ru (T.N.Z.); annazamay@yandex.ru (A.S.K.)

2 Laboratory for Digital Controlled Drugs and Theranostics, Federal Research Center "Krasnoyarsk Science Center of the Siberian Branch of the Russian Academy of Science", 660036 Krasnoyarsk, Russia; d_veprintsev@mail.ru

3 Department of Nephrology, Krasnoyarsk Interdistrict Clinical Hospital of Emergency Medical Care Named after N.S. Karpovich, 660062 Krasnoyarsk, Russia; irina-ler@bk.ru (I.A.L.); mross@mail.ru (M.L.R.); alfasv-ja@list.ru (S.A.V.); sofiaglizer@mail.ru (S.L.G.)

4 Faculty of Medicine, Krasnoyarsk State Medical University Named after Prof. V.F. Voyno-Yasenetsky, 660022 Krasnoyarsk, Russia; stk99@yandex.ru

5 Department of Chemistry and Biomolecular Sciences, University of Ottawa, Ottawa, ON K1N6N5, Canada; zminic@uottawa.ca (Z.M.); Maxim.Berezovski@uottawa.ca (M.V.B.)

* Correspondence: yury.glazyrin@gmail.com

Abstract: Diabetic nephropathy, hypertension, and glomerulonephritis are the most common causes of chronic kidney diseases (CKD). Since CKD of various origins may not become apparent until kidney function is significantly impaired, a differential diagnosis and an appropriate treatment are needed at the very early stages. Conventional biomarkers may not have sufficient separation capabilities, while a full-proteomic approach may be used for these purposes. In the current study, several machine learning algorithms were examined for the differential diagnosis of CKD of three origins. The tested dataset was based on whole proteomic data obtained after the mass spectrometric analysis of plasma and urine samples of 34 CKD patients and the use of label-free quantification approach. The k-nearest-neighbors algorithm showed the possibility of separation of a healthy group from renal patients in general by proteomics data of plasma with high confidence (97.8%). This algorithm has also be proven to be the best of the three tested for distinguishing the groups of patients with diabetic nephropathy and glomerulonephritis according to proteomics data of plasma (96.3% of correct decisions). The group of hypertensive nephropathy could not be reliably separated according to plasma data, whereas analysis of entire proteomics data of urine did not allow differentiating the three diseases. Nevertheless, the group of hypertensive nephropathy was reliably separated from all other renal patients using the k-nearest-neighbors classifier "one against all" with 100% of accuracy by urine proteome data. The tested algorithms show good abilities to differentiate the various groups across proteomic data sets, which may help to avoid invasive intervention for the verification of the glomerulonephritis subtypes, as well as to differentiate hypertensive and diabetic nephropathy in the early stages based not on individual biomarkers, but on the whole proteomic composition of urine and blood.

Keywords: chronic kidney disease; machine learning; differential diagnosis; proteomics; mass spectrometry; label-free quantification

1. Introduction

Chronic kidney disease (CKD) is a supra-nosological concept that unites all patients with signs of kidney damage and/or a decrease in their function [1]. CKD is one of the major health problems with high mortality, because it causes irreversible changes in renal failure. No obvious clinical symptoms appear in early stage disease until severe damage has occurred [2]. Therefore, the need for early diagnosis of CKD is obvious. Diseases leading to CKD can be divided into two groups: (1) processes localized directly in the kidneys and urinary tract (glomerulonephritis, pyelonephritis, etc.), and (2) diseases in which the kidneys are target organs (diabetes, hypertensive disease, systemic diseases, etc.). Diagnosis of the disease causing the damage is paramount in all cases of the CKD presence [3–5]. The most common causes of CKD are diabetic nephropathy, hypertension, and glomerulonephritis [6]. Clinical manifestations, serum creatinine (Scr), and renal histopathology are commonly used to diagnose CKD and determine its different stages. The role of Scr is very limited [2]. Although kidney biopsy for histopathology may be an invasive and painful procedure, it is considered as the gold standard for the diagnosis of renal disease [7]. Bleeding and other surgical complications may follow this procedure. To reduce these risks, it could be safer to use alternative techniques.

The study of proteomic composition of urine and other human bio-fluids is very promising for the diagnosis of different kidney pathologies and for understanding the mechanisms of their occurrence. Proteinuria may reflect abnormal plasma protein loss, as a result of: (a) an increase in glomerular permeability for macromolecular proteins (glomerular proteinuria), (b) incomplete tubular reabsorption of low molecular weight proteins (tubular proteinuria), (c) abnormal loss of proteins of renal origin and urinary tract. Thus, the analysis of the urine proteome potentially allows us to speak about the localization of nephron damage, which greatly facilitates the differential diagnosis [8,9]. Research is currently underway, both in the search for specific proteins found in CKD [10–14] and attempts to highlight individual proteins that would become markers of specific diseases that cause CKD [15,16].

Often, information on changes in the expression level of a single protein is not enough to obtain sufficient accuracy and the sensitivity required for a clinical diagnostic system, and it is necessary to apply several indicators simultaneously. Thus, the use of a panel of 28 urinal proteins has shown the ability to differentiate Immunoglobulin-A nephropathy and primary membranous nephropathy with a sensitivity of 77% and specificity of 100% [17]. The sets of differently expressed urinal proteins were used for the differential diagnosis of lupus nephritis, primary membranous nephropathy, diabetic nephropathy, and focal segmental glomerulosclerosis. The sensitivity of differential diagnosis remained at 70% when using a set of 5 proteins, but the accuracy fell below 50% when using a set of less than 20 proteins [18]. It shows that these indicators are still insufficient for the effective differentiation of CKDs.

However, the most versatile and universal approach for differential diagnosis should consider the full quantitative information about a large number of proteins contained in patient's fluids. Multicomponent proteomics data derived from mass spectrometric analysis of a non-diagnosed patient's sample can be processed in comparison with similar data sets obtained from people with known diagnoses, to assign a new patient to a particular group. For this purpose the mathematical models of machine learning, which take into account the interactions of a large amount of data in a multidimensional space, can be used. Such an approach may become a new concept of an effective and universal test system for both early diagnosis of CKD and post diagnostic differentiation of renal diseases of different origin.

Recent methods of large data sets processing are often based on the principle of "black box", where input data are transformed into decision factors without any additional knowledge of internal working. Mathematical instruments, such as machine learning and data analysis, are increasingly being used in medicine [19,20]. Machine learning is a branch of the data science that trains computers to perform tasks by observing patterns in large datasets and using them to derive rules or algorithms that optimize task performance [21]. It is used for computer-aided diagnosis of acute neurological events [22] and retinal disease [23]. These studies were mainly based on general clinical indicators, whereas the application of the wide-scale method of quantitative proteomics based on a comparison of relative expressions of a large number of proteins can show much greater efficiency.

In this paper, we introduce a new approach to the differential diagnosis of CKDs of different origins, such as diabetic nephropathy, chronic glomerulonephritis and hypertensive nephropathy, which is based on large proteomics data sets obtained by mass spectrometry of blood plasma and urine, by means of several models of machine learning. The tested algorithms showed good abilities to differentiate the various groups of the tested renal patients according to the proteomic data.

2. Results

Plasma and urine samples were collected from 15 patients with diabetic nephropathy (group D), from 14 patients with glomerulonephritis (group G), from 5 patients with hypertensive nephropathy (group H), and from 14 healthy volunteers (group N). Table 1 summarizes the principal characteristics of the CKD patients.

Table 1. Principal characteristics of the chronic kidney diseases (CKD) patients.

Variable	Group D	Group G	Group H
Sex, *n* (%)			
Male	6 (40)	8 (57)	2 (40)
Female	9 (60)	6 (43)	3 (60)
Age, mean ± SD (years)	62.11 ± 17.91	48.46 ± 16.83	60.6 ± 14.15
Stage of renal disease, *n* (%)			
Stage 1	6 (40)	7 (50)	0 (0)
Stage 2 + 3	7 (46.7)	2 (14.3)	0 (0)
Stage 4 + 5	2 (13.3)	5 (35.7)	5 (100)
Level of proteinuria			
Below 30 mg/l, *n* (%)	0 (0)	0 (0)	0 (0)
30 - 300 mg/l, *n* (%)	5 (33.4)	5 (35.7)	1 (20)
Above 300 mg/l, *n* (%)	10 (66.6)	9 (64.3)	4 (80)
Presence of hypertension, *n* (%)	8 (53)	10 (71.4)	5 (100)
eGFR, mean ± SD (mL/min)	39.56 ± 15.27	68.38 ± 48.36	14.8 ± 7.19
Biopsy tested patients, *n* (%)	0 (0)	2 (14.3)	0 (0)
Type of glomerulonephritis			
Chronic glomerulonephritis, *n* (%)		10 (71.4)	
Nephrotic syndrome, *n* (%)		4 (28.6)	

Abbreviations: SD, standard deviation; eGFR, estimated glomerular filtration rate.

The plasma samples were depleted from albumin and immunoglobulin, the urine samples were concentrated by filter columns. All protein samples were prepared for mass spectrometry in duplicates and each duplicate was analyzed twice. These technical replicates were marked as A and B. The total set of plasma probes contained 190 samples (group G—56, group D—58, group H—20, and group N—56). The number of urine samples derived from patients was 97 (group G—40, group D—41, and group H—16); urine from healthy people was not taken due to low normal protein concentrations. The samples were not divided into fractions to limit the resulted data set for the convenience of bioinformatic processing. Two sets of quantitative proteomics data from blood and urine samples (Table S1) were obtained. No specific differences on proteome profiles between different patients groups expressed in the distribution of individual proteins were found by conventional statistical methods. Thus, machine learning algorithms, taking into account the overall contribution of the proteomic composition of the samples, were applied. The data were independently tested in two ways. At first, we distinguished the total CKD patients from the healthy individuals, and then we differentiated three groups of patients from each other without comparison with healthy control.

2.1. *Separation of CKD Patients from the Healthy Individuals by Plasma Proteome*

A total of 246 proteins were identified and quantified by label-free quantification (LFQ) from the plasma probes, and 184 of them were considered as relevant after the quality filtration. Then, the differences in plasma proteome of CKD patients and healthy individuals were estimated by principal component analysis (PCA). After the consistency check and averaging of the replicates, the dataset was reduced to 90 samples (group G—27, group D—28, group H—9, and group N—26) and label-free quantification (LFQ) values of 184 proteins were converted to the 17 principal components providing the cumulative variance of 70%.

The KNeighbors machine learning model (kNN) with the Euclidean distance was used for the separation of the total set of CKD patients (groups G, D, H) from the healthy individuals (group N). The best number of neighbors was found as 3. The mean proportion of correct classifier responses was 97.8%. Thus, the total CKD patients were differentiated from the healthy individuals using proteomics data of plasma with high confidence.

2.2. *Differentiation of the Three Groups of Renal Patients by Plasma Proteome*

The possibility of differentiation of various types of CKD with similar symptoms by proteomics data was tested. At this step, the control samples obtained from healthy people (group N) were discarded and 134 CKD patient's samples were taken; 175 proteins in 131 samples were left after the quality control check.

The PCA analysis showed that 14 principal components were necessary for 70% of cumulative variance, and 64 averaged results were obtained after the consistency check. Three models of machine learning were tested: KNeighbors, logistic regression, and support vector machine (SVM). The optimal hyper parameters were found: number of neighbors (*n*_neighbors = 1) for KNeighbors, constant of regularization (C = 1) for logistic regression, kernel (kernel = 'rbf') and gamma (gamma = 0.5) for SVM. The mean proportions of correct classifier responses were 87.5%, 84.3%, 82.8%, respectively. Based on this cross-validation quality assessment, the KNeighbors classifier was chosen as the best for further calculations. A number of errors of the nearest-neighbors algorithm were found for each class for the entire set. Class D had 2 errors from 28 (7.1%), class G had 2 errors from 27 (7.4%), and class H had 4 errors from 9 (44.4%). Thus, this algorithm works well for differential separation of group D from group G, but does not allow distinguishing class H.

Finally, the class H samples were excluded from the analysis and 55 samples were left in the set. The nearest-neighbor algorithm gave only two errors for this set (the proportions of correct decisions were 96.3% for class G and 96.4% for class D). Thus, this algorithm showed good results for the use in a medical test system that can separate glomerulonephritis from diabetic nephropathy based on plasma proteome.

2.3. *Differential Diagnosis Based on Urine Proteome and Separation of Group H from the Total Patients*

A total of 409 proteins were identified and quantified by LFQ, and 241 proteins in 96 samples left after the quality control.

We found 13 principal components to be optimal after the PCA. The consistency check and averaging resulted in 47 samples (group G—19, group D—20, and group H—8). Four machine learning models were tested. A decision tree was added to the three algorithms mentioned above. None of the tested algorithms with optimized hyper parameters showed high proportion of correct decisions. It was lower than 80% overall, thus showing no evident possibility to differentiate the three tested groups on the basis of urine proteome data, and allowing us to conclude that the urine proteome in comparison with plasma proteome has much less differences in the tested groups of patients.

The capabilities of "one against all" models for the separation of classes were tested. It was found that the classifier 1-nn (nearest-neighbor algorithm) gives an accuracy equal to 100% for class H by the entire set of urine proteomics data. It correctly defined all the samples of class H and had no false definitions. Thus, this model showed good capability to separate patients of group H (hypertensive nephropathy) from the remaining groups of renal patients.

3. Discussion

Focused on efficient processing of proteomics data, this work had two goals: 1) development of the concept of a non-invasive early-stage test system for general kidney malfunctions, and 2) the differentiation by origin of previously diagnosed renal diseases with similar symptoms. For these, using our data set, we first tried to distinguish the total group of CKD patients from the healthy group, and then to differentiate the three groups of patients from each other.

At the first step, it was important to find out whether the common differences in plasma proteome appear in patients with renal disease and in healthy people. This task was not particularly difficult. It turned out that KNeighbors machine learning model (kNN) is able to differentiate CKD patients from healthy individuals with high confidence (97.8% of correct classifier responses).

Glomerular filtration rate (GFR) remains for today the most operating marker of kidney malfunction, which is usually estimated taking into account endogenous filtration markers like serum creatinine and cystatin C [24], but the accuracy of their measuring is still under consideration [25]. It shows that new proteomic biomarkers may facilitate more accurate and earlier detection of renal pathologies [26]. Machine learning has been successfully applied to proteomics data for classification of samples and identification of biomarkers, and can be used across a wide range of diseases [27]. Thus, the high accuracy in separating a group of renal patients from healthy ones that we demonstrated by processing of plasma proteome data using machine learning proved to be effective for the introduction of this approach into clinical diagnosis.

The second goal of our research was to examine the ability of complex differentiation of various CKDs by plasma proteome data. It is difficult to predict in advance the most efficient processing algorithm for analyzing multidimensional data, thus we tested three models. The KNeighbors classifier (Model 1) was chosen as the most effective after comparing with the logistic regression and support vector machine (SVM), because of the best proportion of correct classifier responses (87.5%). After the less represented group of hypertensive patients was excluded, the proportion of correct decisions increased above 96%, thus showing a high ability to separate diabetic patients with indirect kidney damage from patients with autoimmune-caused internal kidney degradation (glomerulonephritis).

Diseases of different origins, which are not only related to kidneys but expressed in symptoms of kidney degradation, may appear in plasma proteomic composition. According to our results, diabetic nephropathy has a specific proteomic signature in blood which is independent of renal degradation. The distinct changes in the expression of individual proteins, such as monocyte chemoattractant protein-1 (MCP-1) and transforming growth factor-β1 (TGF-β1) [28], or even in panels of several proteins [29] noted previously as predicting the rate of renal function decline in diabetes, may also be accompanied by other more complex changes in the plasma proteome. On the other hand, the hypertonic signature of renal degradation with the damage of the tubules and the interstitium was not expressed in specific changes in the blood proteome, according to our data. Therefore, the proposed approach can be recommended for further development as a medical test system based on plasma proteome that can separate glomerulonephritis from other CKD patients, e.g., diabetics.

Urine sampling is even easier compared to venous blood collection and the sample preparation procedure eliminates the extra step of plasma depletion from major proteins. We tried to use both bio-fluids to obtain the proteomics data and compared them to find the most suitable way for differential diagnosis of the three types of kidney diseases. Urine samples obtained from healthy people were not used in this study, due to much lower protein concentrations compared with renal patients.

As well as for the plasma proteome, we tested kNN, SVM, and logistic regression as means for distinguishing the urine proteome datasets. In addition, the decision tree algorithm has been added to the comparison. However, as a result, none of the tested models gave the proportion of correct decisions above the level of 80%, thus showing no clear ability to differentiate simultaneously the three tested groups based on urine proteome data.

The additional "one against all" model showed the best results in the separation of only one tested group of patients. The classifier 1-nn (nearest-neighbor algorithm, Model 2) gives an accuracy of 100% for class H, showing no false definitions across the entire data set. Processing of urine proteome by machine learning showed the ability of distinguishing hypertensive nephropathy from other renal diseases. Since, here, we used a sample set that is not very representative (only 5 hypertensive patients), this approach should be recommended for further testing on larger groups.

Diabetic nephropathy and proliferative forms of glomerulonephritis have a similar histological picture of diffuse glomerulosclerosis, tubulointerstitial fibrosis, and atrophy, and also variable degrees of hyaline arteriolosclerosis and arterial sclerosis. In hypertensive nephropathy, primary pathological changes in afferent arterioles lead to ischemic damage to the glomerular apparatus [30]. Thus, the degradation of various kidney structures can result in a difference in the transmitted proteins that enter the urine of hypertensive patients. Proteinuria of the same origin, associated with glomerular defects probably did not have specific features depending on the genesis of renal degradation, and therefore diabetes and glomerulonephritis did not appear in urinal protein variations according to our study.

To test the differences in pathological renal filtration in the context of protein size, we compared molecular masses of the proteins found in the urine of patients from the three CKD groups. No distinct specificity for a particular disease was found in our case, as shown in Figure 1. Thus, the differences in the total proteome, which can be traced by machine learning, do not concern the molecular masses and sizes of proteins and are manifested in other complex features.

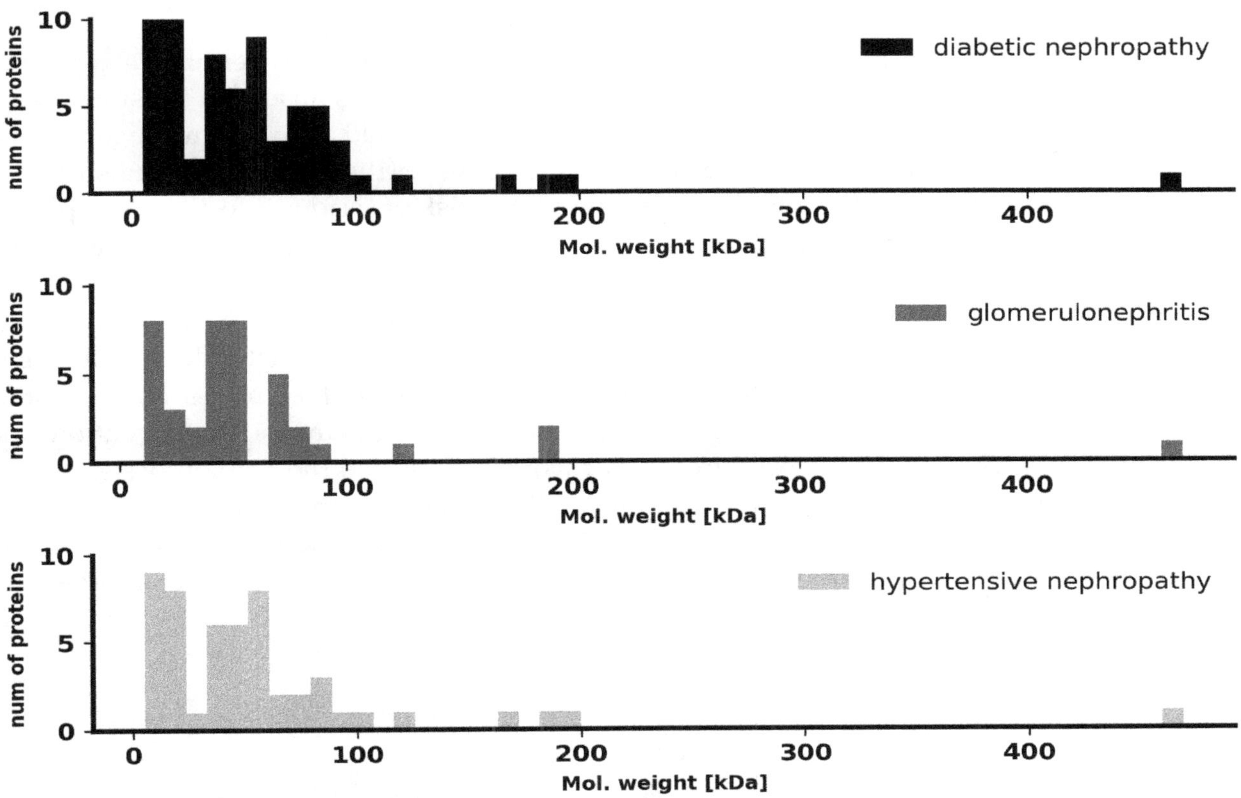

Figure 1. Distribution of urine proteins by molecular weight in the three studied groups of patients.

In this study, we conclude that the urine proteome, compared with the plasma proteome, has much less differences in our tested groups. As a result, urine is not quite suited for universal differential diagnosis in this analytical way, but this approach may remain useful in some cases, for example, to isolate patients with hypertensive nephropathy.

In addition, it is possible to use a two-stage approach to the differential diagnosis of CKD (Figure 2), including a combination of primary proteomic analysis of urine to cut off the hypertensive origin of the disease (using Model 2), followed by proteomic analysis of blood plasma to separate diabetic nephropathy and glomerulonephritis (using Model 1).

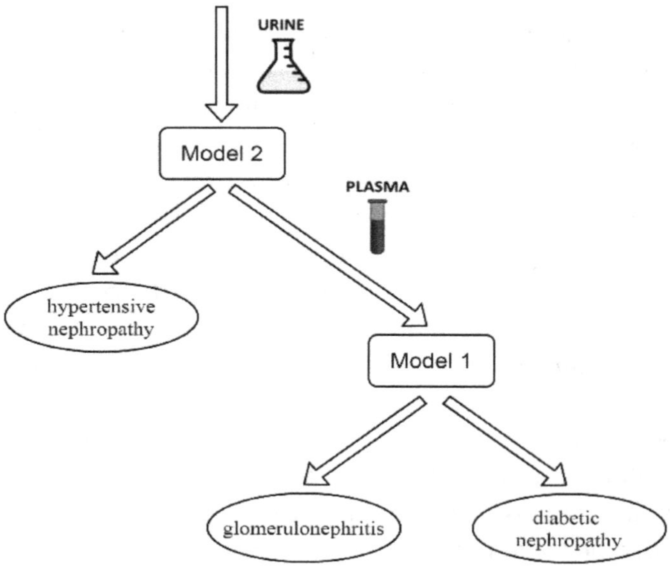

Figure 2. Scheme of two-stage differential diagnosis of chronic kidney disease using proteomic data of urine and plasma.

While the application of the presented strategy can be limited for the hypertensive nephropathy due to the fact that its diagnosis is mostly clinical and proteinuria is absent in most of the cases, for correctly diagnosed diabetic nephropathy, a specific therapy aimed at correcting sugar levels can be more actively applied. Treatment strategies for glomerulonephritis include immunosuppression with glucocorticosteroids and cytostatics, associated with the risk of serious infectious complications. The similar therapy for patients with diabetes can be dangerous, since they have a higher risk of purulent complications. Generally, differential diagnosis between glomerulonephritis and diabetic nephropathy should be carried out on the basis of kidney biopsy. However, several complicating points exist: (1) kidney biopsy is not always unambiguous, (2) this is an invasive method, (3) kidney biopsy should be performed in a specialized center, (4) to assess the dynamics of the process, a second study is required, which in the case of kidney biopsy is associated with repeated invasive intervention, and (5) the patient may refuse an invasive procedure. In this work, we studied the phenotypes expressed in the proteomes that distinguish the presented groups. All associated pathologies, including diabetes, should be undoubtedly reflected in the phenotypic proteomes, which we examined by choosing groups in this way (with and without diabetes) and dividing them using a machine learning approach.

4. Materials and Methods

4.1. Patients

A total of 34 CKD patients participated in the study (Table 1). Diagnosis of diabetic nephropathy patients was made clinically by the presence of diabetes; most patients had hypertension. Hypertensive nephropathy was diagnosed clinically by the presence of hypertension without presence of diabetes; no biopsy was performed in these groups. A group of glomerulonephritis patients were diagnosed by biopsy. All participants signed an informed consent. The study was approved by the Ethical Committee of the Krasnoyarsk State Medical University named after Professor V.F. Voyno-Yasenetsky (ethical code 88/2019 of 27 February 2019).

4.2. Sample Preparation

The plasma samples were depleted from albumin and immunoglobulin using ProteoPrep depletion columns (Sigma-Aldrich, St. Louis, MO, USA) according to the manufacturer's protocol. Proteins from the urine samples were concentrated with Amicon Ultra-4 3 kDa centrifugal filter columns (Merck Millipore, County Cork, Ireland). The protein concentrations were determined by UV-1280 spectrophotometer (Shimadzu, Kyoto, Japan) and samples with 4 μg of protein were taken for mass spectrometry. The proteins were reduced by dithiothreitol, alkylated by iodoacetamide, and digested by trypsin according to the manufacturer's protocols (Thermo Scientific, Waltham, MA, USA). The samples were desalted by 10 μL C18 pipette tips from the same manufacturer in accordance with its protocol and dried before analysis.

4.3. Liquid Chromatography and Mass Spectrometry

The samples were dissolved in phase "A" (0.1% of formic acid) and 2 μg of each sample were injected into the Dionex UltiMate 3000 RSLC nano liquid chromatographer (Thermo Scientific, USA) with Acclaim RSLC PepMap C18 separation column (15 cm length, 75 μm inner diameter, 2 μm particles). The solvent gradient was increased from 0% to 40% of phase "B" (0.1% of formic acid in 80% acetonitrile) for 90 min, maintaining a constant flow rate of 200 nL/min. The Orbitrap Fusion mass spectrometer (Thermo Scientific, USA) was operated in data-dependent mode with scans of parent and fragment ions changing in cycle of 4 s. Full scans were made at a resolution of 60,000 by the Orbitrap mass detector, and fragments generated by high energy collision dissociation (HCD) were registered by ion trap at normal rate.

4.4. Protein Search and Label-Free Quantification

The raw data files were processed by MaxQuant 1.6 software (Max Planck Institute for Biochemistry, Martinsried, Germany) [31]. Label-free quantification (LFQ) parameter was enabled. Unique and razor peptides were chosen for protein quantification. Carbamidomethylation of cysteine was set as a fixed modification, and oxidation of methionine and N-term acetylation were set as variable modifications. Protein search was performed against an actual SwissProt protein database with the human taxonomy restriction. The Orbitrap instrument was chosen and mass tolerance of 20 ppm was set for the first search and 4.5 ppm was set for the main search. Protein false discovery rate (FDR) of 0.01 was set. The obtained values of LFQ intensities (Table S1) were considered as relative indicators of protein expressions over the sample groups.

4.5. Data Analysis

All LFQ data analysis was performed using Anaconda Python 3 with Pandas and Scikit-learn libraries. Two steps of data filtration were made. Non-widespread proteins and low quality samples were excluded from the further analysis. Proteins detected in less than 5 samples and samples in which less than 50 proteins were found were not taken into account. Then, the LFQ normalization procedure was performed as follows: protein LFQ level for each sample was divided to the maximum of LFQ level of the certain protein among all the samples, giving the quantitative values to the range from 0 to 1. Then principal component analysis (PCA) was applied to reduce the data dimensions. We switched to a lower number of features expressed in projections of multiple protein LFQ values to the vectors of principal components. The next step was performed to check the consistency of the samples using data from the pairs of technical replicates. A closest Euclidean neighbor in the space of the principal components was found for each sample. The replicated samples were considered as consistent if a closest neighbor for replicate A was the corresponding replicate B and vice versa. The coordinates in the space of principal components for these replicates were averaged and they were considered as one sample. Samples that were not verified by this method were excluded.

Machine learning algorithms KNeighbors (kNN), logistic regression, support vector machine (SVM) and decision tree were used at the final step of the data analysis. In order to find optimal model hyper parameters, a grid search was used. As the number of experimental samples was not large enough, we did not use the separation of the dataset into training and test sets. We could not select a test set for the final quality verification of the models, since in this case the evaluation of the quality of the trained model would be very unstable, due to the randomness of the division of training and test sets, when marginal measurements may fall into the test set. Instead, we used the leave-one-out cross-validation on the whole dataset to control the model quality.

Accordingly, we excluded each sample from the entire set, trained the model on the remaining set, and then checked it on this extracted sample.

Then, we used mean accuracy metrics, i.e., the average proportion of correct answers to estimate the quality. This metrics seems to be adequate, because the class imbalance is insignificant (the ratio of class sizes does not exceed 3.2).

These procedures allowed us to use all available data as efficiently as possible and to avoid randomness in choosing a test sample.

5. Conclusions

The machine learning algorithms show good abilities to differentiate various groups across large data sets. Full proteomics data obtained by mass spectrometry can be very useful for this approach to medical diagnosis. These data contain general information about changes in normal body processes in those cases when common diagnostic approaches using single biomarkers or even panels of biomarkers do not work well enough. With the testing machine learning models on proteomics data obtained from the plasma and urine of patients of three types of CKD, the best results were obtained using the nearest-neighbor algorithm. In this case, according to the proteomics data of plasma, the two groups of patients with diabetic nephropathy and glomerulonephritis are well separated from the group of healthy people. On the other hand, a less presented group of patients with hypertensive nephropathy is better isolated from groups of patients of the two other CKD types by the "one against all" method based on the urine proteome data set.

The further development of the approach presented here may help to avoid invasive intervention and contraindicated intervention in some cases for the verification of the glomerulonephritis subtypes, which is currently performed only by kidney biopsy and microscopic morphological confirmation. The diagnosis of hypertensive and diabetic nephropathy at an early stage also remains relevant and the capabilities of machine learning methods based on proteomics data may be useful for this purpose.

Author Contributions: Conceptualization, methodology, mass spectrometry, software calculations, writing—original draft preparation, Y.E.G. and D.V.V.; blood and urine samples collection and preparation, medical investigations, I.A.L., M.L.R., S.A.V., and S.L.G.; medical investigations, writing—review and editing, T.N.Z. and M.M.P.; mass spectrometry experiments, Z.M.; supervision, review, and editing of the final version of the manuscript, M.V.B. and A.S.K. All authors have read and agreed to the published version of the manuscript.

Acknowledgments: The authors sincerely thank Ivan Denisov for help in preparing the manuscript.

Abbreviations

CKD	Chronic kidney disease
Scr	Serum creatinine
D	Diabetic nephropathy group
G	Glomerulonephritis group

H	Hypertonic nephropathy group
N	Healthy volunteers group
SD	Standard deviation
PCA	Principal components analysis
LFQ	Label-free quantification
kNN	K nearest neighbors algorithm
SVM	Support vector machine
MCP-1	Monocyte chemoattractant protein-1
TGF-β1	Transforming growth factor-β1
eGFR	Estimated glomerular filtration rate
FDR	False discovery rate

References

1. Levey, A.S.; Eckardt, K.-U.; Tsukamoto, Y.; Levin, A.; Coresh, J.; Rossert, J.; Zeeuw, D.D.E.; Hostetter, T.H.; Lameire, N.; Eknoyan, G. Definition and classification of chronic kidney disease: A position statement from Kidney Disease: Improving Global Outcomes (KDIGO). *Kidney Int.* **2005**, *67*, 2089–2100. [CrossRef]
2. Wang, Y.-N.; Ma, S.-X.; Chen, Y.-Y.; Chen, L.; Liu, B.-L.; Liu, Q.-Q.; Zhao, Y.-Y. Chronic kidney disease: Biomarker diagnosis to therapeutic targets. *Clin. Chim. Acta* **2019**, *499*, 54–63. [CrossRef] [PubMed]
3. Lamb, E.J.; MacKenzie, F.; Stevens, P.E. How should proteinuria be detected and measured? *Ann. Clin. Biochem.* **2009**, *46*, 205–217. [CrossRef] [PubMed]
4. Uchida, S. Differential diagnosis of chronic kidney disease (CKD): By primary diseases. *Jpn. Med. Assoc. J.* **2011**, *54*, 22–26.
5. Vassalotti, J.A.; Centor, R.; Turner, B.J.; Greer, R.C.; Choi, M.; Sequist, T.D. Practical Approach to Detection and Management of Chronic Kidney Disease for the Primary Care Clinician. *Am. J. Med.* **2016**, *129*, 153–162. [CrossRef] [PubMed]
6. Alebiosu, C.O.; Ayodele, O.E. The global burden of chronic kidney disease and the way forward. *Ethn. Dis.* **2005**, *15*, 418–423.
7. Cunningham, A.; Benediktsson, H.; Muruve, D.A.; Hildebrand, A.M.; Ravani, P. Trends in Biopsy-Based Diagnosis of Kidney Disease: A Population Study. *Can. J. Kidney Health Dis.* **2018**, *5*, 205435811879969. [CrossRef]
8. McMahon, G.M.; Waikar, S.S. Biomarkers in Nephrology: Core Curriculum 2013. *Am. J. Kidney Dis.* **2013**, *62*, 165–178. [CrossRef]
9. Bergón, E.; Granados, R.; Fernández-Segoviano, P.; Miravalles, E.; Bergón, M. Classification of Renal Proteinuria: A Simple Algorithm. *Clin. Chem. Lab. Med.* **2002**, *40*, 1143–1150. [CrossRef]
10. Mischak, H.; Delles, C.; Vlahou, A.; Vanholder, R. Proteomic biomarkers in kidney disease: Issues in development and implementation. *Nat. Rev. Nephrol.* **2015**, *11*, 221–232. [CrossRef] [PubMed]
11. Dakna, M.; Harris, K.; Kalousis, A.; Carpentier, S.; Kolch, W.; Schanstra, J.P.; Haubitz, M.; Vlahou, A.; Mischak, H.; Girolami, M. Addressing the Challenge of Defining Valid Proteomic Biomarkers and Classifiers. *BMC Bioinform.* **2010**, *11*, 594. [CrossRef] [PubMed]
12. Good, D.M.; Zürbig, P.; Argilés, À.; Bauer, H.W.; Behrens, G.; Coon, J.J.; Dakna, M.; Decramer, S.; Delles, C.; Dominiczak, A.F.; et al. Naturally Occurring Human Urinary Peptides for Use in Diagnosis of Chronic Kidney Disease. *Mol. Cell. Proteom.* **2010**, *9*, 2424–2437. [CrossRef] [PubMed]
13. Schanstra, J.P.; Zürbig, P.; Alkhalaf, A.; Argiles, A.; Bakker, S.J.L.; Beige, J.; Bilo, H.J.G.; Chatzikyrkou, C.; Dakna, M.; Dawson, J.; et al. Diagnosis and Prediction of CKD Progression by Assessment of Urinary Peptides. *J. Am. Soc. Nephrol.* **2015**, *26*, 1999–2010. [CrossRef] [PubMed]
14. Pontillo, C.; Jacobs, L.; Staessen, J.A.; Schanstra, J.P.; Rossing, P.; Heerspink, H.J.L.; Siwy, J.; Mullen, W.; Vlahou, A.; Mischak, H.; et al. A urinary proteome-based classifier for the early detection of decline in glomerular filtration. *Nephrol. Dial. Transplant.* **2017**, *32*, 1510–1516. [PubMed]
15. Argyropoulos, C.P.; Chen, S.S.; Ng, Y.-H.; Roumelioti, M.-E.; Shaffi, K.; Singh, P.P.; Tzamaloukas, A.H. Rediscovering Beta-2 Microglobulin As a Biomarker across the Spectrum of Kidney Diseases. *Front. Med.* **2017**, *4*, 73. [CrossRef]
16. Wu, J.; Chen, Y.; Gu, W. Urinary proteomics as a novel tool for biomarker discovery in kidney diseases. *J. Zhejiang Univ. Sci. B* **2010** *11*, 227–237. [CrossRef]

17. Haubitz, M.; Wittke, S.; Weissinger, E.M.; Walden, M.; Rupprecht, H.D.; Floege, J.; Haller, H.; Mischak, H. Urine protein patterns can serve as diagnostic tools in patients with IgA nephropathy. *Kidney Int.* **2005**, *67*, 2313–2320. [CrossRef]
18. Varghese, S.A.; Powell, T.B.; Budisavljevic, M.N.; Oates, J.C.; Raymond, J.R.; Almeida, J.S.; Arthur, J.M. Urine Biomarkers Predict the Cause of Glomerular Disease. *J. Am. Soc. Nephrol.* **2007**, *18*, 913–922. [CrossRef]
19. Sajda, P. Machine Learning for Detection and Diagnosis of Disease. *Annu. Rev. Biomed. Eng.* **2006**, *8*, 537–565. [CrossRef]
20. Sun, D. Development of New Diagnostic Techniques—Machine Learning. In *Substance and Non-substance Addiction*; Zhang, X., Shi, J., Tao, R., Eds.; Springer: Singapore, 2017; Volume 1010, pp. 203–215.
21. Lynch, C.J.; Liston, C. New machine-learning technologies for computer-aided diagnosis. *Nat. Med.* **2018**, *24*, 1304–1305. [CrossRef]
22. Titano, J.J.; Badgeley, M.; Schefflein, J.; Pain, M.; Su, A.; Cai, M.; Swinburne, N.; Zech, J.; Kim, J.; Bederson, J.; et al. Automated deep-neural-network surveillance of cranial images for acute neurologic events. *Nat. Med.* **2018**, *24*, 1337–1341. [CrossRef] [PubMed]
23. De Fauw, J.; Ledsam, J.R.; Romera-Paredes, B.; Nikolov, S.; Tomasev, N.; Blackwell, S.; Askham, H.; Glorot, X.; O'Donoghue, B.; Visentin, D.; et al. Clinically applicable deep learning for diagnosis and referral in retinal disease. *Nat. Med.* **2018**, *24*, 1342–1350. [CrossRef] [PubMed]
24. Lopez-Giacoman, S. Biomarkers in chronic kidney disease, from kidney function to kidney damage. *World J. Nephrol.* **2015**, *4*, 57–73. [CrossRef] [PubMed]
25. MacIsaac, R.J.; Tsalamandris, C.; Thomas, M.C.; Premaratne, E.; Panagiotopoulos, S.; Smith, T.J.; Poon, A.; Jenkins, M.A.; Ratnaike, S.I.; Power, D.A.; et al. The accuracy of cystatin C and commonly used creatinine-based methods for detecting moderate and mild chronic kidney disease in diabetes. *Diabet. Med.* **2007**, *24*, 443–448. [CrossRef] [PubMed]
26. Rysz, J.; Gluba-Brzózka, A.; Franczyk, B.; Jabłonowski, Z.; Ciałkowska-Rysz, A. Novel Biomarkers in the Diagnosis of Chronic Kidney Disease and the Prediction of Its Outcome. *Int. J. Mol. Sci.* **2017**, *18*, 1702. [CrossRef]
27. Swan, A.L.; Mobasheri, A.; Allaway, D.; Liddell, S.; Bacardit, J. Application of Machine Learning to Proteomics Data: Classification and Biomarker Identification in Postgenomics Biology. *OMICS J. Integr. Biol.* **2013**, *17*, 595–610. [CrossRef]
28. Verhave, J.C.; Bouchard, J.; Goupil, R.; Pichette, V.; Brachemi, S.; Madore, F.; Troyanov, S. Clinical value of inflammatory urinary biomarkers in overt diabetic nephropathy: A prospective study. *Diabetes Res. Clin. Pract.* **2013**, *101*, 333–340. [CrossRef] [PubMed]
29. Pena, M.J.; Heinzel, A.; Heinze, G.; Alkhalaf, A.; Bakker, S.J.L.; Nguyen, T.Q.; Goldschmeding, R.; Bilo, H.J.G.; Perco, P.; Mayer, B.; et al. A Panel of Novel Biomarkers Representing Different Disease Pathways Improves Prediction of Renal Function Decline in Type 2 Diabetes. *PLoS ONE* **2015**, *10*, e0120995. [CrossRef]
30. Alsaad, K.O.; Herzenberg, A.M. Distinguishing diabetic nephropathy from other causes of glomerulosclerosis: An update. *J. Clin. Pathol.* **2007**, *60*, 18–26. [CrossRef]
31. Cox, J.; Mann, M. MaxQuant enables high peptide identification rates, individualized p.p.b.-range mass accuracies and proteome-wide protein quantification. *Nat. Biotechnol.* **2008**, *26*, 1367–1372. [CrossRef]

8

Glomerular Deposition of Nephritis-Associated Plasmin Receptor (NAPlr) and Related Plasmin Activity: Key Diagnostic Biomarkers of Bacterial Infection-Related Glomerulonephritis

Takahiro Uchida * and Takashi Oda

Kidney Disease Center, Department of Nephrology and Blood Purification, Tokyo Medical University Hachioji Medical Center, Hachioji, Tokyo 193-0998, Japan; takashio@tokyo-med.ac.jp

* Correspondence: tu05090224@gmail.com

Abstract: It is widely known that glomerulonephritis (GN) often develops after the curing of an infection, a typical example of which is GN in children following streptococcal infections (poststreptococcal acute glomerulonephritis; PSAGN). On the other hand, the term "infection-related glomerulonephritis (IRGN)" has recently been proposed, because infections are usually ongoing at the time of GN onset in adult patients, particularly in older patients with comorbidities. However, there has been no specific diagnostic biomarker for IRGN, and diagnosis is based on the collection of several clinical and pathological findings and the exclusion of differential diagnoses. Nephritis-associated plasmin receptor (NAPlr) was originally isolated from the cytoplasmic fraction of group A streptococcus as a candidate nephritogenic protein for PSAGN and was found to be the same molecule as streptococcal glyceraldehyde-3-phosphate dehydrogenase and plasmin receptor. NAPlr deposition and related plasmin activity were observed with a similar distribution pattern in the glomeruli of patients with PSAGN. However, glomerular NAPlr deposition and plasmin activity could be observed not only in patients with PSAGN but also in patients with other glomerular diseases, in whom a preceding streptococcal infection was suggested. Furthermore, such glomerular staining patterns have been demonstrated in patients with IRGN induced by bacteria other than streptococci. This review discusses the recent advances in our understanding of the pathogenesis of bacterial IRGN, which is characterized by NAPlr and plasmin as key biomarkers.

Keywords: poststreptococcal acute glomerulonephritis; infection-related glomerulonephritis; nephritis-associated plasmin receptor; plasmin

---

1. Introduction

A wide variety of bacterial infection-related renal diseases are known, among which the most common is acute kidney injury (AKI) [1], which occurs as part of multiple organ failure. Changes in hemodynamics and cytokine expression are thought to be involved in the pathogenesis of AKI.

Bacterial infections also cause renal injury, partly through immune mechanisms. For example, glomerulonephritis (GN) can develop following streptococcal upper respiratory tract or skin infections with a latent period of approximately 10 days. As streptococcal infections are usually cured when GN is diagnosed and there is a distinct infection-free latent period, the GN has been referred to as poststreptococcal acute glomerulonephritis (PSAGN) [2–4].

In previous years, most cases of AGN were PSAGN in children; however, probably owing to the improvement of living environments and the adequate usage of antibiotics, the incidence of PSAGN has been decreasing, particularly in developed countries [4]. Whereas PSAGN is still the most common cause of pediatric AGN, adult AGN cases have been increasing, and those associated with non-streptococcal infections, particularly infections by *Staphylococcus aureus*, are now as common as PSAGN [5]. Thus, a major shift in the epidemiology of AGN has occurred. In Japan, cases of PSAGN, which accounted for more than two-thirds of AGN cases in the 1970s, decreased to about 30% after the 1980s, whereas AGN cases associated with *S. aureus* infections reached 30% in the 1990s [6].

Furthermore, in adult AGN patients, the infection is usually still present at the time when GN is diagnosed. Based on these backgrounds, instead of "postinfectious AGN", the disease concept of infection-related glomerulonephritis (IRGN) has recently been proposed [5]. Notably, whereas in most patients, PSAGN resolves without any specific therapy, the prognosis of patients with IRGN is poor, and older patients, particularly those with an immunocompromised background, such as diabetes mellitus, malignancies, or alcoholism, are reported to be at high risk [7]. Controlling the underlying infection and managing complications are essential for the treatment of IRGN, and immunosuppressive therapy is generally not recommended. However, the prompt diagnosis of IRGN is often difficult because specific diagnostic biomarkers have not yet been identified.

We herein present an overview of our recent understanding of the pathogenesis of bacterial IRGN. Accumulated data suggest that the disease concept of bacterial IRGN can be further expanded, and glomerular deposition of nephritis-associated plasmin receptor (NAPlr), originally considered to be a candidate nephritogenic protein for PSAGN [8] and related plasmin activity [9], can be used as general diagnostic biomarkers of bacterial IRGN. Although infections of various viruses, mycobacteria, fungi, or protozoa are also known to cause IRGN [1], they are not within the scope of this article.

2. NAPlr and Plasmin Activity in Glomeruli as Biomarkers of PSAGN

NAPlr is a 43-kDa protein that was originally isolated from the cytoplasmic fraction of group A streptococcus as a candidate nephritogenic protein for PSAGN [8]. Glomerular NAPlr deposition is detected by immunostaining, and is frequently observed in the early phase of PSAGN; all patients within 2 weeks of disease onset have been reported to show NAPlr deposition [2].

NAPlr was also found to be the same molecule as streptococcal glyceraldehyde-3-phosphate dehydrogenase (GAPDH) [8]. Although GAPDH is a well-known housekeeping gene, it also has pleiotropic functions, such as energy production (glycolysis), regulation of gene expression, and autophagy [10]. In addition, GAPDH from some bacteria, including streptococci, has been shown to have plasmin-binding activity [11,12].

NAPlr binds plasmin and maintains plasmin activity by protecting it from its physiological inhibitors. Plasmin activity can be detected by *in situ* zymography using a plasmin-sensitive synthetic substrate, which is resistant to the addition of α_2-antiplasmin but is completely abrogated by aprotinin, a serine protease inhibitor [9]. Plasmin is considered to cause glomerular damage directly by degrading extracellular matrix proteins and indirectly by activating pro–matrix metalloproteases. Additionally, plasmin can exert proinflammatory function by activating and accumulating inflammatory cells.

NAPlr is also known to convert complement component C3 to C3b, indicating its involvement in the activation of the alternative complement pathway [8]. However, it should be noted that NAPlr deposition is observed mainly in glomerular neutrophils, mesangial cells, and endothelial cells, and its distribution in glomeruli is different from that of C3 and IgG, which are considered to localize within the subepithelial hump [13]. In this regard, NAPlr, which also contains a urokinase-type plasminogen activator receptor (uPAR)-binding site [11], may bind with uPAR expressed on neutrophils, thereby inducing prominent endocapillary inflammation in early phase PSAGN, or NAPlr may be phagocytosed by neutrophils as exogenous material. Thus, glomerular damage from the disease may initially occur in the inner side of the glomerular capillary walls by NAPlr deposition, rather than subepithelial immune complexes.

Streptococcal pyrogenic exotoxin B (SPEB), which is another potential nephritogenic protein of PSAGN with cationic character, has been considered to pass through the glomerular basement membrane and be deposited in the subepithelial area [14]. However, a subsequent study showed that the glomerular distribution of NAPlr and SPEB were essentially similar and that NAPlr staining was dominant [13]. Importantly, as with NAPlr, SPEB has plasmin-binding activity [5]. Thus, it is possible that these 2 (or more) proteins are cooperatively involved in the disease pathogenesis of PSAGN. Figure 1 shows a scheme of the mechanisms involved in the development of PSAGN.

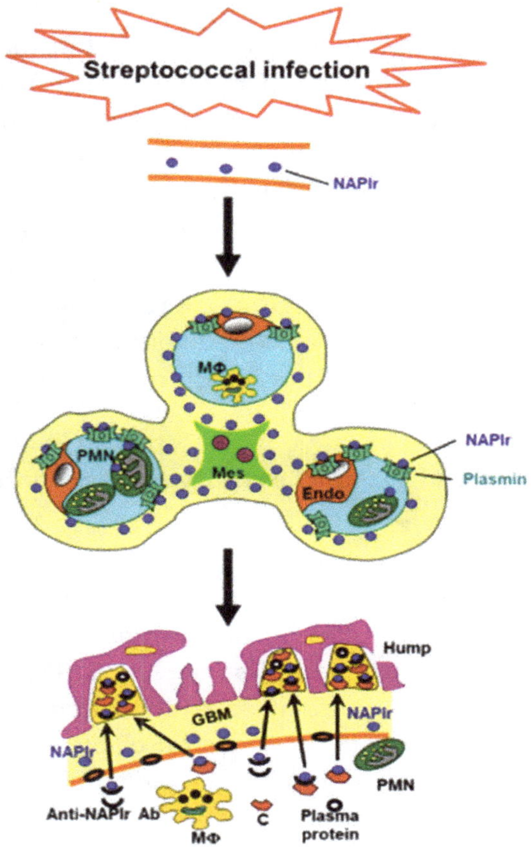

Figure 1. Putative mechanism for the development of poststreptococcal acute glomerulonephritis. Streptococcal infection induces the release of nephritogenic proteins, such as nephritis-associated plasmin receptor (NAPlr), into the circulation. Circulating NAPlr accumulates on the inner side of the glomerular capillary walls, and then traps and maintains the activity of plasmin, which induces glomerular damage by the degradation of extracellular matrix proteins or by activating and accumulating inflammatory cells. Thereafter, immune complexes, formed either *in situ* or in the circulation, pass through the altered glomerular basement membrane (GBM). Accumulation of immune complexes, complements, and plasma proteins forms "humps" on the outer side of the glomerular capillary walls. This scheme is based on the figure from Oda et al. [2]. Ab: antibody; C: complement; Endo: endothelial cell; Mes: mesangial cell; MΦ: macrophage; PMN: polymorphonuclear cell.

Some streptococcal strains have been isolated from PSAGN patients, and such strains have been considered to be "nephritogenic". However, NAPlr, as well as SPEB, have been found in virtually all streptococcal strains [14]. In addition, gene sequences of NAPlr were highly conserved and its protein expression levels were similar between various streptococcal strains [15]. Therefore, it is reasonable to think that any strains expressing NAPlr can be nephritogenic. Another possibility also remains that although NAPlr (and SPEB) are essential molecules, other factors, from both bacteria and the hosts, play important roles in the onset/progression of PSAGN.

There have been several reports showing the occurrence of IRGN in renal transplant recipients, suggesting that IRGN may be a cause of renal allograft injury [16,17]. We have recently encountered a renal transplant recipient who developed PSAGN; notably, NAPlr deposition and plasmin activity were observed in the glomeruli of the patient's transplanted kidney (manuscript in preparation).

3. Streptococcal Infection-related Nephritis (SIRN): Glomerular Diseases with NAPlr Deposition and Related Plasmin Activity Induced by Streptococcal Infection

The unique glomerular staining patterns of NAPlr and plasmin activity were found not only in patients with PSAGN but also in some patients with other glomerular diseases, such as C3 glomerulopathy [18,19], membranoproliferative glomerulonephritis (MPGN) type I [20,21], antineutrophil cytoplasmic antibody (ANCA)-associated vasculitis (both ANCA positive [22] and negative [23]), and IgA vasculitis [24], in which a preceding streptococcal infection is suggested by serological markers, and these cases are referred to as SIRN [2,25]. Although prominent endocapillary proliferation is a common histological feature, the differences in immune responses of the affected hosts may affect the specific histology. In addition, there have been some cases in which patients had a preceding streptococcal infection that initially occurred as PSAGN but later developed into C3 glomerulopathy [26]. It has also been reported that C3 nephritic factor activity is transiently observed in some PSAGN patients during the acute phase of the disease [27]. Thus, the disease concept of SIRN remains to be established, and there are no specific criteria differentiating patients with SIRN from those with the above glomerular diseases. However, it should be noted that streptococcal infections are associated with several forms of GN and that NAPlr and plasmin activity may be biomarkers of these diseases.

4. Glomerular NAPlr Deposition and Plasmin Activity as Candidates of General Biomarkers of Bacterial IRGN

The diagnosis of IRGN is made based on a combination of clinical and pathological findings. Nasr et al. [5] proposed the diagnostic criteria for IRGN as follows, in which at least 3 of the 5 items are required for a positive diagnosis: (1) clinical or laboratory evidence of infection preceding or at the onset of GN, (2) decrease in serum complement levels, (3) endocapillary proliferative and exudative glomerulonephritis, (4) C3-dominant or codominant glomerular immunofluorescence staining, and (5) hump-shaped subepithelial deposits on electron microscopy. The most common pathogen causing bacterial IRGN is staphylococcus, followed by streptococcus and Gram-negative bacteria. Infection sites are diverse, including the upper respiratory tract, skin, lung, and urinary tract, and the identification of foci is sometimes difficult. In addition, disease-specific diagnostic biomarkers have not been identified to date, and there are usually several differential diagnoses that show confounding clinical or pathological characteristics. Therefore, the prompt and accurate diagnosis of IRGN is often difficult.

Interestingly, glomerular NAPlr deposition and plasmin activity have recently been demonstrated in patients with IRGN induced by some bacterial strains, such as *Streptococcus pneumoniae* [28], *Aggregatibacter actinomycetemcomitans* (a Gram-negative coccobacillus that sometimes causes periodontal disease and infectious endocarditis) [29], *Mycoplasma pneumoniae* [30], or *S. aureus* (both methicillin-sensitive and -resistant strains; unpublished observations). The sequences of *S. pneumoniae* GAPDH share high identity with NAPlr, and the C-terminal sequences of *S. pneumoniae* GAPDH, which are most likely to be associated with the plasmin-binding activity, are completely identical to those of streptococcal GAPDH [28]. *M. pneumoniae* GAPDH has been shown to not only have cross-immunoreactivity to the anti-NAPlr antibody but also to have a plasmin-binding function. In addition, *M. pneumoniae* GAPDH has been reported to bind to plasminogen and convert it to plasmin [31]. As shown in Table 1, sequences of GAPDH from *A. actinomycetemcomitans* and *S. aureus* also show high similarity to that of NAPlr at the amino acid level, and *S. aureus* GAPDH has been reported to bind to enzymatically active plasmin [32]. As stated above, GAPDH sequences are highly preserved between streptococcal species [15], and it is, therefore, reasonable that GAPDH from these bacteria have plasmin-binding ability and that its deposition in glomeruli is detected by the anti-NAPlr antibody. However, it should be noted that although the glomerular staining pattern of NAPlr is essentially the same among patients with IRGN, the staining intensity in patients with non-streptococcal IRGN is generally weaker than in those with PSAGN. In this regard, the timing of when a renal biopsy is performed might affect the staining intensity; it could be possible that, in patients with non-streptococcal IRGN, performing renal biopsy during the acute phase is often avoided because of comorbidities or ongoing infection. Another possibility is that positive immunostaining of NAPlr in patients with non-streptococcal IRGN is caused by cross-immunoreactivity to the anti-NAPlr antibody, and is, therefore, weaker than that in patients with PSAGN.

Table 1. Identity and similarity of bacterial GAPDH and streptococcal GAPDH (nephritis-associated plasmin receptor; NAPlr).

Pathogen	Nucleotide		Amino acid	
	Identity	Similarity	Identity	Similarity
Aggregatibacter actinomycetemcomitans	59	59	50	85
Mycoplasma pneumonia	60	60	54	87
Staphylococcal aureus	54	54	67	92

Data are presented as percentages. Nucleotide and amino acid sequences of bacterial GAPDH registered with Kyoto Encyclopedia of Genes and Genomes (http://www.genome.jp/kegg/kegg_ja.html) were used, and identities and similarities were evaluated by Dr. Masayuki Fujino (the AIDS Research Center, National Institute of Infectious Diseases) using genetic information processing software (GENETYX-MAC ver. 18, GENETYX Corporation, Tokyo, Japan).

On the other hand, even if the overall amino acid sequence similarity is not very high, it is possible that some types of bacterial GAPDH, which have a similar steric structure at the antibody-binding site, show cross-immunoreactivity to the anti-NAPlr antibody. Indeed, positive staining for NAPlr and plasmin activity has been used as a marker of IGRN in patients with various forms of glomerulonephritis, such as proliferative glomerulonephritis with monoclonal immunoglobulin G deposits [33] and eosinophilic proliferative glomerulonephritis [34], even if neither the pathogens nor the infection sites could be identified. As the binding site of the anti-NAPlr antibody and that of plasmin in the GAPDH sequence would be different, the GAPDH of some bacteria are expected to bind with plasmin but not react with the anti-NAPlr antibody. In this regard, whether there are IRGN cases in which glomerular plasmin activity is observed without immunoreactivity to the anti-NAPlr antibody needs to be investigated in the future.

Collectively, GAPDH from various bacteria appear to react with the anti-NAPlr antibody and to have plasmin-binding ability, and positivity of the anti-NAPlr antibody and plasmin activity in glomeruli may act as both diagnostic and pathogenetic biomarkers of bacterial IRGN in general. Putative pathogenic mechanisms of IRGN, focusing on NAPlr and plasmin activity as biomarkers, are depicted in Figure 2.

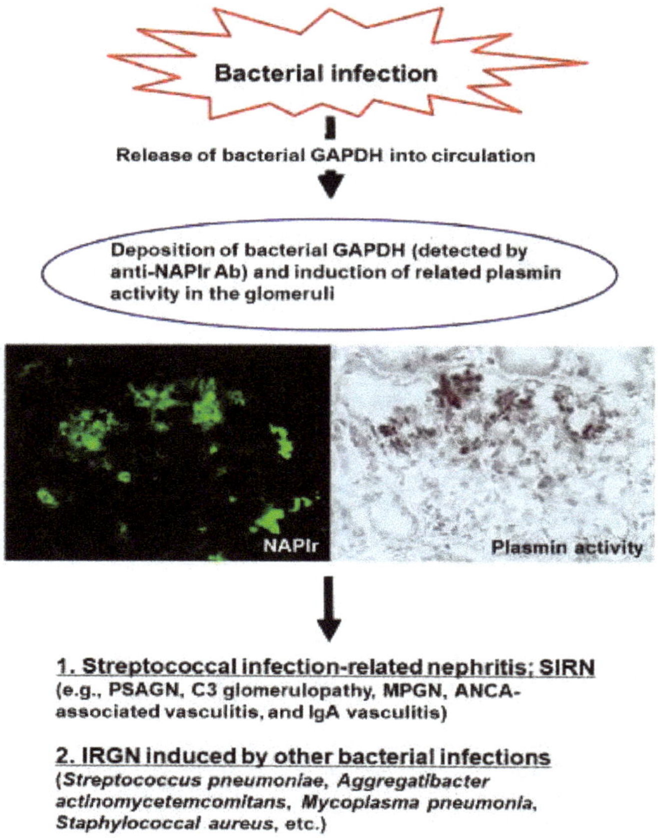

Figure 2. Possible scheme for the pathogenic mechanisms of bacterial infection-related glomerulonephritis (IRGN), focusing on the glomerular deposition of nephritis-associated plasmin receptor (NAPlr) and related plasmin activity. Ab: antibody; ANCA: antineutrophil cytoplasmic antibody; GAPDH: glyceraldehyde-3-phosphate dehydrogenase; MPGN: membranoproliferative glomerulonephritis; PSAGN: poststreptococcal acute glomerulonephritis.

5. NAPlr and Plasmin Activity in Extraglomerular Regions

In the previous study, NAPlr deposition has been observed almost exclusively in the glomeruli of IRGN patients, and the question hence arises as to whether NAPlr deposition is truly limited to the glomeruli. Interestingly, a case of PSAGN complicated by acute interstitial nephritis, in which positive SPEB immunostaining was observed in the interstitium as well as in the glomeruli, has been reported [35]. Although acute tubulointerstitial nephritis after streptococcal infection without obvious GN is rare, such a case has indeed been reported, in which SPEB immunostaining was positive in the affected area [36]. In the former case report [35], the authors also performed immunofluorescence staining of NAPlr using a commercially available antibody but failed to detect its deposition. In this regard, however, it should be noted that immunostaining results can vary depending on the antibodies used and the staining conditions [2]. Thus, whether NAPlr deposition occurs in the tubulointerstitial area or not should be examined more carefully using different antibodies and staining conditions. NAPlr immunofluorescence staining using an original antibody (and *in situ* zymography for plasmin activity) can be performed at the laboratory of Dr. Takashi Oda (Kidney Disease Center, Department of Nephrology and Blood Purification, Tokyo Medical University Hachioji Medical Center; takashio@tokyo-med.ac.jp).

Tubulointerstitial plasmin activity could be found in patients with various renal diseases unrelated to bacterial infection [9,37]. However, NAPlr deposition could not be observed, and plasmin activity was almost exclusively limited to the tubulointerstitial area in the renal tissues of these patients. Although definitive causative roles remain to be solved, this plasmin activity in the tubulointerstitial area may be involved in renal tubulointerstitial inflammation and fibrosis, because plasmin is supposed to induce the infiltration and activation of inflammatory cells and to induce fibrogenesis. Indeed, tubulointerstitial plasmin activity was associated with the degree of tubulointerstitial change, global glomerulosclerosis rate, and estimated glomerular filtration rate [37]. Data regarding tubulointerstitial plasmin activity in patients with IRGN are scarce, and, hence, further accumulation of cases is needed to investigate this matter in more detail.

PSAGN patients rarely show alveolar hemorrhage, and immune complex deposition is suggested in the pathogenesis of alveolar hemorrhage [38]. Therefore, another important issue that remains to be investigated is whether or not NAPlr deposition and related plasmin activity are observed in the lung tissue of patients with PSAGN complicated by alveolar hemorrhage. In this regard, an interesting case of IRGN, in which the causative pathogen was not detected but NAPlr deposition and plasmin activity were observed not only in the glomeruli but also in the renal tubulointerstitial area and pulmonary arteries, has recently been reported [34].

6. Concluding Remarks

NAPlr, isolated from the cytoplasmic fraction of group A streptococcus, has been shown to trap plasmin and maintain its activity and was originally considered as a nephritogenic protein for PSAGN. Indeed, NAPlr deposition and related plasmin activity have been observed to have an almost identical distribution in the glomeruli of early phase PSAGN patients at a high frequency. The interactions among NAPlr, plasmin activity, and SPEB and the association between these elements and complements or immune complexes, both *in vitro* and *in vivo*, should be investigated in future studies.

Some patients with other glomerular diseases, in whom a preceding streptococcal infection is clinically suggested, were found to also show glomerular NAPlr deposition and plasmin activity, and hence, these cases can be referred to as SIRN. Furthermore, such glomerular-staining patterns of NAPlr and plasmin activity are found in some patients with IRGN induced by other bacteria. The amino acid sequence of GAPDH from some types of bacteria show high similarity to the sequence of NAPlr and these bacterial GAPDH molecules appear to have a plasmin-binding ability. Even if the overall similarity is not so high, it is possible that some bacterial GAPDH molecules, which have a similar steric structure at the antibody-binding site, show cross-immunoreactivity to the anti-NAPlr antibody.

It has become evident that bacterial infections are more deeply involved in various renal diseases, including IRGN, than we previously considered. Although the development of noninvasive techniques to detect infections with high sensitivity and high specificity is undoubtedly crucial, the identification of bacterial proteins associated with the pathogenesis of IRGN is also an important ongoing effort. Thus, future studies evaluating the possibility of NAPlr and plasmin activity as common diagnostic biomarkers of bacterial IRGN are anticipated.

Author Contributions: Writing the manuscript draft: T.U.; manuscript revision: T.O. All authors have read and agreed to the published version of the manuscript.

Acknowledgments: We are grateful to Masayuki Fujino at the AIDS Research Center, National Institute of Infectious Diseases, for performing the database searches regarding amino acids and nucleotide sequences of bacterial GAPDH, and to Nobuyuki Yoshizawa at the Hemodialysis Unit, Showanomori Hospital, for his valuable advice and discussions.

References

1. Prasad, N.; Patel, M.R. Infection-Induced Kidney Diseases. *Front. Med.* **2018**, *5*, 327. [CrossRef] [PubMed]
2. Oda, T.; Yoshizawa, N.; Yamakami, K.; Sakurai, Y.; Takechi, H.; Yamamoto, K.; Oshima, N.; Kumagai, H. The role of nephritis-associated plasmin receptor (NAPlr) in glomerulonephritis associated with streptococcal infection. *J. Biomed. Biotechnol.* **2012**, *2012*, 417675. [CrossRef] [PubMed]
3. Soderholm, A.T.; Barnett, T.C.; Sweet, M.J.; Walker, M.J. Group A streptococcal pharyngitis: Immune responses involved in bacterial clearance and GAS-associated immunopathologies. *J. Leukoc. Biol.* **2018**, *103*, 193–213. [CrossRef] [PubMed]

4. Satoskar, A.A.; Parikh, S.V.; Nadasdy, T. Epidemiology, pathogenesis, treatment and outcomes of infection-associated glomerulonephritis. *Nat. Rev. Nephrol.* **2020**, *16*, 32–50. [CrossRef]
5. Nasr, S.H.; Radhakrishnan, J.; D'Agati, V.D. Bacterial infection-related glomerulonephritis in adults. *Kidney Int.* **2013**, *83*, 792–803. [CrossRef]
6. Usui, J.; Tawara-Iida, T.; Takada, K.; Ebihara, I.; Ueda, A.; Iwabuchi, S.; Ishizu, T.; Iitsuka, T.; Takemura, K.; Kawamura, T.; et al. Temporal Changes in Post-Infectious Glomerulonephritis in Japan (1976–2009). *PLoS ONE* **2016**, *11*, e0157356. [CrossRef]
7. Nasr, S.H.; Fidler, M.E.; Valeri, A.M.; Cornell, L.D.; Sethi, S.; Zoller, A.; Stokes, M.B.; Markowitz, G.S.; D'Agati, V.D. Postinfectious glomerulonephritis in the elderly. *J. Am. Soc. Nephrol.* **2011**, *22*, 187–195. [CrossRef]
8. Yoshizawa, N.; Yamakami, K.; Fujino, M.; Oda, T.; Tamura, K.; Matsumoto, K.; Sugisaki, T.; Boyle, M.D. Nephritis-associated plasmin receptor and acute poststreptococcal glomerulonephritis: Characterization of the antigen and associated immune response. *J. Am. Soc. Nephrol.* **2004**, *15*, 1785–1793. [CrossRef]
9. Oda, T.; Yamakami, K.; Omasu, F.; Suzuki, S.; Miura, S.; Sugisaki, T.; Yoshizawa, N. Glomerular plasmin-like activity in relation to nephritis-associated plasmin receptor in acute poststreptococcal glomerulonephritis. *J. Am. Soc. Nephrol.* **2005**, *16*, 247–254. [CrossRef]
10. Butera, G.; Mullappilly, N.; Masetto, F.; Palmieri, M.; Scupoli, M.T.; Pacchiana, R.; Donadelli, M. Regulation of Autophagy by Nuclear GAPDH and Its Aggregates in Cancer and Neurodegenerative Disorders. *Int. J. Mol. Sci.* **2019**, *20*, 2062. [CrossRef]
11. Terao, Y.; Yamaguchi, M.; Hamada, S.; Kawabata, S. Multifunctional glyceraldehyde-3-phosphate dehydrogenase of Streptococcus pyogenes is essential for evasion from neutrophils. *J. Biol. Chem.* **2006**, *281*, 14215–14223. [CrossRef] [PubMed]
12. Bergmann, S.; Rohde, M.; Hammerschmidt, S. Glyceraldehyde-3-phosphate dehydrogenase of Streptococcus pneumoniae is a surface-displayed plasminogen-binding protein. *Infect. Immun.* **2004**, *72*, 2416–2419. [CrossRef] [PubMed]
13. Oda, T.; Yoshizawa, N.; Yamakami, K.; Tamura, K.; Kuroki, A.; Sugisaki, T.; Sawanobori, E.; Higashida, K.; Ohtomo, Y.; Hotta, O.; et al. Localization of nephritis-associated plasmin receptor in acute poststreptococcal glomerulonephritis. *Hum. Pathol.* **2010**, *41*, 1276–1285. [CrossRef]
14. Rodriguez-Iturbe, B.; Batsford, S. Pathogenesis of poststreptococcal glomerulonephritis a century after Clemens von Pirquet. *Kidney Int.* **2007**, *71*, 1094–1104. [CrossRef]
15. Fujino, M.; Yamakami, K.; Oda, T.; Omasu, F.; Murai, T.; Yoshizawa, N. Sequence and expression of NAPlr is conserved among group A streptococci isolated from patients with acute poststreptococcal glomerulonephritis (APSGN) and non-APSGN. *J. Nephrol.* **2007**, *20*, 364–369. [PubMed]
16. Gopalakrishnan, N.; Jeyachandran, D.; Abeesh, P.; Dineshkumar, T.; Kurien, A.A.; Sakthirajan, R.; Balasubramaniyan, T. Infection-related glomerulonephritis in a renal allograft. *Saudi J. Kidney Dis. Transplant.* **2017**, *28*, 1421–1426.
17. Bullen, A.; Shah, M.M. De Novo Postinfectious Glomerulonephritis Secondary to Nephritogenic Streptococci as the Cause of Transplant Acute Kidney Injury: A Case Report and Review of the Literature. *Case Rep. Transplant.* **2018**, *2018*, 2695178. [CrossRef]
18. Sawanobori, E.; Umino, A.; Kanai, H.; Matsushita, K.; Iwasa, S.; Kitamura, H.; Oda, T.; Yoshizawa, N.; Sugita, K.; Higashida, K. A prolonged course of Group A streptococcus-associated nephritis: A mild case of dense deposit disease (DDD)? *Clin. Nephrol.* **2009**, *71*, 703–707. [CrossRef]
19. Suga, K.; Kondo, S.; Matsuura, S.; Kinoshita, Y.; Kitano, E.; Hatanaka, M.; Kitamura, H.; Hidaka, Y.; Oda, T.; Kagami, S. A case of dense deposit disease associated with a group A streptococcal infection without the involvement of C3NeF or complement factor H deficiency. *Pediatric Nephrol.* **2010**, *25*, 1547–1550. [CrossRef]
20. Yamakami, K.; Yoshizawa, N.; Wakabayashi, K.; Takeuchi, A.; Tadakuma, T.; Boyle, M.D. The potential role for nephritis-associated plasmin receptor in acute poststreptococcal glomerulonephritis. *Methods* **2000**, *21*, 185–197. [CrossRef]
21. Okabe, M.; Tsuboi, N.; Yokoo, T.; Miyazaki, Y.; Utsunomiya, Y.; Hosoya, T. A case of idiopathic membranoproliferative glomerulonephritis with a transient glomerular deposition of nephritis-associated plasmin receptor antigen. *Clin. Exp. Nephrol.* **2012**, *16*, 337–341. [CrossRef] [PubMed]
22. Kohatsu, K.; Suzuki, T.; Yazawa, M.; Yahagi, K.; Ichikawa, D.; Koike, J.; Oda, T.; Shibagaki, Y. Granulomatosis With Polyangiitis Induced by Infection. *Kidney Int. Rep.* **2019**, *4*, 341–345. [CrossRef] [PubMed]

23. Yano, K.; Suzuki, H.; Oda, T.; Ueda, Y.; Tsukamoto, T.; Muso, E. Crescentic poststreptococcal acute glomerulonephritis accompanied by small vessel vasculitis: Case report of an elderly male. *BMC Nephrol.* **2019**, *20*, 471. [CrossRef] [PubMed]
24. Kikuchi, Y.; Yoshizawa, N.; Oda, T.; Imakiire, T.; Suzuki, S.; Miura, S. Streptococcal origin of a case of Henoch-Schoenlein purpura nephritis. *Clin. Nephrol.* **2006**, *65*, 124–128. [CrossRef] [PubMed]
25. Iseri, K.; Iyoda, M.; Yamamoto, Y.; Kobayashi, N.; Oda, T.; Yamaguchi, Y.; Shibata, T. Streptococcal Infection-related Nephritis (SIRN) Manifesting Membranoproliferative Glomerulonephritis Type I. *Intern. Med.* **2016**, *55*, 647–650. [CrossRef]
26. Prasto, J.; Kaplan, B.S.; Russo, P.; Chan, E.; Smith, R.J.; Meyers, K.E. Streptococcal infection as possible trigger for dense deposit disease (C3 glomerulopathy). *Eur J. Pediatrics* **2014**, *173*, 767–772. [CrossRef]
27. Fremeaux-Bacchi, V.; Weiss, L.; Demouchy, C.; May, A.; Palomera, S.; Kazatchkine, M.D. Hypocomplementaemia of poststreptococcal acute glomerulonephritis is associated with C3 nephritic factor (C3NeF) IgG autoantibody activity. *Nephrol. Dial. Transplant.* **1994**, *9*, 1747–1750.
28. Odaka, J.; Kanai, T.; Ito, T.; Saito, T.; Aoyagi, J.; Betsui, H.; Oda, T.; Ueda, Y.; Yamagata, T. A case of post-pneumococcal acute glomerulonephritis with glomerular depositions of nephritis-associated plasmin receptor. *CEN Case Rep.* **2015**, *4*, 112–116. [CrossRef]
29. Komaru, Y.; Ishioka, K.; Oda, T.; Ohtake, T.; Kobayashi, S. Nephritis-associated plasmin receptor (NAPlr) positive glomerulonephritis caused by Aggregatibacter actinomycetemcomitans bacteremia: A case report. *Clin. Nephrol.* **2018**, *90*, 155–160. [CrossRef]
30. Hirano, D.; Oda, T.; Ito, A.; Yamada, A.; Kakegawa, D.; Miwa, S.; Umeda, C.; Takemasa, Y.; Tokunaga, A.; Wajima, T.; et al. Glyceraldehyde-3-phosphate dehydrogenase of Mycoplasma pneumoniae induces infection-related glomerulonephritis. *Clin. Nephrol.* **2019**, *92*, 263–272. [CrossRef]
31. Grundel, A.; Pfeiffer, M.; Jacobs, E.; Dumke, R. Network of Surface-Displayed Glycolytic Enzymes in Mycoplasma pneumoniae and Their Interactions with Human Plasminogen. *Infect. Immun.* **2015**, *84*, 666–676. [CrossRef] [PubMed]
32. Modun, B.; Williams, P. The staphylococcal transferrin-binding protein is a cell wall glyceraldehyde-3-phosphate dehydrogenase. *Infect. Immun.* **1999**, *67*, 1086–1092. [CrossRef] [PubMed]
33. Takehara, E.; Mandai, S.; Shikuma, S.; Akita, W.; Chiga, M.; Mori, T.; Oda, T.; Kuwahara, M.; Uchida, S. Post-infectious Proliferative Glomerulonephritis with Monoclonal Immunoglobulin G Deposits Associated with Complement Factor H Mutation. *Intern. Med.* **2017**, *56*, 811–817. [CrossRef] [PubMed]
34. Okabe, M.; Takamura, T.; Tajiri, A.; Tsuboi, N.; Ishikawa, M.; Ogura, M.; Ohashi, R.; Oda, T.; Yokoo, T. A case of infection-related glomerulonephritis with massive eosinophilic infiltration. *Clin. Nephrol.* **2018**, *90*, 142–147. [CrossRef] [PubMed]
35. Ando, F.; Sohara, E.; Ito, E.; Okado, T.; Rai, T.; Uchida, S.; Sasaki, S. Acute poststreptococcal glomerulonephritis with acute interstitial nephritis related to streptococcal pyrogenic exotoxin B. *Clin. Kidney J.* **2013**, *6*, 347–348. [CrossRef]
36. Chang, J.F.; Peng, Y.S.; Tsai, C.C.; Hsu, M.S.; Lai, C.F. A possible rare cause of renal failure in streptococcal infection. *Nephrol. Dial. Transplant.* **2011**, *26*, 368–371. [CrossRef]
37. Uchida, T.; Oda, T.; Takechi, H.; Matsubara, H.; Watanabe, A.; Yamamoto, K.; Oshima, N.; Sakurai, Y.; Kono, T.; Shimazaki, H.; et al. Role of tubulointerstitial plasmin in the progression of IgA nephropathy. *J. Nephrol.* **2016**, *29*, 53–62. [CrossRef]
38. Yoshida, M.; Yamakawa, H.; Yabe, M.; Ishikawa, T.; Takagi, M.; Matsumoto, K.; Hamaguchi, A.; Ogura, M.; Kuwano, K. Diffuse alveolar hemorrhage in a patient with acute poststreptococcal glomerulonephritis caused by impetigo. *Intern. Med.* **2015**, *54*, 961–964. [CrossRef]

9

Circulating Long Noncoding RNA LNC-EPHA6 Associates with Acute Rejection after Kidney Transplantation

Koen E. Groeneweg, Jacques M.G.J. Duijs, Barend W. Florijn, Cees van Kooten, Johan W. de Fijter, Anton Jan van Zonneveld, Marlies E.J. Reinders and Roel Bijkerk *

Department of Internal Medicine (Nephrology) and the Einthoven Laboratory for Vascular and Regenerative Medicine, Leiden University Medical Center, Albinusdreef 2, 2333 ZA Leiden, Zuid Holland, The Netherlands; k.e.groeneweg@lumc.nl (K.E.G.); J.M.G.J.Duijs@lumc.nl (J.M.G.J.D.); b.w.florijn@lumc.nl (B.W.F.); C.van_Kooten@lumc.nl (C.v.K.); J.W.de_Fijter@lumc.nl (J.W.d.F.); A.J.van_Zonneveld@lumc.nl (A.J.v.Z.); M.E.J.Reinders@lumc.nl (M.E.J.R.)

* Correspondence: R.Bijkerk@lumc.nl

Abstract: Acute rejection (AR) of a kidney graft in renal transplant recipients is associated with microvascular injury in graft dysfunction and, ultimately, graft failure. Circulating long noncoding RNAs (lncRNAs) may be suitable markers for vascular injury in the context of AR. Here, we first investigated the effect of AR after kidney transplantation on local vascular integrity and demonstrated that the capillary density markedly decreased in AR kidney biopsies compared to pre-transplant biopsies. Subsequently, we assessed the circulating levels of four lncRNAs (LNC-RPS24, LNC-EPHA6, MALAT1, and LIPCAR), that were previously demonstrated to associate with vascular injury in a cohort of kidney recipients with a stable kidney transplant function (n = 32) and recipients with AR (n = 15). The latter were followed longitudinally six and 12 months after rejection. We found higher levels of circulating LNC-EPHA6 during rejection, compared with renal recipients with a stable kidney function (p = 0.017), that normalized one year after AR. In addition, LNC-RPS24, LNC-EPHA6, and LIPCAR levels correlated significantly with the vascular injury marker soluble thrombomodulin. We conclude that AR and microvascular injury are associated with higher levels of circulating LNC-EPHA6, which emphasizes the potential role of lncRNAs as biomarker in the context of AR.

Keywords: long noncoding RNA; kidney transplantation; rejection; microvascular injury

---

1. Introduction

Acute rejection (AR) is considered to be a prominent cause of graft failure in the first year after transplantation in kidney transplant recipients [1,2], although the long-term consequences of AR remain a subject of discussion. Despite better screening and improved immune suppressive therapies, rejection is still suspected to cause a significant proportion of death censored graft failure after kidney transplantation [3,4]. Previous research showed a prolonged effect on kidney function deterioration as well as graft survival after a rejection episode [2]. Microvascular endothelial cells (ECs) are very susceptible to injury, that can result from episodes of AR. Following the alloimmune response, cytokines and growth factors are produced that can lead to EC activation and microvascular destabilization [5–10]. These rejection-associated events can result in perpetual EC damage and promotion of (aberrant) angiogenesis within the allograft [5,7,9]. Together, these insults can lead to the loss of the microvasculature, chronic ischemia and cell death [11,12], and ultimately, to the development of interstitial fibrosis/tubular atrophy and graft dysfunction [5,6,9]. Therefore, monitoring the course of microvascular injury after rejection could be beneficial in deciding on the best treatment strategies. Previously, we found the vascular injury markers soluble thrombomodulin (sTM) and Angiopoietin-2 (Ang-2) to increase upon AR. sTM normalized in the first year after AR, while Ang-2 remained elevated [13]. Noncoding RNA, such as micro RNAs (miRNA) and long noncoding RNAs (lncRNA)are increasingly recognized to play an important role in vascular injury [14]. The functions of lncRNAs appear to be very diverse as they can bind DNA, proteins, and other RNAs. E.g. lncRNAs have been demonstrated to serve as a scaffold for transcription factors or can assist chromatin-modifying enzymes, thereby regulating gene expression [15]. LncRNAs were also found to be important for miRNA processing, (alternative) splicing, translation and post-transcriptional regulation, for instance via sponging miRNAs [16,17]. In addition, lncRNAs can be promising biomarkers in a variety of vascular diseases and kidney injury [14,16]. Furthermore, lncRNAs have previously been associated with AR [18], but their dynamics after rejection have not been studied before. Earlier, we described that specific lncRNAs (MALAT1, LNC-RPS24, LNC-EPHA6, and LIPCAR) associate with microvascular damage and angiogenic factors in patients with diabetic nephropathy that received simultaneous kidney-pancreas transplantation [19], but their relation with AR and associated vascular damage is unclear. As such, in this study we first explored the relation of AR with local microvascular injury. Then, in a cross-sectional study of patients with T cell mediated AR, we analyzed selected vascular injury related lncRNAs as potential biomarkers for vascular damage in the context of kidney transplant rejection and assess the dynamics in these lncRNAs after rejection.

2. Results

2.1. *Decreased Capillary Density in Acute Rejection Biopsies*

To assess the impact of AR on the local capillary density in the kidney, we quantified the number of endothelial cells (EC) and pericytes in archival acute rejection biopsies by immunohistochemical staining of the EC for CD34 antigen and the pericytes for the CD73 marker (resp. $n = 102$ and $n = 29$). Subsequently, we compared these parameters to the available pre-transplant biopsies (resp. $n = 78$ and $n = 66$) of these patients [20]. Patient characteristics can be found in Supplementary Table S1. As shown in Figure 1, we observed a strong decrease in both the number of endothelial cells (~2.5-fold, mboxemphp < 0.0001) as well as pericytes (~6-fold, $p < 0.0001$) in AR, indicating loss of the peritubular capillary network in AR.

2.2. *Patient Characteristics of Cross Sectional and Longitudinal AR Study Population*

Next, we sought to investigate the relation of circulating lncRNAs with AR. To that end, we included plasma samples of a different cross-sectional study cohort that included patients with acute T cell mediated rejection and a control group of patients with stable kidney transplant function after transplantation (hereafter mentioned as 'stable'). In addition, AR patients were studied longitudinally at 6 and 12 months after rejection to determine the dynamics after AR. The baseline characteristics of the transplant recipients in this cohort are described in Table 1. Most common causes of initial kidney failure before transplantation were autosomal dominant polycystic kidney disease (23%), focal segmental glomerulosclerosis (17%) and IgA nephropathy (13%). The mean time after transplantation (12 months) was comparable. Immunosuppressive regimen did not differ significantly. eGFR was lower and proteinuria higher in patients with AR, compared with stable patients (resp. $p < 0.001$ and $p = 0.003$). Factors that can influence the amount of vascular injury next to rejection, such as donor age, dialysis before transplantation, and months since transplantation, did not differ significantly. Incidence of active smokers was 7% in AR patients and 13% in stable patients. Panel reactive antibodies (PRA), mismatch, immunosuppressive regimen and the presence of previous transplantations did not differ between stable patients and patients with AR. Patients with AR had interstitial rejection, with or without involvement of the vasculature, and were treated with methylprednisolone (67%), ATG alone (13%), or a combination of methylprednisolone and ATG (13%) or alemtuzumab (13%).

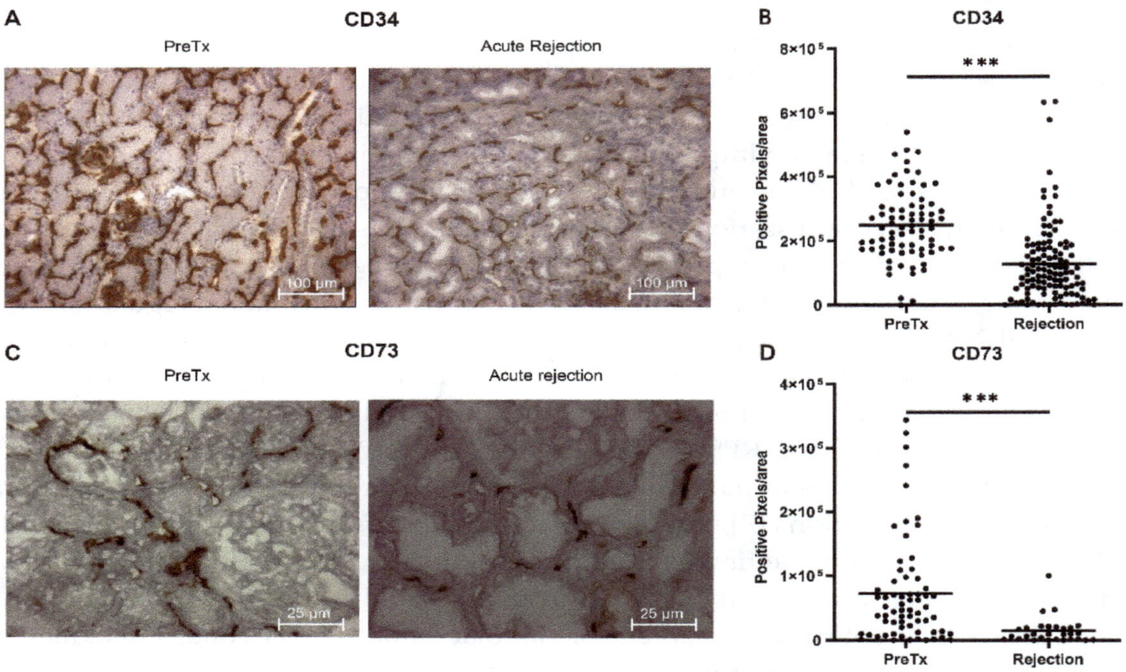

Figure 1. Decreased capillary density after acute rejection. (**A**) Representative images of CD34 staining for pre-transplantation and acute rejection (AR) biopsies. (**B**) Quantification of CD34 staining (PreTx, $n = 78$; AR, $n = 102$). (**C**) Representative images of CD73 staining for pre-transplantation and acute rejection (AR) biopsies. (**D**) Quantification of CD73 staining (PreTx, $n = 66$, AR, $n = 29$). *** p-value < 0.001.

Table 1. Cross-sectional study patient characteristics of patients with a stable kidney transplant function (stable) and patients with acute rejection (AR).

	Stable ($n = 32$)	AR ($n = 15$)	p-Value
Sex, *Male, n* (%)	21 (66%)	10 (67%)	1.00 [1]
Age, *Years ± SD*	51 ± 14	54 ± 12	0.35 [2]
BMI (kg/m^2)	26.4 ± 4.6	24.4 ± 3.5	0.15 [1]
Preemptive, *n* (%)	16 (50%)	5 (33%)	0.36 [1]
Months Since KTx, *Median (IQR)*	12 ± 1	12 ± 15	0.97 [2]
PRA >5%, *n* (%)	6 (19%)	1 (7%)	0.40 [1]
Previous Transplantations, *n* (%)	2 (6%)	3 (20%)	0.31 [1]
Mismatch A/B/DR, *Mean*	1.0/1.2/0.8	0.9/1.3/1.0	0.76/0.81/0.63 [1]
Donor Characteristics			
Sex, *male, n (%)*	11 (34%)	7 (47%)	0.52 [1]
Age, *years ± SD*	50 ± 17	47 ± 12	0.64 [2]
Induction Therapy, *n* (%)			0.54 [1]
Alemtuzumab	3 (9%)	0	
IL-2 receptor inhibitor	29 (91%)	15 (100%)	
Immunosuppressive Drugs, *n* (%)			
Tacrolimus	22 (69%)	8 (53%)	0.20 [1]
Cyclosporine	5 (16%)	3 (20%)	1.00 [1]
Prednisone	32 (100%)	14 (93%)	0.32 [1]
Mycophenolate mofetil	25 (78%)	8 (53%)	0.07 [1]
Everolimus	6 (19%)	1 (7%)	0.40 [1]

Table 1. *Cont.*

	Stable (n = 32)	AR (n = 15)	p-Value
Acute Rejection Therapy, *n* (%)			
ATG		2 (13%)	
methylprednisolone	-	10 (67%)	
methylprednisolone + ATG	-	2 (13%)	
methylprednisolone + alemtuzumab	-	1 (7%)	
eGFR (mL/min/1.73 m²)	54 ± 12	34 ± 14	<0.001 [2]
Proteinuria (g/24 h), Median *(IQR)*	0.17 (0.13–0.25)	0.36 (0.23–1.19)	0.003 [3]

[1] Fisher's exact test, [2] unpaired t-test, [3] Mann-Whitney U test, KTx = kidney transplantation, PRA = panel reactive antibody.

2.3. *Circulating LNC-EPHA6 Levels Directly Correlate with Acute Rejection*

In order to assess the relationship between AR and vascular injury related lncRNAs LNC-RPS24, MALAT1, LNC-EPHA6, and LIPCAR, circulating levels of these lncRNAs were measured in stable patients and AR patients. In this cohort, MALAT1 levels were only detectable in less than 30% of patients and therefore not included in further analyses. Relative expression of circulating LNC-EPHA6 was significantly higher in patients with AR, compared with stable patients (p = 0.017; Figure 2). LNC-RPS24 and LIPCAR showed a similar trend, although these differences did not reach statistical significance (resp. p = 0.11 and p = 0.16).

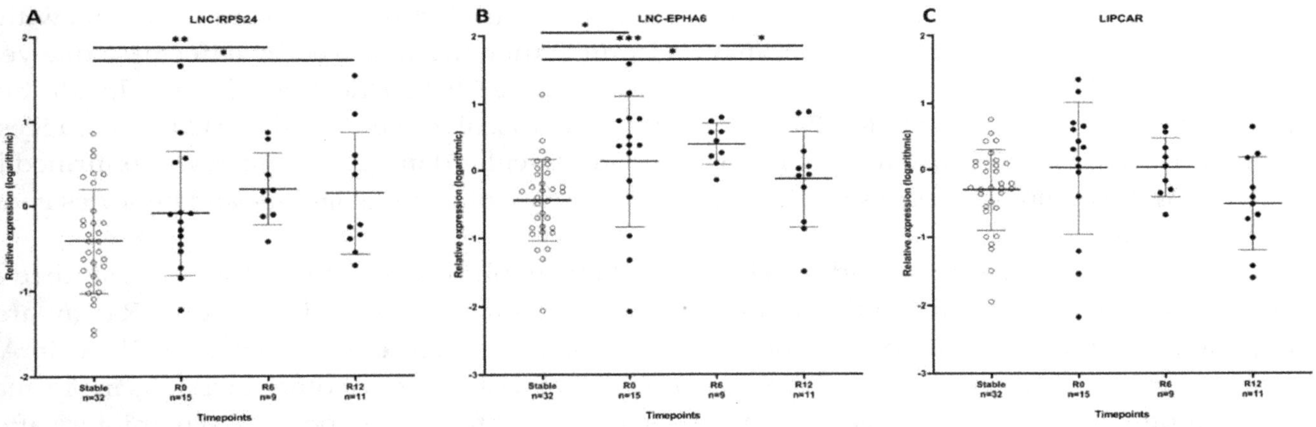

Figure 2. Circulating lncRNA levels are effected by acute rejection. Relative expression of LNC-RPS24 (**A**), LNC-EPHA6 (**B**), and LIPCAR (**C**) in the cross-sectional cohort; kidney recipients with a stable kidney function (Stable; n = 32), kidney recipients with acute rejection at the time of rejection (R0), and 6 and 12 months after rejection (R6 and R12). Data are presented as mean ± SD, * p-value < 0.05, ** p-value < 0.01, *** p-value < 0.001.

2.4. *Circulating LNC-EPHA6 Decreases in the First Year After Acute Rejection*

Since vascular damage persists after a rejection episode, patients with AR were followed longitudinally to study the dynamics of lncRNAs in the first year after AR. Elevated levels of circulating LNC-EPHA6 persisted until six months after AR (p < 0.001) and decreased significantly one year after rejection, although LNC-EPHA6 levels at one year after rejection remained slightly higher levels than in stable patients (p = 0.03; Figure 2). LIPCAR showed a similar pattern without reaching significance (p = 0.16), while LNC-RPS24 increased one year after transplantation (Figure 2). eGFR did not change significantly the year after AR.

2.5. LNC-RPS24, LNC-EPHA6 and LIPCAR Correlate with Soluble Thrombomodulin

In order to analyze the association of lncRNAs with vascular injury due to AR, we studied the correlation of LNC-RPS24, LNC-EPHA6, and LIPCAR with vascular injury markers sTM and Ang-2 that were previously assessed [13]. There, we showed a significant increase of sTM levels in patients with acute rejection, followed by a subsequent normalization one year after transplantation, while the ratio between Ang-2 and Ang-1 (mainly determined by Ang-2) significantly increased during AR without significant changes afterwards. Here, no significant associations were found between LNC-RPS24, LNC-EPHA6, and LIPCAR with Ang-2. However, interestingly, LNC-RPS24, LNC-EPHA6, and LIPCAR correlated positively with sTM (Table 2).

Table 2. Correlation of lncRNAs with vascular injury markers sTM, Ang-2. Values represent correlation coefficient and p-value.

	LNC-RPS24	LNC-EPHA6	LIPCAR
Vascular injury markers			
sTM	0.331 ($p = 0.035$)	0.383 ($p = 0.013$)	0.321 ($p = 0.041$)
Ang-2	ns	ns	ns

sTM = soluble thrombomodulin, Ang-2 = Angiopoietin-2.

3. Discussion

Our study shows that levels of circulating LNC-EPHA6 are significantly higher in patients with T cell-mediated AR after renal transplantation, compared with kidney transplant recipients with a stable allograft function. LNC-EPHA6 remains elevated after AR, followed by a decrease one year after rejection. LIPCAR shows a similar pattern, but did not reach statistical significance. In addition, LNC-EPHA6, LIPCAR, and LNC-RPS24 correlate with the vascular injury marker sTM. This suggests that, in particular, LNC-EPHA6 may be related to microvascular damage, of which we confirmed its relation to AR by demonstrating a significantly lower presence of endothelial cells and pericytes in our renal biopsy study.

LNC-EPHA6 was earlier found to relate to diabetic nephropathy [19], but was not studied in the context of AR before. Our finding of higher LNC-EPHA6 levels in patients with AR compared with patients without AR provided proof of principle of the biomarker potential of lncRNAs in AR. However, here we analyzed four pre-selected lncRNAs, thus analyses of other lncRNAs in AR may yield additional associations and may potentially be important for prediction of (vascular injury after) AR. This is in line with two other studies that showed an association between lncRNAs and AR that suggested their value for diagnosis of AR in kidney transplantation [21,22]. Moreover, in a rat study, the lncRNA PRINS was shown to be significantly up-regulated in kidneys of rats with cold ischemia-elicited allograft rejection, compared with rats without rejection [23]. In addition, lncRNAs may also be of value in predicting the development of chronic damage after kidney transplantation [24].

Interestingly, levels of circulating LNC-EPHA6 decrease after AR, while eGFR remains stable. This substantiates that changes in LNC-EPHA6 are likely not to be related to changes in kidney function, but other factors in the pathogenesis of AR, such as persisting microvascular injury. This suggestion is supported by the strong correlation with sTM. However, although significant differences between immunosuppressive drug regimen were not observed, we cannot exclude that differences in rejection treatment altered levels of circulating lncRNAs. Furthermore, an association with the function of the EPHA6 gene might be possible, since lncRNAs are frequently co-regulated and co-expressed with their neighboring genes [25]. The EPHA6 gene is part of a EPH receptor tyrosine kinases family, and thereby interacts with ephrins which subsequently regulates several cellular processes including angiogenesis [26,27].

LIPCAR showed a similar trend after rejection as LNC-EPHA6. This could suggest a similar association as LNC-EPHA6 with rejection. However, changes in LIPCAR did not reach statistical significance due to a large variation. Analysis of LIPCAR in a larger cohort of patients with AR may confirm the link with vascular injury in rejection, since the size of our groups limits the interpretation of LIPCAR in our study. Circulating LNC-RPS24 was only marginally higher in rejection, but increased six months after year after rejection and remained higher. Although speculative, this may be the result of persistent vascular injury after AR or a consequence of the rejection treatment. Lastly, we found LncRNA MALAT1 to be only detectable in less than 30% of the patients in our cohort. Previously, MALAT1 was however detectable in most diabetes mellitus patients [19], suggesting that diabetes mellitus may increase circulating Malat1 levels. However, next to the previously mentioned limited group size, a relatively large spread of lncRNA levels within groups limits the possibility of drawing robust conclusions. The interpretation of subtle changes (e.g., correlation of lncRNAs with the specific Banff classification score for tubulitis, interstitial inflammation, and intimal arteritis) is difficult and larger groups are necessary for the identification of a specific lncRNA as a novel biomarker. However, differences in lncRNAs levels point out the interesting possible added value of lncRNAs in the context of acute cellular rejection. Identification of lncRNAs in the context of antibody-mediated rejection would be interesting as well, since this rare condition also has major implications for the amount of vascular injury.

In conclusion, LNC-EPHA6 is higher in kidney transplant recipients with rejection, compared with those without. This is the first study that shows changes in vascular injury related lncRNAs the first year after rejection. The results suggest that lncRNAs may reflect (micro)vascular damage in the context of rejection and emphasizes the potential role of lncRNAs as biomarkers to monitor vascular injury in kidney transplant rejection.

4. Materials and Methods

4.1. Renal Biopsy Study

Renal biopsies were selected from patients that had a biopsy proven acute renal allograft rejection, as previously described [20]. Patient and transplantation characteristics are summarized in Supplementary Table S1. Frozen biopsy tissue sections (4 μm) were fixed in acetone, endogenous peroxidase was blocked with H2O2, and slides were blocked with 1% bovine serum albumin and 5% normal human serum in PBS. Sections were then incubated with specific antibodies directed against CD34 (BD Biosciences, Breda, The Netherlands) and CD73 (BD Biosciences, Breda, The Netherlands) followed by appropriate secondary antibodies that were HRP-conjugated (Jackson Immunoresearch, Westgrove, PA, USA). Stainings were visualized using Nova RED (Vector Labs, Peterborough, UK). Quantification of immunohistological staining results was performed using image J software.

4.2. Patient Study Cohort

A total of 47 patients were enrolled in a cross-sectional, observational, single center study. All patients were transplanted between 2006 and 2012 in the Leiden University Medical Center (LUMC) in Leiden, The Netherlands. The cohort consisted of 2 groups, namely renal transplant recipients with AR (n = 15) and a control group consisting of renal recipients 12 months after transplantation without rejection and with a stable kidney transplant function (n = 32). In addition, recipients from the rejection group were followed longitudinally. Plasma samples were obtained at 6 and 12 months after rejection.

The cohort has been described earlier where analysis of circulating Ang-2 and sTM in plasma was performed [13].

All subjects gave their informed consent for inclusion before they participated in the study. The study was conducted in accordance with the Declaration of Helsinki, and the protocol was approved by the Ethics Committee of The Leiden University Medical Center (P09.141).

4.3. Immunosuppressive Drugs, Rejection and Rejection Treatment

All patients received immunosuppressive drug therapy according to the standard of care at the time of transplantation. IL-2 receptor inhibitor as induction therapy was the standard of care and alemtuzumab was administered in case the treating physician expected a higher risk of rejection. The presence and type of rejection was assessed using the Banff classification. The choice for a specific rejection treatment was made according to the standard of care at the time of rejection [13].

4.4. RNA Isolation

The RNeasy Micro Kit (Qiagen, Venlo, The Netherlands) was used with an adapted protocol, to isolate total RNA from 200 μL plasma. In summary, using 800 trizol μL reagent (Invitrogen, Breda, The Netherlands), the plasma/Trizol sample was centrifuged for 15 min (15,000× g) after the addition of 160 μL chloroform. Then, 100% ethanol (1.5 volume) was added to the aqueous phase and transferred to a MinElute Spin column (Qiagen) followed by centrifugation for 15 s (18,000× g). Subsequently, 700 μL RWT buffer and twice 500 μL RPE buffer was used to wash the column. The column was centrifuged (18,000× g) for 15 s after the first two washing steps and 2 min (18,000× g) after the third washing step. 15 μL RNase-free water was added for elution of the RNA.

4.5. RT-qPCR

To quantify circulating lncRNA levels we performed RT-qPCR. Isolated RNA was reverse transcribed using Iscript (Biorad) according to the protocol of the manufacturer. RT-qPCR of target genes was done using SYBR Green Master Mix (Applied Biosystems, Waltham, MA, USA). The primer sequences of target lncRNAs are given in Supplementary Table S2.

4.6. Statistical Analyses

Categorical data are described as total count and percentages, parametric data as mean ±standard deviation (SD), and non-parametric data as median and interquartile range (IQR). Testing for differences of baseline characteristics was performed by using Fishers exact test for categorical data and the unpaired t test and Mann–Whitney U test for parametric and non-parametric data.

Circulating lncRNA levels were normalized by the double delta CT method to miR-16 and subsequently transformed logarithmically (with base 10). The logarithmic relative expression of all three lncRNAs was normally distributed. In the longitudinal study the data was analyzed by using a linear mixed model analysis. Analysis of correlations between the lncRNAs and vascular markers was performed using Spearman rank correlation.

A p-value < 0.05 was considered to be statistically significant. SPSS version 23.0 (SPSS, Inc., Chicago, IL, USA) was used for the data analysis and Graphpad Prism version 8.0 (Graphpad Prism Software, Inc., San Diego, CA, USA).

Author Contributions: Conceptualization, R.B. and A.J.v.Z.; Methodology, R.B.; Software, K.E.G.; Validation K.E.G., R.B. and J.M.G.J.D.; Formal Analysis, K.E.G.; Investigation J.M.G.J.D. and B.W.F.; Resources M.E.J.R.; Data Curation K.E.G.; Writing–Original Draft Preparation K.E.G. and R.B.; Writing–Review & Editing, J.M.G.J.D., B.W.F., C.v.K., J.W.d.F., A.J.v.Z., M.E.J.R. and R.B.; Visualization K.E.G.; Supervision, A.J.v.Z., M.E.J.R. and R.B.; Project Administration K.E.G. and R.B.; Funding Acquisition, A.J.v.Z. and R.B. All authors have read and agreed to the published version of the manuscript.

References

1. Chand, S.; Atkinson, D.; Collins, C.; Briggs, D.; Ball, S.; Sharif, A.; Skordilis, K.; Vydianath, B.; Neil, D.; Borrows, R. The Spectrum of Renal Allograft Failure. *PLoS ONE* **2016**, *11*, e0162278. [CrossRef]
2. Clayton, P.A.; McDonald, S.P.; Russ, G.R.; Chadban, S.J. Long-Term Outcomes after Acute Rejection in Kidney Transplant Recipients: An ANZDATA Analysis. *J. Am. Soc. Nephrol.* **2019**, *30*, 1697–1707. [CrossRef]

3. El-Zoghby, Z.M.; Stegall, M.D.; Lager, D.J.; Kremers, W.K.; Amer, H.; Gloor, J.M.; Cosio, F.G. Identifying specific causes of kidney allograft loss. *Am. J. Transpl.* **2009**, *9*, 527–535. [CrossRef]
4. Park, W.Y.; Paek, J.H.; Jin, K.; Park, S.B.; Choe, M.; Han, S. Differences in Pathologic Features and Graft Outcomes of Rejection on Kidney Transplant. *Transpl. Proc.* **2019**, *51*, 2655–2659. [CrossRef]
5. Bruneau, S.; Woda, C.B.; Daly, K.P.; Boneschansker, L.; Jain, N.G.; Kochupurakkal, N.; Contreras, A.G.; Seto, T.; Briscoe, D.M. Key Features of the Intragraft Microenvironment that Determine Long-Term Survival Following Transplantation. *Front Immunol.* **2012**, *3*, 54. [CrossRef]
6. Contreras, A.G.; Briscoe, D.M. Every allograft needs a silver lining. *J. Clin. Investig.* **2007**, *117*, 3645–3648. [CrossRef]
7. Denton, M.D.; Davis, S.F.; Baum, M.A.; Melter, M.; Reinders, M.E.; Exeni, A.; Samsonov, D.V.; Fang, J.; Ganz, P.; Briscoe, D.M. The role of the graft endothelium in transplant rejection: Evidence that endothelial activation may serve as a clinical marker for the development of chronic rejection. *Pediatr. Transpl.* **2000**, *4*, 252–260. [CrossRef]
8. Reinders, M.E.; Fang, J.C.; Wong, W.; Ganz, P.; Briscoe, D.M. Expression patterns of vascular endothelial growth factor in human cardiac allografts: Association with rejection. *Transplantation* **2003**, *76*, 224–230. [CrossRef]
9. Reinders, M.E.; Rabelink, T.J.; Briscoe, D.M. Angiogenesis and endothelial cell repair in renal disease and allograft rejection. *J. Am. Soc. Nephrol.* **2006**, *17*, 932–942. [CrossRef]
10. Reinders, M.E.; Sho, M.; Izawa, A.; Wang, P.; Mukhopadhyay, D.; Koss, K.E.; Geehan, C.S.; Luster, A.D.; Sayegh, M.H.; Briscoe, D.M. Proinflammatory functions of vascular endothelial growth factor in alloimmunity. *J. Clin. Investig.* **2003**, *112*, 1655–1665. [CrossRef]
11. Bishop, G.A.; Waugh, J.A.; Landers, D.V.; Krensky, A.M.; Hall, B.M. Microvascular destruction in renal transplant rejection. *Transplantation* **1989**, *48*, 408–414. [CrossRef]
12. Long, D.A.; Norman, J.T.; Fine, L.G. Restoring the renal microvasculature to treat chronic kidney disease. *Nat. Rev. Nephrol.* **2012**, *8*, 244–250. [CrossRef] [PubMed]
13. Bijkerk, R.; Florijn, B.W.; Khairoun, M.; Duijs, J.; Ocak, G.; de Vries, A.P.J.; Schaapherder, A.F.; Mallat, M.J.; de Fijter, J.W.; Rabelink, T.J.; et al. Acute Rejection After Kidney Transplantation Associates With Circulating MicroRNAs and Vascular Injury. *Transpl. Direct.* **2017**, *3*, e174. [CrossRef] [PubMed]
14. Lorenzen, J.M.; Thum, T. Long noncoding RNAs in kidney and cardiovascular diseases. *Nat. Rev. Nephrol.* **2016**, *12*, 360–373. [CrossRef]
15. Vierbuchen, T.; Fitzgerald, K.A. Long non-coding RNAs in antiviral immunity. In *Seminars in Cell and Developmental Biology*; Elsevier: London, England, 2020; E4977.
16. Ignarski, M.; Islam, R.; Müller, R.U. Long Non-Coding RNAs in Kidney Disease. *Int. J. Mol. Sci.* **2019**, *20*, 3276. [CrossRef]
17. Geisler, S.; Coller, J. RNA in unexpected places: Long non-coding RNA functions in diverse cellular contexts. *Nat. Rev. Mol. Cell. Biol.* **2013**, *14*, 699–712. [CrossRef] [PubMed]
18. Nafar, M.; Kalantari, S.; Ghaderian, S.M.H.; Omrani, M.D.; Fallah, H.; Arsang-Jang, S.; Abbasi, T.; Samavat, S.; Dalili, N.; Taheri, M.; et al. Expression Levels of lncRNAs in the Patients with the Renal Transplant Rejection. *Urol. J.* **2019**, *16*, 572–577.
19. Groeneweg, K.E.; Au, Y.W.; Duijs, J.M.; Florijn, B.W.; van Kooten, C.; de Fijter, J.W.; Reinders, M.E.; van Zonneveld, A.J.; Bijkerk, R. Diabetic nephropathy alters circulating long noncoding RNA Levels that normalize following simultaneous pancreas-kidney transplantation. *Am. J. Transpl.* **2020**. [CrossRef]
20. Zuidwijk, K.; de Fijter, J.W.; Mallat, M.J.; Eikmans, M.; van Groningen, M.C.; Goemaere, N.N.; Bajema, I.M.; Van Kooten, C. Increased influx of myeloid dendritic cells during acute rejection is associated with interstitial fibrosis and tubular atrophy and predicts poor outcome. *Kidney Int.* **2012**, *81*, 64–75. [CrossRef]
21. Ge, Y.Z.; Xu, T.; Cao, W.J.; Wu, R.; Yao, W.T.; Zhou, C.C.; Wang, M.; Xu, L.W.; Lu, T.Z.; Zhao, Y.C.; et al. A Molecular Signature of Two Long Non-Coding RNAs in Peripheral Blood Predicts Acute Renal Allograft Rejection. *Cell. Physiol. Biochem.* **2017**, *44*, 1213–1223. [CrossRef]
22. Zou, Y.; Zhang, W.; Zhou, H.H.; Liu, R. Analysis of long noncoding RNAs for acute rejection and graft outcome in kidney transplant biopsies. *Biomark Med.* **2019**, *13*, 185–195. [CrossRef] [PubMed]
23. Zou, X.F.; Song, B.; Duan, J.H.; Hu, Z.D.; Cui, Z.L.; Yang, T. PRINS Long Noncoding RNA Involved in IP-10-Mediated Allograft Rejection in Rat Kidney Transplant. *Transpl. Proc.* **2018**, *50*, 1558–1565. [CrossRef] [PubMed]

24. Xu, J.; Hu, J.; Xu, H.; Zhou, H.; Liu, Z.; Zhou, Y.; Liu, R.; Zhang, W. Long Non-coding RNA Expression Profiling in Biopsy to Identify Renal Allograft at Risk of Chronic Damage and Future Graft Loss. *Appl. Biochem. Biotechnol.* **2020**, *190*, 660–673. [CrossRef]
25. Cabili, M.N.; Trapnell, C.; Goff, L.; Koziol, M.; Tazon-Vega, B.; Regev, A.; Rinn, J.L. Integrative annotation of human large intergenic noncoding RNAs reveals global properties and specific subclasses. *Genes Dev.* **2011**, *25*, 1915–1927. [CrossRef]
26. Das, G.; Yu, Q.; Hui, R.; Reuhl, K.; Gale, N.W.; Zhou, R. EphA5 and EphA6: Regulation of neuronal and spine morphology. *Cell Biosci.* **2016**, *6*, 48. [CrossRef]
27. Li, S.; Ma, Y.; Xie, C.; Wu, Z.; Kang, Z.; Fang, Z.; Su, B.; Guan, M. EphA6 promotes angiogenesis and prostate cancer metastasis and is associated with human prostate cancer progression. *Oncotarget* **2015**, *6*, 22587–22597. [CrossRef] [PubMed]

10

Changes in Novel AKI Biomarkers after Exercise

Wojciech Wołyniec [1,*], Wojciech Ratkowski [2], Joanna Renke [3] and Marcin Renke [1]

1 Department of Occupational, Metabolic and Internal Diseases, Institute of Maritime and Tropical Medicine, Medical University of Gdańsk, 9b Powstania Styczniowego Street, 81-519 Gdynia, Poland; mrenke@gumed.edu.pl
2 Department of Athletics, Gdańsk University of Physical Education and Sport, 1 Górskiego Street, 80-336 Gdańsk, Poland; maraton1954@o2.pl
3 Department of General and Medical Biochemistry, University of Gdansk, 59 Wita Stwosza Street, 80-308 Gdańsk, Poland; joanna.renke@biol.ug.edu.pl
* Correspondence: wolyniecwojtek@gmail.com

Abstract: More than 100 substances have been identified as biomarkers of acute kidney injury. These markers can help to diagnose acute kidney injury (AKI) in its early phase, when the creatinine level is not increased. The two markers most frequently studied in plasma and serum are cystatin C and neutrophil gelatinase-associated lipocalin (NGAL). The former is a marker of kidney function and the latter is a marker of kidney damage. Some other promising serum markers, such as osteopontin and netrin-1, have also been proposed and studied. The list of promising urinary markers is much longer and includes cystatin C, NGAL, kidney injury molecule-1 (KIM-1), liver-type fatty-acid-binding protein (L-FABP), interleukin 18, insulin-like growth factor binding protein 7 (IGFBP-7), tissue inhibitor of metalloproteinases-2 (TIMP-2) and many others. Although these markers are increased in urine for no longer than a few hours after nephrotoxic agent action, they are not widely used in clinical practice. Only combined IGFBP-7/TIMP-2 measurement was approved in some countries as a marker of AKI. Several studies have shown that the levels of urinary AKI biomarkers are increased after physical exercise. This systematic review focuses on studies concerning changes in new AKI biomarkers in healthy adults after single exercise. Twenty-seven papers were identified and analyzed in this review. The interpretation of results from different studies was difficult because of the variety of study groups, designs and methodology. The most convincing data concern cystatin C. There is evidence that cystatin C is a better indicator of glomerular filtration rate (GFR) in athletes after exercise than creatinine and also at rest in athletes with a lean mass lower or higher than average. Serum and plasma NGAL are increased after prolonged exercise, but the level also depends on inflammation and hypoxia; therefore, it seems that in physical exercise, it is too sensitive for AKI diagnosis. It may, however, help to diagnose subclinical kidney injury, e.g., in rhabdomyolysis. Urinary biomarkers are increased after many types of exercise. Increases in NGAL, KIM-1, cystatin-C, L-FABP and interleukin 18 are common, but the levels of most urinary AKI biomarkers decrease rapidly after exercise. The importance of this short-term increase in AKI biomarkers after exercise is doubtful. It is not clear if it is a sign of mild kidney injury or physiological metabolic adaptation to exercise.

Keywords: urinary biomarkers; markers of AKI; cystatin-C; NGAL; KIM-1; exercise; acute kidney injury

---

1. Introduction

The analysis of human urine has been a part of medical practice for 6000 years. Uroscopy was "the mirror of medicine" or, in more ordinary terms, the first additional test in medicine, and was widely used to diagnose almost all medical conditions [1]. Now, urinalysis is one of the most common laboratory tests in medical practice.

Two-hundred years ago, the father of modern nephrology, Dr Richard Bright, discovered that patients with dropsy had albuminuria and structural changes in the kidneys. Dr Bright first described the classical nephrological triad and found a correlation between changes in urine (albuminuria) and diseased kidneys at autopsy [2]. Sixty-six years ago, Kenneth D. Gardner Jr. first described changes in urine after physical exercise. The proteinuria and hematuria were found in healthy subjects after relatively gentle exercise, therefore Gardner called these conditions "athletic pseudo-nephritis", assuming that it is a physiological, transient and benign condition [3]. Those two observations defined the limits of our understanding of the significance of proteinuria. On the one hand, albuminuria is one of the most important markers of severe and sometimes fatal kidney diseases with well-described structural changes. But on the other hand, the list of physiological conditions in which transient proteinuria is observed is quite long. Protein in urine is found after exercise, exposure to cold or heat and protein-rich food (alimentary proteinuria), and proteinuria can also occur in pregnancy, fever, heart failure and in a vertical position (orthostatic, postural proteinuria) [4].

In recent decades, new methods of urine examination have been proposed: tubular enzymes, novel biomarkers of acute kidney injury (AKI), metabolomics, proteomics, transcriptomics and genomics [5–7]. The very promising new AKI biomarkers were called "kidney troponins" and hinted at the possibility of early diagnosis of kidney diseases. Some of the markers showed high sensitivity in AKI diagnosis. Numerous studies concerned urinary neutrophil gelatinase-associated lipocalin (NGAL), kidney injury molecule-1 (KIM-1), cystatin C (Cyst-C), liver-type fatty-acid-binding protein (L-FABP), interleukin 18, insulin-like growth factor binding protein 7 (IGFBP-7) and tissue inhibitor of metalloproteinases-2 (TIMP-2) [5,8,9]. Nevertheless, the only AKI biomarker test which is currently FDA (Food and Drug Administration)-approved for clinical use in the USA, and which is also used in some European countries, is NephroCheck, which combines TIMP-2 and IGFBP-7 [10].

The history of serum examination in kidney diseases is relatively short. In the last 100 years, creatinine established its position as the best marker of glomerular filtration rate (GFR) [11,12]. 22 years ago, Cyst-C was considered as an equal or even better marker of GFR than creatinine. Due to its higher price and lower availability, it is not widely used. Interestingly, although serum concentrations of both substances correlate strictly, they are eliminated by kidneys in two different ways. Both are freely filtered in the glomeruli, but creatinine is never reabsorbed and secreted, while cystatin C in healthy individuals is reabsorbed and metabolized in the proximal tubule. Therefore, in normal conditions, excretion of Cyst-C is very low [13]. Some other novel biomarkers of AKI, like NGAL and osteopontin, can be measured in serum [5].

The serum and urine markers of kidney injury were mainly studied in AKI. The aim of this review was to analyze changes of those markers after physiological condition—exercise. All but one of the studies analyzed were conducted in the last 10 years. The high number of proposed markers of AKI is sometimes confusing. Consequently, this review was ordered according to the classification suggested by Oh in a state-of-the-art review published this year (Table 1) [5]. The purpose of this review was to describe the newest markers of AKI, which is why conventional markers—creatinine, albuminuria, tubular enzymes—were not in the scope of the paper.

Table 1. Biomarkers of acute kidney injury (AKI) studied in exercise discussed in this review—classification according to Oh et al. [5].

Functional Biomarkers	Damage Biomarkers	Pre-Injury Phase Biomarkers
sCyst-C	uCyst-C uNGAL, sNGAL, pNGAL uKIM-1 uL-FABP uIL-6, uIL-8, uIL-18, uTTF uCalbindin uTNFα uYKL-40 uMCP-1	uIGFBP-7 uTIMP-2

Abbreviations: u—urinary, s—serum, p—plasma, Cyst-C—cystatin C, NGAL—neutrophil gelatinase-associated lipocalin, KIM-1—kidney injury molecule-1, L-FABP—liver-type fatty-acid-binding protein, IL—interleukin, TTF3—trefoil factor-3, TNFα—tumor necrosis factor α, YKL-40—chitinase 3-like protein 1, MCP-1—monocyte chemoattractant protein-1, IGFBP-7—insulin-like growth factor binding protein 7, TIMP-2—tissue inhibitor of metalloproteinases-2.

Repeated episodes of acute kidney failure may lead to chronic kidney disease (CKD); therefore, proper diagnosis of AKI is important [14]. There is no evidence that sport practicing can lead to chronic kidney problems; nevertheless, after marathon run and other endurance events, an acute renal failure requiring renal replacement therapy was observed [15]. The possible factors causing post-exercise AKI are dehydration, sub-clinical rhabdomyolysis, inflammation, increased energy demanding renal sodium uptake, reduced renal perfusion and nonsteroidal anti-inflammatory drugs (NSAIDs) frequently used by runners [16,17]. There is evidence that dehydration and soft drink intake during and following exercise may lead to acute kidney dysfunction [18] and that physical work in heat is leading to chronic kidney disease [19].

2. Results: Studies Concerning Novel Biomarkers of AKI after Exercise

2.1. *Functional Biomarker—Serum Cystatin C*

Cystatin C is a non-glucosylated 13 kD basic protein which belongs to the cysteine protein inhibitors family and is produced at a constant rate by all nucleated cells. Cystatin C is an inhibitor of lysosomal proteinases and one of the most important extracellular inhibitors of cysteine proteases [5,9]. Cystatin C is freely filtered in glomeruli and then reabsorbed and metabolized in the proximal tubule. Studies on diabetes, protein-induced glomerular hyperfiltration and extreme exercise demonstrated that acute changes in serum (s)Cyst-C provide a better approximation of GFR than serum creatinine (sCr). sCyst-C is affected by sex and race and to a small degree, by inflammation [20]. In clinical studies on acute kidney injury, an increase in serum and urine cystatin C levels is observed earlier than an increase in creatinine [5,9,20,21].

2.1.1. Changes in sCyst-C after a Marathon

There were several studies dedicated to study changes in sCyst-C level after exercise. The increase in sCyst-C after a marathon was first noticed by Mingels et al. In this study of 70 recreational runners, the authors showed that the increase in sCyst-C is lower than the increase in sCr after exercise. This increase after a marathon was half that of creatinine (34% vs 53% increase, and after correction for the effect of dehydration, 21% vs 42%). Serum Cyst-C was increased above the upper reference limit in 46% of runners (in 26% after correction) [20]. Very similar changes—a significant increase in the sCyst-C level immediately after a marathon run—were observed by Scherr [22], McCullough [23] and Hewing [24] (Table 2).

Table 2. Changes in sCyst-C level after a marathon.

Study	sCyst-C Before a Marathon (mg/L)	sCyst-C after a Marathon (mg/L)	The Relative Increase in sCyst-C (%)	sCyst-C in Follow-Up (mg/L)
Mingels et al. [20]	0.71 (0.56–0.95)	0.95 (0.63–1.45)	34% (21% after correction of effect of dehydration)	0.73 (0.6–0.93) (day after, measured only in 18/70 subjects)
Scherr et al. [22]	0.77 (0.71–0.85)	0.94 (0.86–1.01)	22%	0.9 (0.81–1.00) (24 h after the race) 0.81 (0.72–0.86) (72 h after the race)
McCullough et al. [23]	0.8 ± 0.1	1.0 ± 0.2	25%	0.8 ± 0.1 (24 h after the race)
Hewing et al. [24]	0.68 (0.75–0.93)	0.85 (0.69–0.99)	25%	0.66 (0.59–0.78) (14 days after the race)

Abbreviations: sCyst-C—serum cystatin-C.

The main differences in these studies concerned changes in the follow-up, but the time of the follow-up was defined in different ways. Therefore, it is difficult to compare those data. Nevertheless, all studies showed a rapid decrease in sCyst-C at rest.

2.1.2. Changes in sCyst-C after Exercises Shorter than a Marathon

Poortmans et al. found that after a 30-min treadmill test at 80% of the maximal oxygen capacity, sCyst-C increased significantly by 13% (from 0.91 ± 0.06 to 1.03 ± 0.09 mg/L) and eGFR -Cyst-C decreased significantly by 19.8% [25]. Another study concerning subjects performing a submaximal test on a cycle ergometer at an exercise intensity of 80% of the maximal heart rate was performed by Bongers et al. In contrast to Poortmans, they did not find any changes in eGFR -Cyst-C after 30 min of exercise (eGFR 118 vs. 116 mL/min/1.73 m^2), but after 150 min of exercise, a significant decrease in eGFR -Cyst-C to 103 mL/min/1.73 m^2 was observed [26]. In Poortmans' and Bongers' studies, only males of the similar age (25 and 23 years) were studied. The difference between these two studies can be related to the type of exercise—in Poortmans' study, a run on a treadmill, and in Bongers' study, cycling on an ergometer [25,26].

2.1.3. Changes in sCyst-C after Longer Exercise than a Marathon

Serum cystatin C was also measured after very long exercise—a 120 km "Infernal trail" race. Surprisingly, there was no change in sCyst-C (0.8 vs. 0.8 mg/L) and eGFR Cyst-C value even increased after the race—from 113.5 to 118.5 mL/min ($p = 0.04$). This could be due to the very low intensity of physical activity. The exercise was very long—a 120 km race with 5700 m positive elevation. The speed was very low (5.2 km/h) and the median time was 23.1 h [27].

2.1.4. sCyst-C is a Better Marker of eGFR than sCr

Interesting observations were made in nine professional cyclists during the Giro d'Italia. In this study, blood was taken before, on the 12th and on the 22nd day of the race. The mean sCyst-C remained very stable: 0.61 ± 0.06 vs 0.62 ± 0.07 vs. 0.63 ± 0.06 mg/L. In this very interesting study, which is described in detail in two papers [28,29], blood was not taken immediately after the single race. Therefore, the study is not exactly in the scope of this review. Nevertheless, it provided evidence that even one of the most exhausting multistage efforts does not lead to an eGFR decrease in healthy, well-trained sportsmen [28,29]. Studies published by Banfi and Colombini showed that in athletes, sCyst-C is a better marker of eGFR than serum creatinine (sCr), also at rest. Some athletes, like cyclists, have a creatinine level that is lower than the reference values, due to a low lean mass (e.g., 9/9 cyclists taking part in the Giro d'Italia), while 12/15 professional rugby players had serum creatinine above the reference values due to their high body mass. In both of these studies, athletes had levels of serum Cyst-C in the normal range [28–30].

sCyst-C is also more precise than a sCr marker of eGFR in studies in which lean body mass is changing. In a study of a 6-month physical activity program in obese boys, serum creatinine increased, but sCyst-C remained unchanged. In the subjects, the lean mass and height increased, while their weight did not change [31].

2.1.5. Summary of Changes in sCyst-C

In summary, the main advantages of sCyst-C over creatinine in studies concerning exercise is that sCyst-C is not correlated with lean mass [28–30,32]. Therefore, sCyst-C may be more suitable for assessing renal function in individuals with a higher muscle mass when mild kidney impairment is suspected [33]. The studies performed after single exercise may suggest that sCyst-C elevation is dependent on intensity and duration. Long and intensive exercises such as a marathon will cause an increase [20,22–24], while short exercises or exercises with lower intensity will not [26,27].

2.2. *Plasma and Serum Damage Markers*

Damage markers can help in early AKI diagnosis even before elevation of sCr and sCyst-C levels [5]. Only a few damage markers are measured in serum or plasma: NGAL, KIM-1, osteopontin and netrin-1. The most studies concerned changes in NGAL.

NGAL, also known as siderocalin or lipocalin 2, is a member of the lipocalin superfamily of carrier proteins, which are approximately 25 kDa in size. NGAL has a bacteriostatic function related to its ability to bind iron-siderophore complexes and thereby prevents iron uptake by bacteria. NGAL also provides an antiapoptotic effect and enhances proliferation of renal tubular cells [8]. It is produced by activated neutrophils in the proximal tubules. NGAL is filtered in the glomerulus and reabsorbed in the proximal tubule. After ischemic, septic or toxic kidney injury, NGAL is dramatically upregulated at the transcript and protein level. Plasma and urinary NGAL levels are significantly increased in those with early structural renal tubular damage caused by various factors [5,8,9].

2.2.1. Changes in Plasma NGAL (pNGAL) after Short Exercises

Changes in pNGAL after exercise were first investigated by Junglee et al. in 2012. In this study dedicated to AKI in exercise, after relatively short exercise (an 800 m run), pNGAL was decreased, which was interpreted by the authors as an effect of increased NGAL renal clearance [34].

In another study performed by Junglee, the pNGAL level increased after a 40-min heat stress run (running on a treadmill on a 1% gradient for 40 min at 65% VO_{2max} (maximal oxygen consumption) in an environmental chamber maintained at a dry bulb temperature of 33 °C with 50% relative humidity (RH)). In this study, the heat stress run was preceded by a 60-min downhill muscle-damaging run (EIMD group) or a 60-min flat run (CON group) and a 30-min seated rest. pNGAL increased in both groups, but the increase was greater in the EIMD group [35].

There were also three studies dedicated to investigating a pNGAL as a marker of inflammation, neutrophil degranulation and organ damage, but not an AKI biomarker [36–38].

Bender et al. studied pNGAL as an inflammatory marker of hand osteoarthiritis (OA) after mechanical exercise of the OA hand. pNGLA increased during the first 15 min after exercising the index hand within the venous blood of the ipsilateral forearm [36]. Kanda et al. studied 9 untrained men during a one leg, calf-rise exercise. pNGAL was studied as a marker of organ damage, muscle disruption and neutrophil mobilization and migration. The authors did not find any changes in pNGAL [37]. Rullman et al., found no significant changes in pNGAL after 27 and 57 min of cycle exercise. During the first 20 min, the subjects exercised at 50% of VO_{2max} and during the next 40 min, at 65% VO_{2max}. In the Rullman study, pNGAL was investigated as a marker of neutrophil degranulation [38].

2.2.2. Changes in pNGAL or Serum NGAL (sNGAL) Levels after Long Exercises

Chapman et al. studied the impact of soft drink consumption during long exercise in heat. Twelve healthy subjects drank two liters of a beverage (soft drink or water) during four hours of exercise in 35.1 °C heat. pNGAL increased post-exercise in both groups [18].

McDermott et al. found a 2-fold significant increase in sNGAL (from 68.51 to 139.12 ng/mL) after a 6-h endurance cycling event during heat (33.2 ± 5.0 °C, 38.4 ± 10.7% RH). Moderate ibuprofen ingestion of 600 mg ibuprofen had no influence on the sNGAL level [39]. Moreover, Lippi et al., found a significant 1.6-fold increase in sNGAL (from 105 to 196 ng/mL) after a 60-km run in a group of trained male athletes [40].

Furthermore, Andrezzoli et al. found only a mild increase in pNGAL in a group of professional cyclists after the mountain stages of two major European professional cycling competitions (Giro D'Italia and Tour de France). Post-competition NGAL values of all the variables investigated remained within the physiological range. The results suggest that even if NGAL values rose slightly and not significantly after competition, no kidney injury occurred in these highly trained athletes during the mountain stages of professional competitions [41].

NGAL, which is an acute phase protein and is upregulated in the lungs during inflammation, was also studied as a marker of inflammation and oxidative stress after long exercise. Mellor et al. found a non-significant NGAL rise after an ascent from sea level to 1085 m over 6 h [42]. In this study, two other cohorts were also studied. There were no changes in NGAL after 3 h exposure to normobaric hypoxia with a 5-min step test, but there was an increase in NGAL after trekking in Nepal [42].

2.2.3. Changes in pNGAL after Work in Heat

Chapman et al. analyzed changes in pNGAL and other biomarkers in two interesting studies. In the first, the impact of different beverage consumption (soft drink or water) during exercise in heat was studied. Twelve healthy subjects drank two liters of fluid during four hours of exercise in 35.1 °C heat [18]. In the second study, thirteen healthy adults (3 women, 10 men, age 23 ± 2 years) exercised for 2 h in a 39.7 ± 0.6 °C, 32% ± 3% relative humidity environmental chamber. In four trials, the subjects received water to remain hydrated (*Water group*), were exposed to continuous upper-body cooling (*Cooling group*), a combination of both (*Water + Cooling group*), or no intervention (*Control group*) [43]. In the first study, in both groups, pNGAL was increased post-exercise and returned to pre-exercise levels after 24 h [18]. In the second study, an increase in pNGAL was also observed and was greater in the control group (without hydration and cooling) compared with the other conditions [43].

2.2.4. Summary of Changes in s/pNGAL

The importance of s/pNGAL in the diagnosis of AKI in exercise is questionable. NGAL is released by respiratory epithelium, liver and heart, and therefore changes in the s/pNGAL level could be caused by inflammation, hypoxia or muscle damage, conditions which are integral to exercise [35,42]. Therefore, it is unclear to which degree, if any, an increase in NGAL after exercise is related to kidney injury. The methodological problem is that a huge difference between athletes is observed [40].

2.3. Urinary Damage Markers

2.3.1. Urinary Cystatin C (uCyst-C)

Since Cyst-C is freely filtered by the glomerulus, reabsorbed and metabolized in the renal tubule, even a small elevation of urinary Cyst-C (uCyst-C) reflects proximal tubule injury [13].

Bongers et al. studied subjects performing submaximal exercise at an 80% HR rate and found a significant increase in uCyst-C with higher values after prolonged exercise (150 min) compared to acute (30 min) exercise [26]. In 2012, the same authors studied urinary markers after single and repetitive bouts of exercise. They examined participants of the International Four Day Marches Nijmegen. Subjects walked at 70% intensity over 30, 40 or 50 km for 3 consecutive days. Bongers studied several urinary markers and found that uCyst-C increased 1.8 times after the first day (from 0.05 to 0.09 mg/L), but this effect disappeared on day 3 (uCyst-C = 0.06 mg/L) [44]. Interestingly, in these studies, uCyst-C was measured mainly to normalize uKIM-1 and uNGAL levels [26,44]. The increase in uCyst-C was also found by Wolyniec after 10 and 100 km runs. There was a 2.56-fold increase after 10 km and a 4.96-fold increase after 100 km. When normalized to creatinine, these increases were 1.39- and 1.95-fold, respectively [45].

The number of studies coming from only two centers is small, but it seems that uCyst-C is a very sensitive marker of proximal tubule dysfunction after exercise.

2.3.2. Changes in uNGAL and uKIM-1 after a Marathon

KIM-1 is a 38.7 kDa type 1 transmembrane glycoprotein member of the TIM family of immunoglobulin superfamily molecules. KIM-1 plays a role in kidney recovery and tubular regeneration because it acts as a phosphatidylserine receptor and thereby mediates the phagocytosis of apoptotic cells. KIM-1 protects kidney against ischemic-reperfusion injury [8]. KIM-1 was found to be expressed at low to undetectable levels in normal kidney tissue but is markedly expressed after ischemic or toxic injury in proximal tubule cells. KIM-1 can serve as a urine and blood AKI biomarker. KIM is elevated in early stages of AKI and its urinary concentration is closely related to the severity of renal damage [5,8,9].

The first study concerning changes in urinary NGAL and KIM-1 after a marathon was performed by McCullough and published in 2010 [23]. The authors showed a 5.7-fold increase in uNGAL and a minor rise in uKIM-1 after a marathon [23]. According to the authors, those were changes "supporting a pathobiologic case for AKI" [23]. Changes in uKIM-1 and uNGAL levels after a marathon were also studied by Mansour et al. [46] The results concerning uNGAL were very similar to these from McCullough's study (a 4.71-fold increase in uNGAL), but the increase in uKIM-1 was much higher. The decrease in uKIM-1 was slower than the other markers studied (uNGAL, uTNF-alfa [tumor necrosis factor α], uIL-18, uIL6, uIL8, uYKL-40, uMCP-1) and 24 h after a marathon, the level was still increased (Table 3) [46].

Table 3. Changes in uNGAL and uKIM-1 after a marathon.

Study	uNGAL before a Marathon (ng/mL)	uNGAL after a Marathon	Fold Increase	KIM-1 before a Marathon	uKIM-1 after a Marathon	Fold Increase
McCullough et al. [23]	8.2 ± 4.0	47.0 ± 28.6 (10.6 ± 7.2 after 24 h)	5.73× (1.29×)	2.6 ± 1.6 ng/mL	3.5 ± 1.6 (2.7 ± 1.6 after 24 h) ng/mL	1.35× (1.03×)
Mansour et al. [46]	8.00 (4.15–30.48)	37.64 (19.03–84.61) (day 2: 18.49 (9.25–33.69))	4.71× (2.31×)	132.59 (67.61–219.98) pg/mL	723.32 (459.36–1970.64) (day 2: 702.42 (123.27–1098.67)) pg/mL	5.46× (5.3×)

Abbreviations: uNGAL—urinary neutrophil gelatinase-associated lipocalin, uKIM-1—urinary kidney injury molecule-1.

2.3.3. Changes in uNGAL after Exercises Shorter than a Marathon

No changes were found in the uNGAL level in Kanda's study on 9 untrained males during a one leg calf-rise exercise [37] and in the Wołyniec study of amateur runners after a submaximal test on a treadmill [47]. In contrast, in two other studies, uNGAL was increased after very short exercise. Junglee et al. noticed an increase in uNGAL and uNGAL/uCr immediately and 25 min after an 800 m run. The uNGAL level returned to the baseline levels after two hours [34]. Spada et al. also noticed an increase in uNGAL after 4 min of an high-intensity interval resistance training (HIIT) session (eight sets of squats performed with the fastest speed and the highest number of repetitions achievable in 20 s with 10 s of rest between sets). In this study, uNGAL was increased in women 2 after exercise and returned to values similar to the baseline 24 h after exercise. In 5/29 females, uNGAL/uCr exceeded 100 ng/mgCr, the value of which is compatible with clinical AKI. In men, the increase in uNGAL and uNGAL/uCr was not statistically significant [48].

Junglee et al. found an 8-fold uNGAL increase after a 40-min heat stress run (65% VO_{2max}, 33 °C): 80% of subjects from the muscle-damaging group and 30% from the flat-run group had uNGAL above the normal range after exercise [35]. Bongers, who studied uNGAL after 30 and 150 min of exercise, found that uncorrected uNGAL and uNGAL corrected to osmolality were increased, while there were no changes in uNGAL corrected to creatinine and cystatin-C [26]. After a 10-km run, both uNGAL and uNGAL/Cr increased significantly (3.9- and 2.9-fold, respectively) in the Wołyniec study [45]. Otherwise, in Semen et al.'s study, a 10 km run caused an increase in uNGAL only when combined with ibuprofen/naproxen use [49]. In the same study, a significant increase in uNGAL was observed in the half-marathon runners [49].

In another study, Semen et al. found that completion of a half marathon after use of a 400 mg single dose ibuprofen led to a 2-fold increase in uNGAL. However, this increase was smaller and not significant in the group supplemented with monomeric and oligomeric flavanols (MOF-VVPP) [50]. In the Wolyniec study, the increase in uNGAL was higher than in Semen's study, although the exercise was shorter. This difference could be partially explained by the higher intensity of a 10-km run but could also be related to the methodology. In the first study, urine samples were collected immediately after the run and in the second, urine samples were collected within 2 h after the run [45,50].

2.3.4. Changes in uNGAL after Exercises Longer than a Marathon

The uNGAL level was elevated after all exercises longer than a marathon run. Bongers found that prolonged walking exercise at 70% intensity caused a 2.25-fold increase in uNGAL on day 1, and a 1.54-fold increase on day 3 compared to the baseline levels [44]. An uNGAL increase was also found by Lippi et al. after a 60-km run (7.7- fold increase in uNGAL) [40], by Jouffroy et al. after an 80-km run (5-fold increase after 53 km, and 2.5-fold after 80 km, without significant changes in uNGAL/uCr) [51], by Wolyniec et al. after 100 km (6.82-fold increase in uNGAL, and only a 2.94-fold increase in uNGAL/uCr) [45] and by Poussel el al. after a 120-km run (2.6-fold increase in uNGAL and a 1.5-fold in uNGAL/uCr) [27]. Only 6.25% of the participants in the Wołyniec study and 12.5 % in the Poussel study had uNGAL/uCr above the reference value [27,45].

2.3.5. Changes in uNGAL after Exercise in Heat

Chapmen et al., performed two exciting studies, as mentioned above [18,43]. In the first, they found that 24 h after exercise in heat, uNGAL was elevated above the pre-exercise level in subjects drinking soft drinks, although uNGAL corrected to uCr osmolality did not produce any changes [18]. In the second study, uNGAL was elevated after 2 h of exercise in heat, and this increase was greater in the control group compared with the other conditions (hydration or/and cooling) [43].

2.3.6. Summary of Changes in uNGAL

Changes in uNGAL were typically found after long exercise. It seems that uNGAL is frequently increased, but rarely exceeds normal values when normalized to creatinine. Some factors, like environmental temperature, type of cooling and hydration, are related to changes in uNGAL. Interpreting these changes is difficult. Machado found elevated levels of uNGAL in endurance cycling athletes 48 h after exercise and suggested that the increase in uNGAL is related to metabolic adaptation to endurance exercise, or possibly predisposition to acute kidney injury over time [52]. In Bongers' study, uNGAL was elevated after the first day of marching and then decreased, which also suggested some kind of kidney adaptation to exercise [44].

2.3.7. Changes in Urinary KIM

Except for the two studies after a marathon mentioned above [23,46], uKIM was studied only in 5 studies coming from 3 centers. In all these studies, uKIM-1 was increased.

Bongers et al. found an increase in uKIM-1 after 30- and 150-min submaximal exercise [26] and after one day of walking, with a subsequent decrease in its level after 3 consecutive days of marching [44]. In the first study, the uKIM-1 corrected to uCr, uCyst-C and urine osmolality showed no significant changes [26]. In the second study, uKIM- 1 corrected to osmolality was increased, while uKIM-1/uCr and uKIM/uCyst-C ratios were unchanged [44]. Wolyniec found an increase in uKIM-1 but not in the uKIM/uCr ratio after a treadmill test, 10 and 100 km runs [45,47]. Jouffroy found a significant increase in uKIM-1 but not in uKIM/uCr during an 80-km run. Interestingly, nine days after the race, uKIM-1 remained significantly higher than the baseline level [51].

2.3.8. Summary of Changes in uKIM-1

uKIM-1 was increased after all exercises, but when normalized to uCr, it was unchanged. The changes in uKIM-1 were long-lasting, uKIM-1 was elevated 2 days after a marathon [46] and 9 days after an 80 km run [51]. At the same time, uNGAL decreased more rapidly.

2.3.9. Changes in Urinary L-FABP after Exercise

L-FABP belongs to the fatty acid-binding protein superfamily and has a molecular mass of about 14 kDa. The function of the members of the FABP family is the regulation of fatty acids uptake and the intracellular transport. L-FABP binds fatty acids and transports them to the mitochondria and peroxisomes. L-FABP also protects renal cells from oxidative stress [8]. The urinary L-FABP level is correlated with the peritubular capillary flow and ischemia. It appears to be a promising biomarker for both the diagnosis and prediction of AKI and its outcomes among critically ill patients [5,8,9]. L-FABP is localized in the proximal tubule and secreted into urine in response to a number of different intrarenal stresses, such as proteinuria, hypoxia, hyperglycemia, hypertension and oxidative stress [37,53,54].

Only two studies in healthy populations concerning changes in uL-FABP after exercise have been published. uL-FABP was significantly increased after incremental short maximal exercise on a cycling ergometer in a group of 116 adults of variable age (24–83 years) in a study published by Kosaki et al. In this experiment, uL-FABP/uCr changes were independently correlated with albuminuria, which supported previous observations that protein overload in the proximal tubule may cause an increase in uL-FABP [53]. After short exercise (one leg calf-rise exercise), Kanda et al. did not find any changes in uL-FABP [37].

2.3.10. Other Studies Concerning Changes in uL-FABP

Hiraki showed that after a single case of a 20-min moderate intensity exercise (20-min treadmill walking, 40–60% exercise intensity) session in 31 adults with chronic kidney disease (CKD), there was no change in uL-FABP. This exercise was rather gentle and even albuminuria was not increased [55]. Kosaki studied individuals aged 50–83 without CKD and found that uL-FABP was the lowest in participants with a higher level of aerobic fitness and muscular strength [56,57] and that 12-week aerobic exercise training significantly decreases uL-FABP levels [57]. Relative changes in uFABP were significantly correlated with the relative changes in physical activity and the mean arterial pressure after intervention. The authors concluded that "habitual exercise appears to be associated with the degree of several stresses on the proximal tubule and to be beneficial for kidney health in middle-aged and older adults" [57]. Uchiyama et al. found a decrease in uL-FABP after a 12-week, home-based exercise program involving 47 patients undergoing peritoneal dialysis [58].

2.3.11. Urinary Interleukins

Urinary interleukins, Il-1, Il-6, IL-8 and Il-18, were proposed as markers of AKI. Interleukins are important mediators of the immune reaction in the innate immune system response and adaptive immunity [8]. All these cytokines are freely filtered and then reabsorbed and metabolized in the proximal tubule; therefore, tubular injury leads to an elevation in their levels in urine [5,6,8,9,48].

Manosur et al. studied changes in urinary interleukins after a marathon and found a 19.2-fold increase in uIL-6, a 9.13-fold increase in uIL-8 and a 7.13-fold increase in uIL-18 [46]. Similarly, Semen et al. observed significant increases of urinary interleukins after a half marathon and the use of 400 mg ibuprofen. There was a 10-fold increase in uIL-6, a 2.87-fold increase in uIL-8 and a non-significant increase in IL-18. The elevations of uIL-6 and uIL-8 were smaller in runners supplemented with MOF-VVPP (5.8- and 1.49-fold, respectively) [50]. Elevation of uIL-6 and uIL-8 was also found by Sugama et al. after a duathlon [59]. Spada et al. found an increase in uIL-18 after a HIIT session [48]. Dutheil et al. found an increase in uIL-8 after a 24 h work shift and, according to the author, this elevation was related to stress [60].

2.4. Pre-Injury Phase Biomarkers IGFBP-7/TIMP-2

Insulin-like growth factor binding protein 7 (IGFBP-7) is a 29 kDa protein, a member of IGFBPs. It is a kind of glycoprotein with a molecular weight of 30 kDa. IGFBP-7 is known to bind and inhibit signaling through IGF-1 receptors [8]. Urinary IGFBP-7 is increased in kidney damage caused by sepsis or ischemia [8,9].

TIMP-2 is a 21 kDa protein, a member of the TIMP family. TIMP2 is a member of the tissue inhibitor of matrix metalloproteinase family. TIMP2 is an endogenous inhibitor of metalloproteinase activities and participates in the regulation of cell growth and apoptosis [8,9].

Combined urinary IGFBP-7 and TIMP-2 predict the occurrence of AKI better than other markers (NGAL KIM, IL19) [8,9]. NephroCheck, which combines TIMP-2 and IGFBP-7, is the only FDA-approved AKI biomarker test for use in the USA and is also used in some European countries [10].

Surprisingly, IGFBP-7 and TIMP-2 were studied only in one study after exercise. Chapman et al. studied thirteen healthy adults exercising in heat (the study is described above) and found elevated levels of uIGFBP-7 and uTIMP-2. There was a greater increase in the urinary biomarkers of AKI in the *Control* group. The differential findings between IGFBP7 (preferentially secreted in the proximal tubules) and TIMP-2 (secreted in the distal tubules) suggested that the proximal tubules are the location of potential renal injury [43].

2.5. Other Promising Markers of AKI (YKL-40, MCP-1 and TNF-alfa, Trefoil Factor 3 (TTF3), Calbindin)

There are over 100 biomarkers of AKI [61]. The urinary biomarkers which have been assessed in numerous studies are: chitinase 3-like protein 1 (YKL-40), MCP-1, TNF-alfa, osteopontin, DKK-1, micro RNAs, hemojuvelin, clusterin, CYR-61, cytochrome-C, epidermal growth factor, malondialdehyde, calprotectin, urine AGT angiotensinogen, matrix metalloproteinase 9, urine cysteine-rich 61, Na^+/H^+ exchanger isoform 3 protein, netrin-1, fetuin-A and trefoil factor 3 (TFF3) [5,8,9]. Most of these markers were not studied after exercise.

In one of the most interesting and largest studies concerning AKI biomarkers after exercise, Mansour et al. found increases in several urinary markers: a 4.5-fold increase in TNFα, a 6.69-fold increase in MCP-1 and an 8.99-fold increase in YKL-40 after a marathon [46]. Sugama et al. found increased uMCP-1 after a duathlon, but this change was not significant when normalized to uCr [59]. Semen et al. found a significant uTNFα increase after a half marathon [50]. Calbindin and TTF3 were studied in one study, and both of these markers increased after HIIT training [48]. The TTF3 family is a group of small molecule polypeptides, and uTTF3 was significantly reduced following renal tubular damage [9]; therefore, the increase in uTTF3 after exercise was surprising.

3. Discussion

Studies concerning new markers of AKI after physical exercise combine two different entities. Markers of AKI were introduced to diagnose the early phase of kidney injury in critically ill patients with sepsis or shock [5,6,8,9], but in these studies, they were measured in healthy subjects during physical activity, like walking, running or cycling. The increase in new AKI biomarkers was anticipated in these studies, because even much less sensitive markers, like serum creatinine and urinalysis, show changes after exercise [3,23].

Although many markers of AKI were described, only a minority were studied after exercise. Some markers are classified as injury markers (e.g., uKIM-1, uTNFalfa, uIL-6, uIL-8, uIL-18, uNGAL) and others as repair biomarkers (e.g., uYKL-40, uMCP-1) [46]. Another classification is based on the site of injury. There are markers of tubular (e.g., NGAL, IL-18, L-FABP, KIM-1, IGFBP-7) and glomerular (e.g., matrix metallopeptidase 9 [MMP-9]) injury [9]. The authors of this review used the classification proposed by Oh et al. [5] (Table 1), which has practical implications.

3.1. Limitations of the Studies Presented

There are several limitations to the studies presented in this review. Twenty-seven studies were analyzed. All but one were published during the last 10 years and 15/27 in the last 5 years. The number of subjects studied ranged from 9 to 167, although most of the studies had a small number of participants: in 16 studies, fewer than 30 participants were investigated and only in 3 studies were there more than 100 participants studied. In 12 studies, only males were analyzed, and only in 7 studies were both sexes represented to the same or very similar degree. In three studies, all concerning marathons, more females were analyzed. The mean age of the participants differed greatly, ranging from 20 to 60 years. There were many different study designs proposed by the researchers, although the most common was a marathon (distance 42,195 m), which was used in 5 studies (Figure 1, Table 4).

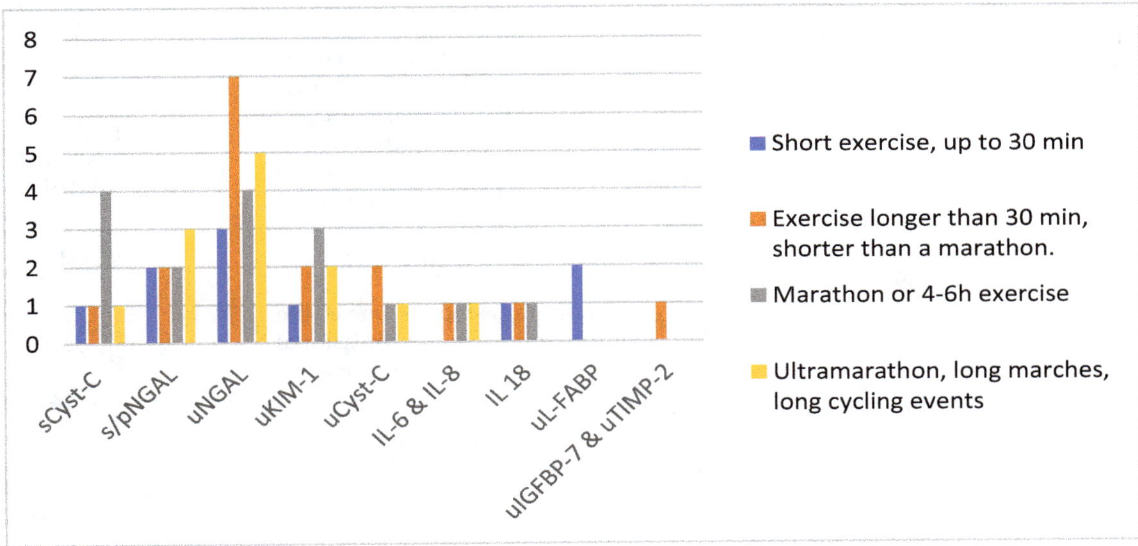

Figure 1. Number of studies in different types of exercise. Abbreviations: u—urinary, s—serum, p—plasma, Cyst-C—cystatin C, NGAL—neutrophil gelatinase-associated lipocalin, KIM-1—kidney injury molecule-1, L-FABP—liver-type fatty-acid-binding protein, IL—interleukin, IGFBP-7—insulin-like growth factor binding protein 7, TIMP-2—tissue inhibitor of metalloproteinases-2.

Table 4. Studies on changes in new AKI markers after single exercise in healthy subjects—ordered according to the year of publication.

Author (Year of Publication)	Study Group	Exercise/Study Design	Markers
Mingels et al. (2009) [20]	70 recreational male runners age 47 (range 30–68) years	marathon	sCyst-C
Scherr et al. (2011) [22]	102 healthy male runners age 42 ± 9.5 y	Marathon	sCyst-C
McCullough et al. (2011) [23]	25 healthy runners age 38.7 ± 9.0 years (13 females, 12 males)	Marathon	sCyst-C uNGAL uKIM-1
Poortmans et al. (2012) [25]	12 male physical educators age 25 ± 5 years	30-min treadmill exercise at 80% of VO_2max	sCyst-C
Junglee et al. (2012) [34]	20 healthy active adults age 24 ± 4 years (7 females, 13 males)	800-m sprint	pNGAL uNGAL uNGAL/uCr
Rullman et al. (2012) [38]	10 healthy men age 25 (range 18–37) years	60-min cycle ergometer test (20 min at 50% of VO_2max; +40 min at 65% of VO_2max)	pNGAL
Lippi et al. (2012) [40]	16 trained male athletes age 42 (range 34–52) years	60-km ultramarathon	sNGAL, uNGAL, uNGAl/uCr
Junglee et al. (2013) [35]	10 active healthy men age 20 ± 2 years	1. 60-min running downhill at a −10% gradient + 40-min run on the treadmill at a 1% gradient at 65% VO_2max in a temp. of 33 °C with 50% RH 2. 60-min flat run + 40-min run on the treadmill at a 1% gradient at 65% VO_2max in a temp. of 33 °C with 50% RH	pNGAL uNGAL uNGLA/u.f.
Mellor et al. (2013) [42]	22 subjects age 36 ± 2.4 years (7 females, 15 males)	ascent from sea level to 1085 m over 6 h	pNGAL
Sugama et al. (2013) [59]	14 male triathletes age 28.7 ± 7.9 years	duathlon race: 5 km of running + 40 km of cycling + 5 km of running	uIL-6 uIL-8
Kanda et al. (2014) [37]	9 untrained healthy men age 24.8 ± 1.3 years	One leg calf-raise exercise 10 sets of 40 repetitions of exercise at 0.5 Hz with 3 min rest between sets	pNGAL uNGAL uFABP
Hewing et al. (2015) [24]	167 recreational runners age 50.3 ± 11.4 years (89 females, 78 males)	marathon	sCyst-C
Andreazzoli et al. (2017) [41]	18 professional male cyclists age 31.5 ± 4 years	mountain stage of one of the major European professional cycling competitions	pNGAL uNGAL
Mansour et al. (2017) [46]	22 heathy amateur runners age 44 (range 22–63) years (13 females, 9 males)	marathon	uNGAL uKIM-1 uIL-6, uIL-8, uIL-18, uTNFα, uYKL-40, uMCP-1
Bongers et al. (2017) [44]	60 marchers age 29 ± 78 years (30 females, 30 males)	30, 40 or 50 km for three consecutive days	uCyst-C, uNGAL, uNGAL/uCyst-C, uNGAL/Cr, uNGAL/uOsm uKIM-1, uKIM-1/uCyst-C, uKIM-1/uCr, uKIM-1/uOsm

Table 4. *Cont.*

Author (Year of Publication)	Study Group	Exercise/Study Design	Markers
Bongers et al. (2018) [26]	35 active healthy males age 23 ± 3 years	150-min cycle ergometer test at 80% of HRmax until 3% hypohydration (samples taken after 30 and 50 min)	sCyst-C, uCyst-C uNGAL, uNGAL/uCyst-C, uNGAL/uCr, uNGAL/uOsm uKIM-1, uKIM/uCyst-C, uKIM-1/uCr, uKIM-1/uOsm
Spada et al. (2018) [48]	58 healthy volunteers age 24 (range 21–28) years (29 males, 29 females)	4 min of HIIRT	uNGAL, uNGAL/uCr uIL-18, uIL-18/uCr uCalbindin, uCalbindin/uCr uTTF, uTTF/uCr
Wołyniec et al. (2018) [47]	19 healthy amateur runners age 35.74 ± 6.99 years (9 females, 10 males)	treadmill run test	uNGAL, uNGAL/uCr uKIM-1, uKIM-1/uCr
McDermott et al. (2018) [39]	40 healthy cyclists age 52 ± 9 years	endurance cycling event (5.7 ± 1.2 h) in heat (33.2 ± 5.0 °C, 38.4 ± 10.7% RH)	sNGAL
Chapman et al. (2019) [18]	12 healthy adults age 24 ± 5 years (3 females, 9 males)	4 h exercise in heat (35,1 °C, 61% RH)	pNGAL uNGAL, uNGAL/u.f.
Wolyniec et al. (2019) [45]	16 Healthy amateur runners age 36.7 ± 8.2 years (2 females, 14 males)	10- and 100-km runs	uCyst-C uNGAL, uNGAL/uCr uKIM-1, uKIM-1/uCr
Jouffroy et al. (2019) [51]	47 healthy males age 43 ± 7 years	80-km ultramarathon	uNGAL, uNGAL/uCr uKIM-1, uKIM-1/uCr
Poussel et al. (2020) [27]	24 healthy runners age 36.5 (range 24–57) years (1 female, 23 males)	120-km ultramarathon with 5700 m of positive elevation gain	sCyst-C uNGAL, uNGAL/uCr
Chapman et al. (2020) [43]	13 healthy adults age 23 ± 2 years (3 females, 10 males)	2 h exercise in a heat (temp 39 °C, 32 % RH)	uNGAL uIGFBP-7 uTIMP-2
Kosaki et al. (2020) [53]	116 adults without chronic kidney disease age 62 (range 24–83) years (31 females, 85 males)	incremental short maximal exercise using a cycling ergometer	uL-FABP/uCr
Semen et al. (2020) [50]	54 healthy runners age 47 ± 15 years (21 females, 33 males)	half marathon after use of 400 mg single-dose ibuprofen: two groups: 1. supplemented with MOF-VVPP 2. Control	uNGAL, uCyst-C uIL-6, uIL-8, uIL-18, uTNFα
Semen et al. (2020) [49]	1. 35 runners age 44 ± 2 years (17 females, 18 males) 2. 45 runners age 55 ± 2 years (24 females, 21 males)	1. 10 km run 2. half marathon	uNGAL

Abbreviations: u—urinary, s—serum, p—plasma, Cyst-C—cystatin C, NGAL—neutrophil gelatinase-associated lipocalin, KIM-1—kidney injury molecule-1, L-FABP—liver-type fatty-acid-binding protein, Il—interleukin, TTF3—trefoil factor-3, TNFα—tumor necrosis factor α, YKL-40—chitinase 3-like protein 1, MCP-1—monocyte chemoattractant protein-1, IGFBP-7—insulin-like growth factor binding protein 7, TIMP-2—tissue inhibitor of metalloproteinases-2, Cr—creatinine, Osm—osmolality, u.f.—urine flow, uMarker/uCyst-C—urinary marker normalized to cystatin C, uMarker/uCr—urinary marker normalized to creatinine, uMarker/uOsm—urinary marker normalized to osmolality, uMarker/u.f.—urinary marker normalized to urine flow, HIIRT—high-intensity interval resistance training, VO_2max—maximal oxygen consumption, HRmax—maximal heart rate, RH—relative humidity, monomeric and oligomeric flavanols (MOF-VVPP).

The diagnosis of AKI was never confirmed by kidney biopsy, which is completely understandable. The studies were performed in relatively small groups and no cases of AKI requiring HD or rhabdomyolysis were observed, because both of these severe complications are extremely rare after exercise. There is insufficient data to describe changes in AKI biomarkers in such severe complications of exercise.

The follow-up was defined in a different way in the studies presented, and in some, there was no follow-up at all.

Suggestions: Studies in larger groups, preferably multicenter, are needed. It could be reasonable to study all markers after a marathon, which is the classical distance, relatively long and intensive. Indeed, it is the most commonly studied type of exercise. More studies in females are also required. Studies with a precisely defined follow-up with several time points, as well as observational case studies on changes in AKI biomarkers in subjects with severe complications could be very interesting.

3.2. Serum or Plasma Markers

Reasonable data only concern cystatin C and NGAL. The results of the studies presented provided enough information to consider cystatin C as a better marker of eGFR than creatinine after exercise and at rest in athletes with high or low lean mass [28–30]. The information concerning plasma or serum NGAL is more questionable. In fact, after some exercises, NGAL is elevated. However, NGAL is also a marker of inflammation, organ damage and hypoxia, and in exercise, it seems to have low specificity for AKI. One practical problem is the huge variability of levels between studies and subjects. One of the possible implications of p/sNGAL measurement is diagnosis of subclinical AKI in uncomplicated rhabdomyolysis, when creatinine and cystatin levels are within the normal range [62].

The general problem with serum measurement after exercise is hemoconcentration. In many publications, the authors used a correction of the effect of dehydration according to Dill and Costill's method [63], on the basis of changes in pre- and post-blood morphology. This approach is reasonable in experimental studies, but in clinical practice, it is difficult to use, because pre-injury blood morphology results are unknown.

Suggestion: We suggest measuring sCyst-C instead of creatinine in future studies of kidney function in exercise. It is reasonable to check sNGAL in the risk group with rhabdomyolysis.

3.3. Urinary Markers

The urinary markers are increased after almost every exercise. The increment is rather small but consistent with individuals. The changes are dependent on the duration and intensity of exercise. Most studies investigated changes in uKIM-1 and uNGAL. After short exercise, an increase in uKIM-1, but not uNGAL, was observed. Elevated uKIM-1 was observed 2 and even 9 days after prolonged exercise. It is difficult to discuss the utility of uL-FABP, uCyst-C and other markers, because only few studies were performed. L-FABP is a marker of hypoxia, therefore it could be an ideal marker for studies in exercise but was used only in very few studies from one study group. What is also surprising is that uIGFBP-7 and uTIMP-2 were only analyzed in one study, and were the only markers approved for early diagnosis of AKI. The methodological problem with interpreting the changes in urinary markers is normalization. It is known that all urinary markers can be diluted, and, e.g., normalization of albuminuria is a standard procedure. In some studies, un-normalized values are used, but most authors normalized AKI markers to creatinine, osmolality, urine flow or cystatin C [18,23,26,27,34,35,40,44–48,51,53]. All these approaches had some limits. The most common was normalization to creatinine.

Suggestion: There is a need for studies on follow-up. Studies showing changes in urine markers shortly after exercise are interesting but have little practical value. In clinical practice, AKI is suspected and diagnosed several hours after exercise. What is most important is what levels of markers are typical for AKI 3, 6, 12 or 24 h after exercise. Although normalization to creatinine has some limits, it is the most common approach, and therefore it is reasonable to use this kind of normalization in subsequent studies.

There is no biomarker specific enough to assess AKI as a single biomarker. There is also no panel assessment using a couple of biomarkers, except combined urinary IGFBP-7 and TIMP-2. Taking into account the results presented in this review, combined uKIM-1/uCr and uNGAL/uCr could be the best to exclude or diagnose AKI after exercise.

3.4. Interpretation

In the presented studies, changes in AKI biomarkers were common. The main problem is how to implement the knowledge from these studies in clinical practice. There are several facts concerning AKI biomarkers, AKI and CKD in athletes:

1. Exercise-induced renal impairment is commonly present but temporary,
2. Severe complications of exercise, like AKI requiring hemodialysis, are rare,
3. Repeated episodes of AKI lead to CKD,
4. There is no data showing that CKD could be related to sports activity,
5. There is a growing body of evidence that exhausting work in heat leads to CKD [19,58–64] and the same risk factors—dehydration and muscle damage, soft drink consumption—are present, for example, in marathon runners.

Suggestion: We suggest that further studies on the physiological role of biomarkers are needed. Epidemiological studies and studies on athletes who have completed several dozen marathons or other long forms of exercise and studies on the impact of work and soft drinks on kidney function are awaited.

4. Materials and Methods

The authors researched the PubMed/MEDLINE electronic database by using terms consisting of the following: (AKI biomarker or cystatin C or NGAL or KIM-1 or urinary interleukin-18 or urinary interleukin or urinary liver-type fatty acid-binding protein or urinary L-FABP or urinary insulin-like growth factor-binding protein 7 or urinary IGFBP7 or urinary tissue inhibitor of metalloproteinases-2 or urinary TIMP-2 or nephrocheck or urinary osteopontin or urinary calbindin or urinary TTF) (nordic walking or physical activity or exercise or marathon or ultramarathon or swimming or cycling or games or football). The search was repeated regularly, and the database was updated until the last update on 13 July 2020, prior to manuscript submission. An additional search was conducted according to a reference list of read papers and by using investigators' names. As the initial selection was done through titles and abstracts, it is possible that some important papers might have been omitted, although the authors tried to identify all that were important. A total of 27 papers were retrieved from 629 titles and abstracts identified in the PubMed database (Figure 2).

In this review, results of 13 additional studies were also shortly discussed. These papers did not consider single exercise in healthy subjects, but revealed important information, and the authors decided to present their results. There was no possibility to perform any statistical analysis because of the high variability of schedules, experimental conditions and different study groups described in the papers cited. Ethical approval was not necessary, because the study did not involve participants.

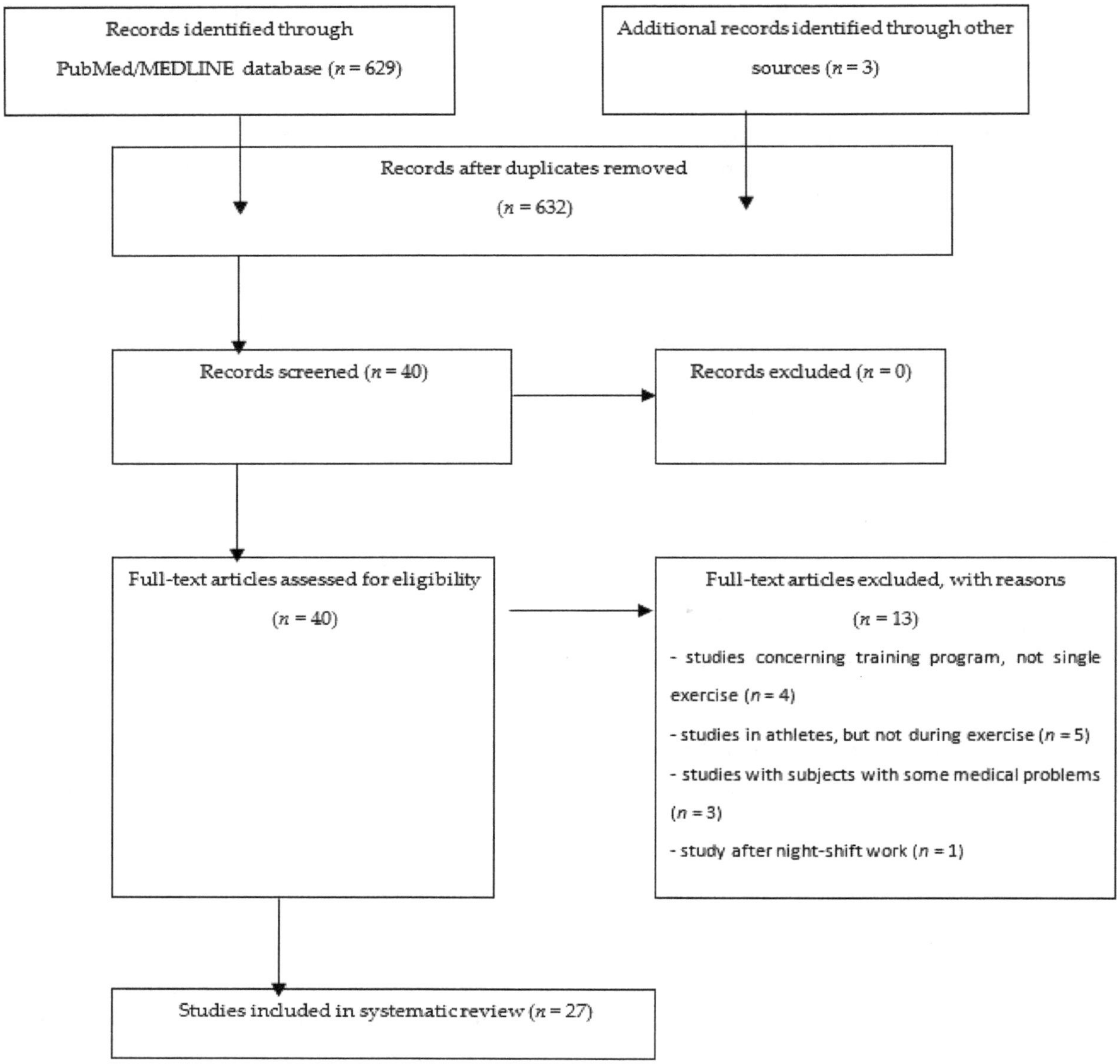

Figure 2. Flow chart illustrating the procedure for article inclusion and exclusion in a systematic review of changes in AKI biomarkers after exercise.

Author Contributions: Conceptualization, W.W. and W.R.; resources W.W., W.R. and J.R.; writing—original draft preparation, W.W.; writing—review and editing, W.R., M.R. and J.R.; visualization W.W.; supervision, M.R. All authors have read and agreed to the published version of the manuscript.

Abbreviations

AKI	acute kidney injury
u	urinary
s	serum
p	plasma
NGAL	neutrophil gelatinase-associated lipocalin
KIM-1	kidney injury molecule-1
Cyst-C	cystatin C
Cr	creatinine
L-FABP	liver-type fatty-acid-binding protein

IL	interleukin
TTF3	trefoil factor-3
TNFα	tumor necrosis factor α
YKL-40	chitinase 3-like protein 1
MCP-1	monocyte chemoattractant protein-1
IGFBP7	insulin-like growth factor binding protein 7
TIMP-2	tissue inhibitor of metalloproteinases-2
uMarker/uCyst-C	urinary marker normalized to cystatin C
uMarker/uCr	urinary marker normalized to creatinine
uMarker/uOsm	urinary marker normalized to osmolality
uMarker/u.f.	urinary marker normalized to urine flow
eGFR	estimated glomerular filtration rate
CKD EPI	Chronic Kidney Disease Epidemiology Collaboration equation
HIIRT	high-intensity interval resistance training
VO_2max	maximal oxygen consumption
HRmax	maximal heart rate
RH	relative humidity
OA	osteoarthiritis
MOF-VVPP	monomeric and oligomeric flavanols
VO_{2max}	maximal oxygen consumption
MMP-9	matrix metallopeptidase 9

References

1. Armstrong, J.A. Urinalysis in Western culture: A brief history. *Kidney Int.* **2007**, *71*, 384–387. [CrossRef] [PubMed]
2. MacKenzie, J.C. Dr Richard Bright—A man of many parts. His bicentenary year—1789–1858. *Bristol Med. Chir. J.* **1989**, *104*, 63–67. [PubMed]
3. Gardner, K.D. Athletic pseudonephritis; alteration of urine sediment by athletic competition. *J. Am. Med. Assoc.* **1956**, *161*, 1613–1617. [CrossRef] [PubMed]
4. Floege, J.; Feehally, J. Introduction to Glomerular Disease: Clinical Presetation. In *Comprehensive Clinical Nephrology*, 4th ed.; Floege, J., Johnson, R.J., Feehally, J., Eds.; Elsevier Inc.: New York, NY, USA, 2010; pp. 15–28. ISBN 978-0-323-05876-6.
5. Oh, D.J. A long journey for acute kidney injury biomarkers. *Ren. Fail.* **2020**, *42*, 154–165. [CrossRef]
6. Wasung, M.E.; Chawla, L.S.; Madero, M. Biomarkers of renal function, which and when? *Clin. Chim. Acta* **2015**, *438*, 350–357. [CrossRef]
7. Rhee, E.P. How omics data can be used in nephrology. *Am. J. Kidney Dis.* **2018**, *72*, 129–135. [CrossRef]
8. Kashani, K.; Cheungpasitporn, W.; Ronco, C. Biomarkers of acute kidney injury: The pathway from discovery to clinical adoption. *Clin. Chem. Lab. Med.* **2017**, *55*, 1074–1089. [CrossRef]
9. Liu, X.; Guan, Y.; Xu, S.; Li, Q.; Sun, Y.; Han, R.; Jiang, C. Early Predictors of Acute Kidney Injury: A Narrative Review. *Kidney Blood Press Res.* **2016**, *41*, 680–700. [CrossRef]
10. Guzzi, L.M.; Bergler, T.; Binnall, B.; Engelman, D.T.; Forni, L.; Germain, M.J.; Gluck, E.; Göcze, I.; Joannidis, M.; Koyner, J.L.; et al. Clinical use of [TIMP-2]•[IGFBP7] biomarker testing to assess risk of acute kidney injury in critical care: Guidance from an expert panel. *Crit. Care* **2019**, *23*, 225. [CrossRef]
11. Jamieson, H.C. Some newer tests of renal function. *Can. Med. Assoc. J.* **1933**, *29*, 598–604.
12. Narayanan, S.; Appleton, H.D. Creatinine: A review. *Clin. Chem.* **1980**, *26*, 1119–1126. [CrossRef] [PubMed]
13. Randers, E.; Kristensen, J.H.; Erlandsen, E.J.; Danielsen, H. Serum cystatin C as a marker of the renal function. *Scand. J. Clin. Lab. Investig.* **1998**, *58*, 585–592. [CrossRef] [PubMed]
14. Rangaswamy, D.; Sud, K. Acute kidney injury and disease: Long-term consequences and management. *BMJ Open Sport Exerc. Med.* **2017**, *3*, e000093. [CrossRef] [PubMed]
15. Hodgson, L.E.; Walter, E.; Venn, R.M.; Galloway, R.; Pitsiladis, Y.; Sardat, F.; Forni, L.G. Acute kidney injury associated with endurance events-is it a cause for concern? A systematic review. *Nephrology* **2018**, *23*, 969–980. [CrossRef] [PubMed]

16. Lima, R.S.A.; Junior, G.B.D.S.; Liborio, A.B.; Daher, E.D.F. Acute kidney injury due to rhabdomyolysis. *Saudi J. Kidney Dis. Transplant.* **2008**, *19*, 721–729.
17. Lipman, G.S.; Shea, K.; Christensen, M.; Phillips, C.; Burns, P.; Higbee, R.; Koskenoja, V.; Eifling, K.; Krabak, B.J. Ibuprofen versus placebo effect on acute kidney injury in ultramarathons: A randomized controlled trial. *Emerg. Med. J.* **2017**, *34*, 637–642. [CrossRef] [PubMed]
18. Chapman, C.L.; Johnson, B.D.; Sackett, J.R.; Parker, M.D.; Schlader, Z.J. Soft drink consumption during and following exercise in the heat elevates biomarkers of acute kidney injury. *Am. J. Physiol. Integr. Comp. Physiol.* **2019**, *316*, R189–R198. [CrossRef]
19. Kupferman, J.; Ramírez-Rubio, O.; Amador, J.J.; López-Pilarte, D.; Wilker, E.H.; Laws, R.L.; Sennett, C.; Robles, N.V.; Lau, J.L.; Salinas, A.J.; et al. Acute Kidney Injury in Sugarcane Workers at Risk for Mesoamerican Nephropathy. *Am J Kidney Dis.* **2018**, *72*, 475–482. [CrossRef]
20. Mingels, A.; Jacobs, L.; Kleijnen, V.; Wodzig, W.; Dieijen-Visser, M. Cystatin C a marker for renal function after exercise. *Int. J. Sports Med.* **2009**, *30*, 668–671. [CrossRef]
21. Odutayo, A.; Cherney, D. Cystatin C and acute changes in glomerular filtration rate. *Clin. Nephrol.* **2012**, *78*, 64–75. [CrossRef]
22. Scherr, J.; Braun, S.; Schuster, T.; Hartmann, C.; Moehlenkamp, S.; Wolfarth, B.; Pressler, A.; Halle, M. 72-h kinetics of high-sensitive troponin T and inflammatory markers after marathon. *Med. Sci. Sports Exerc.* **2011**, *43*, 1819–1827. [CrossRef] [PubMed]
23. McCullough, P.A.; Chinnaiyan, K.M.; Gallagher, M.J.; Colar, J.M.; Geddes, T.; Gold, J.M.; Trivax, J.E. Changes in renal markers and acute kidney injury after marathon running. *Nephrology* **2011**, *16*, 194–199. [CrossRef] [PubMed]
24. Hewing, B.; Schattke, S.; Spethmann, S.; Sanad, W.; Schroeckh, S.; Schimke, I.; Halleck, F.; Peters, H.; Brechtel, L.; Lock, J.; et al. Cardiac and renal function in a large cohort of amateur marathon runners. *Cardiovasc. Ultrasound* **2015**, *13*, 13. [CrossRef] [PubMed]
25. Poortmans, J.R.; Gulbis, B.; De Bruyn, E.; Baudry, S.; Carpentier, A. Limitations of serum values to estimate glomerular filtration rate during exercise. *Br. J. Sports Med.* **2013**, *47*, 1166–1170. [CrossRef] [PubMed]
26. Bongers, C.C.W.G.; Alsady, M.; Nijenhuis, T.; Tulp, A.D.M.; Eijsvogels, T.M.H.; Deen, P.M.T.; Hopman, M.T.E. Impact of acute versus prolonged exercise and dehydration on kidney function and injury. *Physiol. Rep.* **2018**, *6*, e13734. [CrossRef] [PubMed]
27. Poussel, M.; Touzé, C.; Allado, E.; Frimat, L.; Hily, O.; Thilly, N.; Rousseau, H.; Vauthier, J.C.; Chenuel, B. Ultramarathon and Renal Function: Does Exercise-Induced Acute Kidney Injury Really Exist in Common Conditions? *Front. Sports Act. Living* **2020**, *1*, 17. [CrossRef]
28. Colombini, A.; Corsetti, R.; Machado, M.; Graziani, R.; Lombardi, G.; Lanteri, P.; Banfi, G. Serum creatine kinase activity and its relationship with renal function indices in professional cyclists during the Giro d'Italia 3-week stage race. *Clin. J. Sport Med.* **2012**, *22*, 408–413. [CrossRef]
29. Colombini, A.; Corsetti, R.; Graziani, R.; Lombardi, G.; Lanteri, P.; Banfi, G. Evaluation of creatinine, cystatin C and eGFR by different equations in professional cyclists during the Giro d'Italia 3-weeks stage race. *Scand. J. Clin. Lab. Investig.* **2012**, *72*, 114–120. [CrossRef]
30. Banfi, G.; Del Fabbro, M.; D'Eril, G.M.; Melegati, G. Reliability of cystatin C in estimating renal function in rugby players. *Ann. Clin. Biochem.* **2009**, *46*, 428. [CrossRef]
31. Lousa, I.; Nascimento, H.; Rocha, S.; Catarino, C.; Reis, F.; Rêgo, C.; Santos-Silva, A.; Seabra, A.; Ribeiro, S.; Belo, L. Influence of the 6-month physical activity programs on renal function in obese boys. *Pediatr. Res.* **2018**, *83*, 1011–1015. [CrossRef]
32. Beetham, K.S.; Howden, E.J.; Isbel, N.M.; Coombes, J.S. Agreement between cystatin-C and creatinine based eGFR estimates after a 12-month exercise intervention in patients with chronic kidney disease. *BMC Nephrol.* **2018**, *18–19*, 366. [CrossRef] [PubMed]
33. Baxmann, A.C.; Ahmed, M.S.; Marques, N.C.; Menon, V.B.; Pereira, A.B.; Kirsztajn, G.M.; Heilberg, I.P. Influence of muscle mass and physical activity on serum and urinary creatinine and serum cystatin C. *Clin. J. Am. Soc. Nephrol.* **2008**, *3*, 348–354. [CrossRef] [PubMed]
34. Junglee, N.A.; Lemmey, A.B.; Burton, M.; Searell, C.; Jones, D.; Lawley, J.S.; Jibani, M.M.; Macdonald, J.H. Does proteinuria-inducing physical activity increase biomarkers of acute kidney injury? *Kidney Blood Press Res.* **2012**, *36*, 278–289. [CrossRef] [PubMed]

35. Junglee, N.A.; Di Felice, U.; Dolci, A.; Fortes, M.B.; Jibani, M.M.; Lemmey, A.B.; Walsh, N.P.; Macdonald, J.H. Exercising in a hot environment with muscle damage: Effects on acute kidney injury biomarkers and kidney function. *Am. J. Physiol. Ren. Physiol.* **2013**, *305*, F813–F820. [CrossRef] [PubMed]
36. Bender, A.; Kaesser, U.; Eichner, G.; Bachmann, G.; Steinmeyer, J. Biomarkers of Hand Osteoarthritis Are Detectable after Mechanical Exercise. *J. Clin. Med.* **2019**, *8*, 1545. [CrossRef] [PubMed]
37. Kanda, K.; Sugama, K.; Sakuma, J.; Kawakami, Y.; Suzuki, K. Evaluation of serum leaking enzymes and investigation into new biomarkers for exercise-induced muscle damage. *Exerc. Immunol. Rev.* **2014**, *20*, 39–54. [PubMed]
38. Rullman, E.; Olsson, K.; Wågsäter, D.; Gustafsson, T. Circulating MMP-9 during exercise in humans. *Eur. J. Appl. Physiol.* **2013**, *113*, 1249–1255. [CrossRef] [PubMed]
39. McDermott, B.P.; Smith, C.R.; Butts, C.L.; Caldwell, A.R.; Lee, E.C.; Vingren, J.L.; Munoz, C.X.; Kunces, L.J.; Williamson, K.; Ganio, M.S.; et al. Renal stress and kidney injury biomarkers in response to endurance cycling in the heat with and without ibuprofen. *J. Sci. Med. Sport* **2018**, *21*, 1180–1184. [CrossRef]
40. Lippi, G.; Sanchis-Gomar, F.; Salvagno, G.L.; Aloe, R.; Schena, F.; Guidi, G.C. Variation of serum and urinary neutrophil gelatinase associated lipocalin (NGAL) after strenuous physical exercise. *Clin. Chem. Lab. Med.* **2012**, *50*, 1585–1589. [CrossRef]
41. Andreazzoli, A.; Fossati, C.; Spaccamiglio, A.; Salvo, R.; Quaranta, F.; Minganti, C.; Di Luigi, L.; Borrione, P. Assessment of pN-GAL as a marker of renal function in elite cyclists during professional competitions. *J. Biol. Regul. Homeost. Agents* **2017**, *31*, 829–835.
42. Mellor, A.; Boos, C.; Stacey, M.; Hooper, T.; Smith, C.; Begley, J.; Yarker, J.; Piper, R.; O'Hara, J.; King, R.; et al. Neutrophil gelatinase-associated lipocalin: Its response to hypoxia and association with acute mountain sickness. *Dis. Markers* **2013**, *35*, 537–542. [CrossRef] [PubMed]
43. Chapman, C.L.; Johnson, B.D.; Vargas, N.T.; Hostler, D.; Parker, M.D.; Schlader, Z.J. Both hyperthermia and dehydration during physical work in the heat contribute to the risk of acute kidney injury. *J. Appl. Physiol.* **2020**, *128*, 715–728. [CrossRef] [PubMed]
44. Bongers, C.C.W.G.; Alsady, M.; Nijenhuis, T.; Hartman, Y.A.W.; Eijsvogels, T.M.H.; Deen, P.M.T.; Hopman, M.T.E. Impact of acute versus repetitive moderate intensity endurance exercise on kidney injury markers. *Physiol. Rep.* **2017**, *5*. [CrossRef] [PubMed]
45. Wołyniec, W.; Kasprowicz, K.; Giebułtowicz, J.; Korytowska, N.; Zorena, K.; Bartoszewicz, M.; Rita-Tkachenko, P.; Renke, M.; Ratkowski, W. Changes in Water Soluble Uremic Toxins and Urinary Acute Kidney Injury Biomarkers After 10- and 100-km Runs. *Int. J. Environ. Res. Public Health* **2019**, *16*, 4153. [CrossRef] [PubMed]
46. Mansour, S.G.; Verma, G.; Pata, R.W.; Martin, T.G.; Perazella, M.A.; Parikh, C.R. Kidney Injury and Repair Biomarkers in Marathon Runners. *Am. J. Kidney Dis.* **2017**, *70*, 252–261. [CrossRef]
47. Wołyniec, W.; Ratkowski, W.; Urbański, R.; Bartoszewicz, M.; Siluk, D.; Wołyniec, Z.; Kasprowicz, K.; Zorena, K.; Renke, M. Urinary Kidney Injury Molecule-1 but Not Urinary Neutrophil Gelatinase Associated Lipocalin Is Increased after Short Maximal Exercise. *Nephron* **2018**, *138*, 29–34. [CrossRef]
48. Spada, T.C.; Silva, J.M.R.D.; Francisco, L.S.; Marçal, L.J.; Antonangelo, L.; Zanetta, D.M.T.; Yu, L.; Burdmann, E.A. High intensity resistance training causes muscle damage and increases biomarkers of acute kidney injury in healthy individuals. *PLoS ONE* **2018**, *13*, e0205791. [CrossRef]
49. Semen, K.O.; van der Doelen, R.H.A.; van der Lugt, M.; van Dam, D.; Reimer, J.; Stassen, F.R.M.; Janssen, L.; Janssen, P.; Janssen, M.J.W.; Bast, A.; et al. Non- steroidal anti-inflammatory drugs increase urinary neutrophil gelatinase-associated lipocalin in recreational runners. *Scand. J. Med. Sci. Sports* **2020**. [CrossRef]
50. Semen, K.O.; Weseler, A.R.; Janssen, M.J.W.; Drittij-Reijnders, M.J.; le Noble, J.L.M.L.; Bast, A. Effects of Monomeric and Oligomeric Flavanols on Kidney Function, Inflammation and Oxidative Stress in Runners: A Randomized Double-Blind Pilot Study. *Nutrients* **2020**, *12*, 1634. [CrossRef]
51. Jouffroy, R.; Lebreton, X.; Mansencal, N.; Anglicheau, D. Acute kidney injury during an ultra-distance race. *PLoS ONE* **2019**, *14*, e0222544. [CrossRef]
52. Machado, J.C.Q.; Volpe, C.M.O.; Vasconcellos, L.S.; Nogueira-Machado, J.A. Quantification of NGAL in Urine of Endurance Cycling Athletes. *J. Phys. Act. Health* **2018**, *15*, 679–682. [CrossRef] [PubMed]
53. Kosaki, K.; Kamijo-Ikemori, A.; Sugaya, T.; Kumamoto, S.; Tanahashi, K.; Kumagai, H.; Kimura, K.; Shibagaki, Y.; Maeda, S. Incremental short maximal exercise increases urinary liver-type fatty acid-binding protein in adults without CKD. *Scand. J. Med. Sci. Sports* **2020**, *30*, 709–715. [CrossRef] [PubMed]

54. Yamamoto, T.; Noiri, E.; Ono, Y.; Doi, K.; Negishi, K.; Kamijo, A.; Kimura, K.; Fujita, T.; Kinukawa, T.; Taniguchi, H.; et al. Renal L-type fatty acid—Binding protein in acute ischemic injury. *J. Am. Soc. Nephrol.* **2007**, *18*, 2894–2902. [CrossRef] [PubMed]
55. Hiraki, K.; Kamijo-Ikemori, A.; Yasuda, T.; Hotta, C.; Izawa, K.P.; Watanabe, S.; Sugaya, T.; Kimura, K. Moderate-intensity single exercise session does not induce renal damage. *J. Clin. Lab. Anal.* **2013**, *27*, 177–180. [CrossRef]
56. Kosaki, K.; Kamijo-Ikemori, A.; Sugaya, T.; Tanahashi, K.; Kumagai, H.; Sawano, Y.; Akazawa, N.; Ra, S.G.; Kimura, K.; Shibagaki, Y.; et al. Relationship between exercise capacity and urinary liver-type fatty acid-binding protein in middle-aged and older individuals. *Clin. Exp. Nephrol.* **2017**, *21*, 810–817. [CrossRef]
57. Kosaki, K.; Kamijo-Ikemori, A.; Sugaya, T.; Tanahashi, K.; Sawano, Y.; Akazawa, N.; Ra, S.G.; Kimura, K.; Shibagaki, Y.; Maeda, S. Effect of habitual exercise on urinary liver-type fatty acid-binding protein levels in middle-aged and older adults. *Scand. J. Med. Sci. Sports* **2018**, *28*, 152–160. [CrossRef]
58. Uchiyama, K.; Washida, N.; Morimoto, K.; Muraoka, K.; Nakayama, T.; Adachi, K.; Kasai, T.; Miyashita, K.; Wakino, S.; Itoh, H. Effects of exercise on residual renal function in patients undergoing peritoneal dialysis: A post-hoc analysis of a randomized controlled trial. *Ther. Apher. Dial.* **2020**. [CrossRef]
59. Sugama, K.; Suzuki, K.; Yoshitani, K.; Shiraishi, K.; Kometani, T. Urinary excretion of cytokines versus their plasma levels after endurance exercise. *Exerc. Immunol. Rev.* **2013**, *19*, 29–48.
60. Dutheil, F.; Trousselard, M.; Perrier, C.; Lac, G.; Chamoux, A.; Duclos, M.; Naughton, G.; Mnatzaganian, G.; Schmidt, J. Urinary interleukin-8 is a biomarker of stress in emergency physicians, especially with advancing age—The JOBSTRESS* randomized trial. *PLoS ONE* **2013**, *8*, e71658. [CrossRef]
61. Pryor, R.R.; Pryor, J.L.; Vandermark, L.W.; Adams, E.L.; Brodeur, R.M.; Schlader, Z.J.; Armstrong, L.E.; Lee, E.C.; Maresh, C.M.; Casa, D.J. Acute Kidney Injury Biomarker Responses to Short-Term Heat Acclimation. *Int. J. Environ. Res. Public Health* **2020**, *17*, 1325. [CrossRef]
62. Apeland, T.; Danielsen, T.; Staal, E.M.; Åsberg, A.; Thorsen, I.S.; Dalsrud, T.O.; Ørn, S. Risk factors for exertional rhabdomyolysis with renal stress. *BMJ Open Sport Exerc. Med.* **2017**, *3*, e000241. [CrossRef] [PubMed]
63. Matomäki, P.; Kainulainen, H.; Kyröläinen, H. Corrected whole blood biomarkers—The equation of Dill and Costill revisited. *Physiol. Rep.* **2018**, *6*, e13749. [CrossRef] [PubMed]
64. Yang, X.; Wu, H.; Li, H. Dehydration-associated chronic kidney disease: A novel case of kidney failure in China. *BMC Nephrol.* **2020**, *21*, 159. [CrossRef] [PubMed]

11

Contribution of Predictive and Prognostic Biomarkers to Clinical Research on Chronic Kidney Disease

Michele Provenzano [1,*], Salvatore Rotundo [2], Paolo Chiodini [3], Ida Gagliardi [1], Ashour Michael [1], Elvira Angotti [4], Silvio Borrelli [5], Raffaele Serra [6], Daniela Foti [2], Giovambattista De Sarro [7] and Michele Andreucci [1,*]

1 Renal Unit, Department of Health Sciences, "Magna Graecia" University of Catanzaro, I-88100 Catanzaro, Italy; ida_88@libero.it (I.G.); ashourmichael@yahoo.com (A.M.)

2 Department of Health Sciences, "Magna Graecia" University of Catanzaro, I-88100 Catanzaro, Italy; srotundo91@gmail.com (S.R.); foti@unicz.it (D.F.)

3 Medical Statistics Unit, University of Campania Luigi Vanvitelli, I-80138 Naples, Italy; paolo.chiodini@unicampania.it

4 Clinical Biochemistry Unit, Azienda Ospedaliera Universitaria Mater Domini Hospital, I-88100 Catanzaro, Italy; e.angotti@materdominiaou.it

5 Renal Unit, University of Campania "Luigi Vanvitelli", I-80138 Naples, Italy; dott.silvioborrelli@gmail.com

6 Interuniversity Center of Phlebolymphology (CIFL), "Magna Graecia" University of Catanzaro, I-88100 Catanzaro, Italy; rserra@unicz.it

7 Pharmacology Unit, Department of Health Sciences, School of Medicine, "Magna Graecia" University of Catanzaro, I-88100 Catanzaro, Italy; desarro@unicz.it

* Correspondence: michiprov@hotmail.it (M.P.); andreucci@unicz.it (M.A.)

Abstract: Chronic kidney disease (CKD), defined as the presence of albuminuria and/or reduction in estimated glomerular filtration rate (eGFR) < 60 mL/min/1.73 m^2, is considered a growing public health problem, with its prevalence and incidence having almost doubled in the past three decades. The implementation of novel biomarkers in clinical practice is crucial, since it could allow earlier diagnosis and lead to an improvement in CKD outcomes. Nevertheless, a clear guidance on how to develop biomarkers in the setting of CKD is not yet available. The aim of this review is to report the framework for implementing biomarkers in observational and intervention studies. Biomarkers are classified as either prognostic or predictive; the first type is used to identify the likelihood of a patient to develop an endpoint regardless of treatment, whereas the second type is used to determine whether the patient is likely to benefit from a specific treatment. Many single assays and complex biomarkers were shown to improve the prediction of cardiovascular and kidney outcomes in CKD patients on top of the traditional risk factors. Biomarkers were also shown to improve clinical trial designs. Understanding the correct ways to validate and implement novel biomarkers in CKD will help to mitigate the global burden of CKD and to improve the individual prognosis of these high-risk patients.

Keywords: end-stage kidney disease (ESKD); cardiovascular disease; epidemiology; CKD; biomarkers

---

1. Introduction

A biomarker is defined, by a collaborative working group involved with both the United States National Institutes of Health (NIH) and the Food and Drug Administration (FDA), as "a characteristic that is measured as an indicator of normal biological processes, pathogenic processes, or responses to an exposure or intervention, including therapeutic interventions" [1]. This working group definition was formed on the initiative of the NIH with the aim of accelerating the development and clinical application of reliable biomarkers based on shared definitions. Indeed, an "ideal" biomarker is defined with the presence of some analytic features: (1) it should be measured and readily available in biological samples, such as blood or urine; (2) it should be reproducible, non-invasive, and not expensive [2]. In addition, several clinical features should also be provided to complete the biomarker's definition; it needs to allow for an early detection of a disease status, while it also needs to have high sensitivity and specificity, i.e., the biomarker needs to differentiate the pathologic status from the normal one and from other clinical conditions, as accurately as possible [3]. The effort made by the NIH–FDA working group is considerable ever since it forecasted and tried to solve the problems of biomarker development, from discovery to clinical application. Indeed, once a biomarker is found to be involved in one or more pathophysiological mechanisms of a disease, it may be introduced into clinical practice to see whether it offers advantages in clinical management and after completion of the validation phase that is considered a crucial step [4]. An important example of the pitfalls of biomarker development is illustrated in the chronic kidney disease (CKD) scenario. CKD is a chronic disease characterized by a poor prognosis, due to the strong association with the development of cardiovascular events, all-cause mortality, and renal events such as renal replacement therapies (RRT, i.e., dialysis or kidney transplantation) [5,6]. The Kidney Disease Improving Global Outcomes Work Group (KDIGO), in 2012, defined CKD with the presence of either decreased kidney function (estimated glomerular filtration rate (eGFR) < 60 mL/min/1.73 m^2) and/or albuminuria, namely, an abnormal amount of protein excretion with urine, for at least three months [7]. The global dimension of the disease is so important that CKD started to be considered a relevant public health problem. Indeed, according to the Global Burden of Kidney Disease, the CKD incidence and prevalence increased by 88.76% and 86.95%, respectively, from 1990 to 2016 [8]. Moreover, the mortality attributed to CKD increased by 41.5% between 1990 and 2017, a percentage that exceeded the mortality due to several neoplasms or cardiovascular (CV) disease [9]. Hence, great effort is advocated toward improving clinical decision-making and reinforcing treatment and prevention of CKD. The KDIGO working group proposed a classification called "CGA" that incorporates the cause (C) of kidney disease, as well as the eGFR (G) and albuminuria (A) levels, to stratify risk in patients with CKD and to better address the importance of the underlying disease. However, considering eGFR and albuminuria levels in cross-tabs, like those reported in KDIGO guidelines, does not take into consideration the complex mechanisms of CKD. In fact, all patients are stratified on the basis of eGFR and albuminuria and allocated in risk categories for prognostic estimations. This approach was also defined as "reductionist", since it does not consider the different etiologies of CKD and many other parameters, including serum or urine biomarkers, which could help clinical management of CKD [10]. Moreover, although the KDIGO also suggested considering the causes of kidney disease to predict poor outcomes in CKD patients, how to incorporate these parameters remains unclear [11]. Few studies included renal diagnoses in risk prediction models and, when diagnoses are present, they are classified in different ways (i.e., four, five, or even six categories) with large heterogeneity between studies, thus making an univocal interpretation difficult [12,13]. There is also a growing debate regarding the question whether an eGFR reduction below the threshold of 60 mL/min/1.73 m^2 represents the consequence of a physiologic senescence or a marker of renal pathology [14,15]. In fact, despite the evidence that eGFR reduction foresees both the onset of end-stage kidney disease (ESKD) and the all-cause death regardless of age, in large general and high-risk populations, other human studies showed that kidneys undergo structural and functional change with aging such as nephrosclerosis and a reduction in measured GFR [14,16]. At the same time, these changes are not associated with a reduction in single-nephron GFR; this is the likely reason why, in the absence of albuminuria, the GFR reduction alone determines only a small increased risk for age-standardized mortality and ESKD [16]. Owing to these important controversies and in an attempt to improve risk stratification and care of CKD patients, as well as to share clinical findings with the nephrology community, the International Society of Nephrology

(ISN) started an international project called "closing the gaps", which encompasses a set of activities that have to be performed to improve the prognosis of CKD patients [17]. The core of this project is about the development, implementation, and clinical application of novel biomarkers in CKD patients. It indeed emerged that, with the exception of cystatin C, which is a filtration marker useful to estimate the eGFR and to improve risk prediction in CKD, the vast majority of previously tested biomarkers in CKD did not reach any clinical application [18]. The aim of this review is to report the principal pieces of evidence regarding biomarker development in CKD, the contribution of these biomarkers to both observational and interventional (i.e., randomized controlled trials) studies, and the possible strategies that could be followed to ameliorate this important branch of clinical research.

2. General Classification of Biomarkers

Depending on the intended use, biomarkers are classified as diagnostic, pharmacodynamic/ response, monitoring, prognostic, or predictive [19]. We focus, in the present review article, on prognostic and predictive biomarkers, as they represent the most developed biomarkers in CKD patients, while they also incorporate characteristics from other categories of biomarkers. A prognostic biomarker is used to identify the probability of a clinical outcome in patients who are already suffering from the disease of interest [1,20]. Furthermore, prognostic biomarkers measure the association between the disease and clinical outcome in the absence of therapy or with standard therapy that all patients are likely to receive. On the other hand, predictive biomarkers are used to determine whether a patient is likely to benefit from a particular therapy. The clinical benefit could be either a good response to a drug if the biomarker is positive or, alternatively, a lack of benefit from the same drug, which can save a patient from drug toxicity or unnecessary side effects [1].

3. Prognostic Biomarkers in CKD

The importance of prognostic biomarkers in the CKD setting is crucial. Indeed, CKD is a multifactorial disease in which risk factors play different roles in different individuals and in different stages of the disease. It was demonstrated, for example, that the presence of type 2 diabetes leads to the development of CKD in up to 30% of subjects. This means that, in these patients, the deleterious pathogenetic mechanisms of diabetes mellitus are sufficient to damage the kidneys with the onset of typical diabetic glomerulosclerosis. Conversely, it is also possible that, in a portion of diabetic patients, the kidneys are injured by the co-existence of arterial hypertension, which causes different lesions (mainly injuring the kidney vessels), with a completely different prognosis.

3.1. Kidney Biomarkers

The assessment of correct risk stratification, i.e., the allocation of CKD patients to the true risk-of-event categories, always represents a difficult challenge for nephrologists and researchers, due to the large variability in etiology and prognosis of CKD [21,22]. In order to accomplish this aim, a growing number of risk prediction models in CKD patients were developed over the past several years. They show how kidney measures, such as albuminuria (or proteinuria) and eGFR, are strong prognostic biomarkers. Indeed, an eGFR reduction to levels below 60 mL/min/1.73 m^2 or even a small increase in albuminuria levels is associated with a significantly increased risk for CV events (CV mortality, coronary heart disease, stroke, heart failure), all-cause mortality, and ESKD (the most advanced stage of CKD that requires referral to renal replacement therapies such as hemodialysis), both in the general population and in patients with an already established CKD (Figure 1) [23–25].

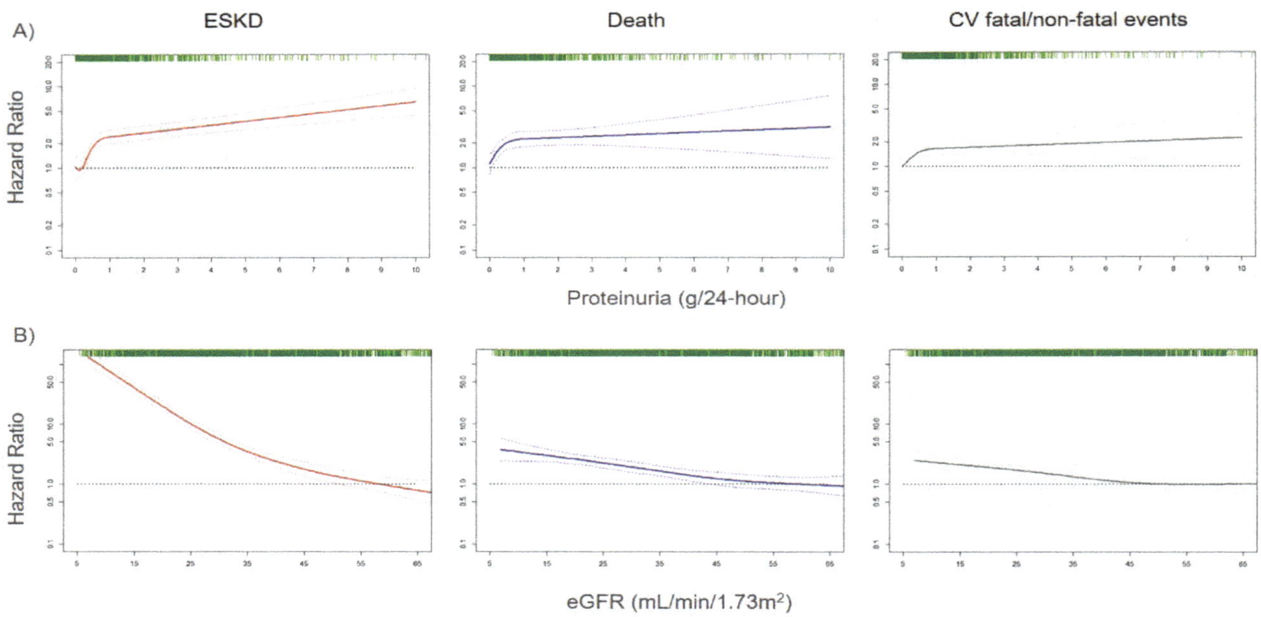

Figure 1. Adjusted risks for end-stage kidney disease (ESKD), death, and cardiovascular (CV) fatal and non-fatal events, by 24-h proteinuria (panel **A**) or estimated glomerular filtration rate (eGFR) (panel **B**) levels. Solid lines represent hazard ratios, whereas dashed lines the 95% confidence intervals. Hazard ratios were modeled by means of restricted cubic spline (RCS) due to the non-linear association with the endpoints. Knots are located at the zeroth, 25th, 50th, and 75th percentiles for proteinuria and 15, 30, 45, 60 mL/min/1.73 m^2 for eGFR. Risks are adjusted for the four-variable Tangri equation [26]: age, gender, eGFR, and proteinuria. Rug plots on the x-axis at the top (colored green) represent the distribution of observations. Data source: pooled analysis of six cohorts of CKD patients referred to Italian nephrology clinics [27].

Albuminuria and eGFR were also recently used to develop individual risk prediction models for both CV and renal risk in CKD patients. These models employ statistical measures (such as calibration, discrimination, and validation) that represent an essential step before applying risk estimates at the individual level [25,26,28,29]. Moreover, risk prediction models are available for patients with early, moderate, and severe stages of CKD. The addition of albuminuria and eGFR to traditional risk factors included in the model (such as age, gender, presence of diabetes, blood pressure, serum cholesterol) was associated with a significant improvement in risk prediction. Even more importantly, the contribution of albuminuria and eGFR to the prediction of CV events (CV mortality, coronary heart disease, stroke, and heart failure) was found to be greater than traditional CV risk factors [24]. This notwithstanding, a main limitation of available risk score is the insufficient, even absent, consideration of underlying causes of renal disease, which is a crucial point when considering that CKD is a set of multiple etiologies rather than a single disease [12,13]. However, these first prediction models established that measuring albuminuria and eGFR is a central step for assessing risk stratification in CKD patients. Mechanisms of damage of albuminuria and eGFR were partially explained. Albuminuria was shown to exert a direct harmful effect on renal glomeruli and tubules [30]. Moreover, it can also be considered as a systemic marker of endothelial dysfunction, and this explains the reason for which the presence of proteinuria strictly forecasts the onset of CV events in the general population, as well as CKD patients [31]. Similarly, eGFR reduction is linked to an increase of uremic toxins that are responsible for kidney and systemic damage. A drop in eGFR was also associated with the development of coronary atherosclerosis, regardless of the presence of diabetes mellitus, dyslipidemia, previous CV disease, and other comorbidities [32]. Several studies showed that an eGFR decrease is associated with the onset of sudden cardiac death (SCD), with the data being confirmed from the early stage of CKD, i.e., from eGFR < 60 mL/min/1.73 m^2 [33–35]. For each 10 mL/min decrement in eGFR, SCD risk increased by 11% [33]. SCD accounts for the vast majority of deaths in CKD patients and is also mediated by metabolic and electrophysiological abnormalities [36]. However, both eGFR and albuminuria have limitations in risk prediction. Albuminuria is not specific for any kidney disease, occurring in ischemic, diabetic, and tubulointerstitial nephropathies, as well as in the vast majority of glomerulonephritis and autoimmune diseases [13]. Albuminuria also presents a random variability, since urine protein excretion follows a circadian rhythm that is influenced by posture, exercise, or dietary factors [37]. The eGFR, albeit associated with a poor prognosis, could also be altered by temporary or reversible clinical conditions, such as volume depletions or sub-acute tubulointerstitial diseases [11]. Taken together, proteinuria and eGFR share the limitation of detecting kidney damage often when it is already established and is, thus, not reversible [15]. Furthermore, urine protein excretion is strictly dependent on eGFR levels, which are an expression of the number of functional nephrons in the kidney. In fact, we recently demonstrated that, in a model in which proteinuria is replaced by F-Uprot (proteinuria/eGFR × 100), an expression of the combination of the two biomarkers, the latter allowed refining risk stratification for ESKD outcome in all CKD stages, even in more advanced CKD [27]. Albuminuria levels are strictly dependent and, thus, modified by both systolic and diastolic blood pressure (BP). As long as the eGFR decreases, a given increase in BP is accompanied by an increase in urine protein excretion. This phenomenon was observed in both animal and human studies and is caused by the "remnant nephron effect", namely, the transmission of systemic hydrostatic pressure to the glomerular microcirculation [38,39]. Moreover, BP is a clinical parameter characterized per se by high variability, which is also detectable during 24-h ambulatory BP measurements (short-term variability) [40]. It was demonstrated that both systolic and diastolic BP variability influence albuminuria levels [41]. Hence, a number of variables were shown to influence albuminuria levels, and this could lead to biased risk estimation, particularly if the risk prediction is based on a single measurement of albuminuria. The ISN indeed highlighted that a consensus needs to be found on how often albuminuria should be measured to warrant a true prediction of cardiovascular and renal endpoints, as well as to monitor the course of CKD [18]. Owing to the evidence that eGFR and albuminuria are able to provide a strong but incomplete prediction of cardiorenal endpoints in CKD patients, the next step of prognostic research focused on the development and assessment of biomarkers that provide useful prognostic information beyond proteinuria and eGFR. A number of markers of inflammation, oxidative stress, or tissue remodeling aroused interest in improving CV and renal risk prediction in CKD patients.

3.2. Markers of Oxidative Stress, Tissue Remodeling, and Metabolism

Myeloperoxidase (MPO) is a biomarker of oxidative stress that fosters nitic oxide consumption and which is associated with the development of atherosclerotic lesions, CV disease, and eGFR decline in CKD [42,43]. A recent observational analysis of the Chronic Renal Insufficiency Cohort (CRIC), which enrolled approximately 4000 patients with CKD in the United States (US), showed that serum MPO levels were associated with the risk of renal outcome, defined as initiation of RRT, 50% eGFR decline, or eGFR $\leq$ 15 mL/min/1.73 m^2 [44]. The key element of this analysis was that the effect of MPO was significant even after adjustment for main confounders, such as baseline eGFR and proteinuria levels. Matrix metalloproteinases (MMPs), endopeptidases involved in tissue development, and homeostasis through the regulation of cell differentiation, apoptosis, and angiogenesis were shown to intervene in inflammatory and fibrotic processes across the kidneys [45,46]. Blood and urine levels of MMPs were linked to renal and CV disease in previous clinical studies in humans. Serum and urine MMP-2, -8, and -9 levels are increased in patients with diabetic CKD, with MMP-9 being significantly associated with the severity of albuminuria [47,48]. Increased plasma levels of TIMP-1 (tissue inhibitor of metalloproteinases-1) predicted the incidence of CKD regardless of inflammatory markers such as C-reactive protein [49]. MMPs and TIMPs also play a role in accelerating the atherosclerotic process by increasing cell migration to the plaque fibrous cap that in turn determines plaque inflammation and rupture [50]. Indeed, the levels of several MMPs (MMP-1, -2, -8, -9) and TIMP-1 were found to be increased in patients with peripheral arterial disease, including those with aneurysms of the arterial wall [51]. Fibroblast growth factor-23 (FGF-23), a hormone involved in phosphorus metabolism that increases progressively as kidney function declines, was significantly associated with mortality, atherosclerotic events, heart failure (HF), and ESKD in CKD patients [52,53].

3.3. Cardiac Biomarkers

Several cardiac biomarkers were investigated, mainly for establishing their role in CV and renal risk prediction in CKD patients. Cardiac troponins (high-sensitivity cardiac troponin (hs-cTnT)) and natriuretic peptides (N-terminal pro-B-type natriuretic peptide (NT-proBNP)) are largely used in CV medicine to diagnose coronary artery disease (CAD) and heart failure (HF), respectively. Both these biomarkers are, thus, an expression of subclinical abnormalities in the heart [54,55]. However, one major problem that makes their introduction in individual risk prediction difficult is that cardiac markers are an expression of both cardiac and kidney dysfunction and cannot discern these two conditions. Natriuretic peptides act by promoting the tubular natriuresis across the kidney and counteracting the effects of renin–angiotensin–aldosterone system, which is triggered by heart failure, as well as renal dysfunction [56]. Concerns about the interpretation of hs-cTnT and natriuretic peptides also derive from the evidence that these marker concentrations are influenced by kidney function levels [56,57]. So far, cardiac markers found more application in the context of prognostic estimation of cardiorenal syndromes (CRS), clinical disorders where an acute or chronic dysfunction of one organ may lead to an acute or chronic dysfunction of the other, thus testifying the strict relationship between the heart and the kidney [58]. In the general population, hs-cTnT and NT-proBNP were shown to be strong predictors for incident HF over time [59,60]. In the setting of CKD, an attempt to evaluate, with appropriate statistical tools, the contribution of cardiac markers to the development of CV events was made using the Atherosclerosis Risk in Communities study (ARIC) population. In this study, examining 7682 non-CKD and 970 patients with CKD stage 1–5, hs-cTnT and NT-proBNP were associated with the development of CV events (defined as the composite of coronary heart disease, stroke, and HF) independently of kidney measures (eGFR and albuminuria) [61]. The finding was confirmed for both CKD and non-CKD patients, as well as for patients with or without previous CV disease. However, the interpretation of these results should be done with caution since the ARIC cohort was stratified, for this analysis, by the presence/absence of CKD, thus limiting the influence of kidney measures on CV risk prediction [61]. Results of the association between cardiac markers and renal outcomes in CKD patients are even more conflicting. The CRIC investigators found, in a cohort of over 3000 CKD patients, that increased plasma levels of growth differentiation factor-15 (GDF-15, a member of the transforming growth factor (TGF)-β cytokine family), hs-cTnT, and NT-proBNP were associated with CKD progression. defined as the onset of ESKD or 50% eGFR decline [62]. However, when all these parameters were added to the prediction model including traditional CV risk factors, the model discrimination (i.e., the ability of the model to separate individuals who develop events from those who do not; see more details in Section 5) did not improve, meaning that their clinical utility was scarce. Moreover, in the Framingham cohort, hs-cTnT was not associated with a faster eGFR decline or with incident CKD [63]. There is, overall, a need for future work to assess the role of cardiac markers in CV and renal risk prediction [61–63].

3.4. Filtration and Urinary Biomarkers

Filtration biomarkers and urinary markers were also investigated. The use of cystatin C to estimate GFR ($eGFR_{cys}$) improved the risk stratification for death, death from CV causes, and ESKD with a large proportion (23%) of patients being reclassified toward true risk estimates when compared with eGFR estimated from serum creatinine ($eGFR_{crea}$) [64]. $eGFR_{cys}$ was also shown to predict the onset of SCD in elderly CKD patients [35]. The combination of serum creatinine and cystatin C for estimating eGFR ($eGFR_{cys\text{-}crea}$) allowed clinicians to anticipate the risk prediction of worse outcomes at 85 mL/min, which is well above the 60 mL/min threshold defined by $eGFR_{crea}$. β2-microglobulin, another filtration marker, showed a statistical power similar to cystatin C in improving prediction of ESKD, all-cause mortality, and new onset of CV disease beyond $eGFR_{crea}$ [65]. With respect to urinary markers, some evidence, albeit controversial, was provided for the association of urinary markers of tubule damage (interleukin (IL)-18, kidney injury molecule-1 (KIM-1), neutrophil gelatinase-associated lipocalin (NGAL)), repair (human cartilage glycoprotein-40 (YKL-40)), and inflammation (monocyte chemoattractant protein-1 (MCP-1)) with the risk of ESKD [66,67]. In fact, when risk prediction models were adjusted for baseline eGFR and albuminuria, the associations of these biomarkers with clinical outcome were consistently attenuated. However, the highest values of KIM-1, MCP-1, and YKL-40 also provided useful risk estimation beyond eGFR and albuminuria in a post hoc analysis of the Systolic Blood Pressure Intervention Trial SPRINT trial [68]. Interestingly, urinary IL-18 and NGAL levels were shown to predict linear eGFR decline over time, an endpoint of growing interest in clinical research [68].

3.5. Prognostic Role of Proteomics, Metabolomics, and Genomics

Proteomics metabolomics and genomics recently provided great input to the implementation of novel biomarkers [69–71]. The advantage of these "omics" techniques is to provide a combination of informative peptides/metabolites that are able to classify patients (hence, the appellation of classifiers) into significant clinical or risk categories. A well-depicted classifier in CKD patients is the CKD273, a panel of 273 urine peptides shown to predict, in long-term follow-up cohort studies, eGFR decline with a strong and independent effect to the onset of albuminuria, particularly in diabetic patients [72–74]. In further risk prediction models, CKD273 was also able to reclassify about 30% of patients compared with the standard equation that considers eGFR and albuminuria, for the risk of CKD progression [75]. The CRIC investigators described, in a recent manuscript, the association between a panel of 13 urine metabolites and CKD progression [76]. Results of this analysis are encouraging since the levels of four metabolites, namely, 3-hydroxyisobutyrate (3-HIBA), 3-methylcrotonyglycine, citric acid, and aconitic acid, were associated with eGFR decline, with 3-HIBA and aconitic acid levels also significantly associated with the hard endpoint ESKD. Of particular interest is the prognostic role of the genetic causes of CKD. Of all CKD cases diagnosed at a young age (<25 years), an actual 30% are determined by monogenic disorders, and inherited CKD is globally more prevalent (prevalence ranged between 30% and 75%) than previously thought, particularly in the presence of a family history of CKD [77,78]. More importantly, the advent of genome-wide association studies (GWAS) allowed the discovery of several single-nucleotide polymorphisms (SNPs) associated with an increased risk for CKD or with a worse prognosis in patients already affected by CKD [78]. Polymorphisms in the Uromodulin (UMOD) gene region rs4293393, which codifies the most abundant urinary protein in healthy subjects, namely, uromodulin (also called Tamm–Horsfall protein), are associated with an increased risk of incident CKD [79]. A similar role in predicting the onset of CKD was exerted by other SNPs such as Protein Kinase AMP-Activated Non-Catalytic Subunit Gamma 2 (PRKAG2), Longevity Assurance Gene Homologs (LASS2), Disabled Homolog 2 (alias DAB Adaptor Protein 2, DAB2), Dachshund Family Transcription Factor 1 (DACH1), and Stanniocalcin 1 (STC1) [80]. Apolipoprotein L1 (APOL1) gene variants were also studied in CKD patients. APOL1 encodes apolipoprotein L1, which is involved in the lysis of *Trypanosoma brucei* and other trypanosomes [81]. The G1 and G2 variants of APOL1 were associated with an increased risk of eGFR decline and disease progression to ESKD in CKD populations [82]. Interestingly, information derived from the SNPs were recently combined into a genetic risk score [78]. This score was shown to be associated with eGFR decline and kidney outcome regardless of albuminuria and other renal risk factors encompassing diabetes, history of CV disease, and hypertension. A number of studies assessing the associations between SNPs and kidney measures were carried-out by the United Kingdom (UK) biobank, a large cohort of over 500,000 participants enrolled in 2006–2010, from which genotypic information was widely collected [83]. Analyses of the UK biobank provided a great contribution to the prognostic research in CKD. For example, genetically predicted testosterone and fasting insulin, with the latter being an expression of insulin resistance, were found to be associated with CKD and worse kidney function in men, thus highlighting the possible reasons for discrepancy in CKD prevalence and CKD progression among men and women [84,85]. Intriguingly, a genome-wide association study of UK biobank showed that albumin-to-creatinine ratio (ACR) is dependent on multiple pathways and that an ACR genetic risk score may improve the prediction of hypertension and stroke [86].

4. Predictive Biomarkers in CKD

Predictive biomarkers are used in disparate fields of medicine to assess the likelihood of response to treatments and the individual pathophysiology of the disease. One major example of this strategy is represented by the large use of predictive biomarkers in oncology. Causative mutations of the breast cancer genes 1 and 2 (BRCA1/2) were found to be predictive biomarkers for identifying the response to poly(ADP-ribose) polymerase (PARP) inhibitors [87]. Such a discovery is crucial as BRCA1/2 provide information on the best drug for the individual patient in order to improve their prognosis. While, in oncology, a set of pathophysiological mechanisms is crucial for tumor development, what complicates the application of predictive biomarkers in chronic diseases is that different mechanisms are active in different stages of the disease itself and in different patients [88]. This means that, if a treatment is started on the basis of a blood/urine biomarker level, the individual prognosis may remain unchanged or even worsen, due to the presence of other active mechanisms of damage, as well as, most importantly, different disease entities that cause the chronic decline of renal function through diverse pathophysiological pathways. Notwithstanding, in chronic disease, great research effort was also started with the aim of personalizing treatments following the methodological concept of "the right drug for the right patient". Hence, the implementation of predictive biomarkers represents a topic of increasing importance.

4.1. Kidney Biomarkers

In nephrology, the most used predictive biomarkers are eGFR and albuminuria. Both these biomarkers can be considered as "dynamic" predictive biomarkers. In fact, their levels change over time with the effects of treatment, such that they can be efficiently used for monitoring the course of CKD and the appropriateness of the therapy followed by the patient. In the past few decades, several interventional studies were carried out testing the effect of nephroprotective drugs on hard endpoints such as mortality, CV events, and ESKD in patients with CKD [89–96]. Although interventions differed between studies, with principally antihypertensive drugs and albuminuria-lowering agents being tested, all these trials pointed out that the CV, mortality, and ESKD risk reductions were strictly associated with a reduction in albuminuria after the start of treatment. Moreover, the magnitude of treatment effect was greater in patients with higher albuminuria levels at the time of the initial visit [95,96]. These findings are reinforced by the evidence that albuminuria changes also played a potentially beneficial role in negative clinical trials. In the Aliskiren Trial in Type 2 Diabetes Using Cardiorenal Endpoints (ALTITUDE), which failed in demonstrating the advantage of adding Aliskiren to an angiotensin-converting enzyme inhibitor (ACEi) or an angiotensin-receptor blocker (ARB) on CV and renal outcomes, patients who showed an albuminuria reduction in the Aliskiren arm (37%) were largely protected against CKD progression compared with those who did not show a reduction in albuminuria levels [97]. All these pieces of evidence testified that albuminuria has great predictive and prognostic power in CKD patients and, although further studies are needed to find the correct threshold of albuminuria reduction that can confer CV and renal risk protection after an appropriate treatment, there is a general consensus that a 30% reduction in its levels from baseline to six months could be acceptable [98]. With respect to eGFR, it was demonstrated that a doubling of serum creatinine level, which corresponds approximately to a 57% eGFR decline, was able to predict CKD progression in previous clinical trials in diabetic CKD patients [99]. The importance of that evidence is highlighted by the fact that, in these previous trials, eGFR decline correlated with renal outcomes after exposure to nephroprotective treatments, thus affirming its role as a predictive biomarker, in addition to a prognostic biomarker [100]. Since then, the association of lesser eGFR declines with CKD outcomes was tested. A post hoc analysis of the Reduction of End Points in Non-Insulin-Dependent Diabetes with the Angiotensin II Antagonist Losartan (RENAAL) and Irbesartan Diabetic Nephropathy Trial (IDNT) clinical trials, two studies that evaluated the efficacy of ARB treatment in patients with diabetes mellitus and nephropathy, showed that 30% and 40% eGFR declines may improve the power of clinical trials if the drug investigated does not determine an acute (within three months of the start of treatment) drop in eGFR [101]. A larger meta-analysis of 37 clinical trials in CKD patients documented a strong association between 30% and 40% eGFR decline in the first 12 months of treatment and the onset of kidney disease progression [100].

4.2. *Biomarkers of Tissue Remodeling*

In addition to proteinuria and eGFR, other promising predictive biomarkers in CKD were described. A change in serum levels of MMPs after exposure to BB-1101, a synthetic hydroxamic acid-based inhibitor of MMP, was associated with a reduction in proteinuria in experimental models of glomerular damage [102]. A similar effect was observed in diabetic CKD patients who underwent treatment with doxycycline, an antibiotic from the tetracycline family, and who were already treated with renin–angiotensin–aldosterone inhibitors (RAAS-i) [103]. Moreover, MMPs are also involved in the mechanism that leads to CV risk reduction exerted by sodium–glucose cotransporter 2 inhibitors (SGLT2-i) through the activation of RECK (reversion-inducing cysteine-rich protein with kazal motifs), an endogenous inhibitor of MMPs [104]. That mechanism appeared to be independent of proteinuria levels and could also be useful for selecting high-risk normoalbuminuric CKD patients to be enrolled in future clinical trials, who represent a non-trivial proportion of the CKD cohort [21].

4.3. *Ultrasound Biomarkers*

Evidence is also emerging for a possible role of the renal resistive index (RRI) as a dynamic predictive biomarker. RRI is a Doppler ultrasonographic index, whose increase reflects both renal and systemic vascular impairment [105]. RRI was also found to predict the onset of CV and kidney outcomes in patients with CKD or essential hypertension [106,107]. RRI values are changed over time by different drug classes, such as RAAS-i and SGLT2-i; novel studies will hopefully reveal in the future if these treatment-induced modifications could also predict hard CV and renal endpoints [108,109].

4.4. *Predictive Role of Proteomics, Metabolomics, and Genomics*

A polymorphism of the angiotensin-converting enzyme gene caused by an insertion/deletion (ACE/ID) modifies the systemic and renal activity of the RAAS, which was recognized to be a trigger of kidney damage [110]. The ACE/DD–ACE/ID polymorphism was able to predict the response to losartan in type 2 diabetic patients enrolled in the RENAAL trial, that is, patients with worse prognosis (D allele carriers) had the best response to losartan [111]. Complex biomarkers and classifiers have a predictive role, in addition to a prognostic role. A set of 21 serum metabolites were selected from a larger panel through a penalized regression analysis, and they were shown to correctly predict the albuminuria response to ARB treatment in type 2 diabetic patients [112]. This classifier revealed that the enzyme nitric oxide synthase 3 (NOS3) is crucial to forecast the response to ARB therapy in diabetic CKD, since it is involved in the molecular mechanism of action of these drugs. A proteomic predictive classifier was developed from the Prevention of REnal and Vascular ENd-stage Disease (PREVEND) study, using plasma proteomics profiles of fibrosis and kidney damage that allowed predicting the albuminuria change in patients treated with RAAS-i [113]. The principal characteristics of prognostic and predictive biomarkers are depicted in Table 1.

Table 1. Summary of the principal prognostic and predictive biomarkers in chronic kidney disease patients.

Biomarkers	Characteristics	Prognostic/Predictive values
Cystatin C	Low-molecular-weight protein, produced by all types of nucleated cells, which acts as a cysteine protease inhibitor. It is freely filtered by the renal glomeruli, then 99% reabsorbed and metabolized in the renal proximal tubule; it is not secreted.	Cystatin C improves the estimation of eGFR and risk prediction of CV and renal events. It also allows a more precise stratification of patients according to their CV and renal risk [64].
β2-microglobulin	Protein present on the surface of immune cells, as a constant subunit of class I histocompatibility antigens. It is also found in blood and other biological fluids, as an expression of cell turnover. It is filtered by the renal glomerulus and reabsorbed at the tubular level.	It improves the prediction of ESKD, all-cause mortality, and new onset of CV disease [65].
hs-cTnT	Cardiac troponins are enzymes present in both skeletal and cardiac muscles. They regulate muscle contraction by controlling the calcium-mediated interaction of actin and myosin.	It improves the risk prediction of CV events, particularly heart failure regardless of the level of kidney function [55,57,114,115], as well as the risk prediction of microvascular events (nephropathy or retinopathy) in diabetic patients and the risk prediction of CKD progression.
NT-proBNP	Amino terminal fragment of the natriuretic type B peptide, normally produced in the heart and released in the case of cardiac stresses consequent to water overload conditions.	It improves the risk prediction of CV events, particularly heart failure regardless of the level of kidney function [55,57,114,115], as well as microvascular events (nephropathy or retinopathy) in diabetic patients and CKD progression. In the SONAR trial, it was used as a predictive biomarker in order to exclude patients with sodium retention after treatment with atrasentan [94]
sST2	A soluble form of the ST2 protein. It is a member of the interleukin 1 receptor family. In the case of myocardial stress, there is an upregulation of the ST2 gene and an increase in sST2 levels; by interacting with IL-33 (ligand for ST2), it counteracts the cardioprotective effect deriving from the ST2-IL 33 bond.	It showed an incremental prediction ability (over NT-proBNP) of death and hospitalizations due to HF in CKD patients [62,116]. It does not predict the risk of CKD progression.
GDF-15	Member of TGF-β cytokine family that is released in response to cellular stress. It appears to have a role in regulating inflammatory processes, apoptosis, cell repair, and cell growth.	It improves the risk prediction of both CV and microvascular events [62,116].
FGF-23	A protein belonging to the family of fibroblast growth factors, involved in the metabolism of phosphates. It is secreted in response to increased serum phosphate or calciprotein particles (colloidal nanoparticles of calcium phosphate dispersed in the blood), from osteocytes/osteoblasts. It acts on the kidneys by reducing the expression of a sodium phosphate transporter located in the renal proximal tubule, thus increasing the urinary excretion of phosphates.	It was significantly associated with mortality, atherosclerotic events, HF, and ESKD in CKD patients [52,53].
MMPs	Calcium-dependent endopeptidases that contain zinc and that are involved in the various processes of tissue development and cellular homeostasis.	Serum MMP-2, -8, and -9 and TIMP-1 are associated with atherogenesis, the severity of kidney damage, and the onset of left-ventricular hypertrophy and peripheral vascular disease [45–51]. MMPs levels are modified by selective and nonselective drugs. Changes in MMP levels are associated with a reduction of CV risk [102–104].

Table 1. *Cont.*

Biomarkers	Characteristics	Prognostic/Predictive values
Urinary markers	Urinary markers of tubule damage (IL-18, KIM-1, NGAL), repair (YKL-40), and inflammation (MCP-1)	Increased urinary concentrations of these biomarkers predict a linear decline in eGFR over time [65–67].
$eGFR_{crea}$	$eGFR_{crea}$ is an estimation of the kidney function level, based on serum creatinine levels, age, gender, and race.	A reduction of eGFR is a potent predictor of CV and renal endpoints [21–23]. A treatment-induced reduction of eGFR (30% and 40% reduction) is considered to be a surrogate endpoint of ESKD [73–75].
Proteinuria	Presence of an abnormal quantity of proteins in urine. It is considered the principal marker of kidney damage.	The increase in proteinuria levels is strongly associated with the onset of fatal and non-fatal CV events [23–25]. In clinical trials, patients who developed a significant reduction in proteinuria levels, during the first months after treatment, were protected against CV and renal events over time [89–97].
F-Uprot	Proteinuria/eGFR × 100. It combines the prognostic/predictive power of two biomarkers (proteinuria and eGFR).	It improves risk stratification for ESKD outcomes at all the stages of CKD [27].
MPO	It is an enzyme belonging to the class of oxide reductase, with bactericidal and pro-inflammatory action.	It is a prognostic marker of cardiovascular risk, and it is associated with the risk of renal outcome (RRT, 50% eGFR decline, eGFR $\leq$ 15 mL/min/1.73 m^2) [42–44].
RRI	Renal resistive index (RRI) is a ultrasonographic index of intrarenal arteries, defined as (peak systolic velocity − end diastolic velocity)/peak systolic velocity.	Raised RI levels above have been shown to reflect renal and systemic vascular impairment and predict CV events in hypertensive and CKD patients [105–107]. Medications as RAAS inhibitors and SGLT2-i reduce RRI levels over time and improve vascular damage [108,109].
ACE ID/DD	Insertion (I)/deletion (D) polymorphism of the angiotensin-converting enzyme (ACE) gene influences the circulating and renal activity of RAAS.	The D allele patients showed a poor CV prognosis in the RENAAL trial [110,111]. Patients with the DD genotype, despite being at a high risk of CV events, showed the better response to losartan in the RENAAL study [110,111].
Classifiers	A classifier is a combination of the informative markers able to classify patients according to their risk of developing an outcome or likelihood of response to a treatment.	13 metabolites predicted CKD progression in the CRIC cohort [76]. A panel of 21 metabolites was shown to predict the proteinuric response to ARBs [112].
CKD273	It is the combination of 273 urinary peptides identified as early indicators of molecular changes that predict the development or progression of CKD. The main components of CKD273 are collagen fragments and protein fragments, including proteins involved in inflammation.	It predicts the risk of development or progression of CKD, allowing the implementation of preventive attitudes. It is used in clinical trials to predict the development of CKD in response to a therapeutic approach [72–75].

eGFR, estimated Glomerular Filtration Rate; CV, Cardiovascular; ESKD, End-Stage-Kidney-Disease; hs-cTnT, high-sensitivity cardiac troponin; CKD, Chronic Kidney Disease; NT-proBNP, N-terminal pro-B-type natriuretic peptide; SONAR, study of diabetic nephropathy with the endothelin receptor antagonist atrasentan; sST2, soluble form of ST2; IL, interleukin; HF, Heart Failure; GDF-15, growth differentiation factor-15; TGF-β, transforming growth factor β; FGF-23, Fibroblast Growth Factor 23; MMP, Matrix metalloproteinases; TIMP, tissue inhibitor of metalloproteinases; KIM-1, Kidney Injury Molecule-1; NGAL, neutrophil gelatinase-associated lipocalin; YKL-40, repair human cartilage glycoprotein-40; MCP-1, monocyte chemoattractant protein-1; MPO, Myeloperoxidase; RRT, Renal Replacement Therapies; RAAS, Renin–Angiotensin–Aldosterone System; SGLT2-i, sodium–glucose cotransporter 2 inhibitors; RENAAL, Reduction of End Points in Non-Insulin-Dependent Diabetes with the Angiotensin II Antagonist Losartan; CRIC, Chronic Renal Insufficiency Cohort; ARBs angiotensin-receptor blockers.

5. Implementation of Biomarkers in Observational Studies

Owing to the importance of improving risk stratification beyond traditional kidney measures and to help clinical decision-making in CKD patients, the evaluation of novel biomarkers acquired great emphasis in clinical research, as witnessed by the growing number of publications on this topic [114]. However, before a biomarker can find full application in clinical practice, several steps need to be satisfied and reported. The first questions that should be addressed are the following: What will be the clinical intended use of the biomarker? Is the assay analytic performance acceptable for the intended use? To answer these important questions, the development process should start with assessing the analytic and clinical validity of the biomarker. Analytic validity refers to evaluating whether the characteristics of the measured biomarker are acceptable in term of precision, accuracy, and reproducibility [115]. It is indeed important to be aware that biomarker levels may vary in clinical practice due to factors not linked to the disease of interest being classified as pre-analytical and analytical factors [116]. Pre-analytical variation depends on several factors that include lifestyle (exercise, smoking habit, obesity), age, race, influence of gender, specimen collections (fasting, time, and temperature of storage) [117]. For instance, albuminuria, measured with the available methods, such as 24-h urine collection or albumin-to-creatinine ratio, is extremely influenced by physical exercise and other conditions that determine a day-by-day variation, defined as random variation [37]. Urinary NGAL concentration is stable in urine for up to seven days, but it is increased by the presence of white blood cells that are an important confounder [118]. Analytic variation is mainly defined by two parameters, which are bias and precision [119]. Bias is the amount by which an average of many repeated measurements made using the assay systematically over- or underestimates the true value. Precision represents the repeatability of measurements under unchanged assay conditions in a laboratory. While analytic validation is often discussed, it is seldom handled in a proper fashion. It was suggested to deepen analytic validation, while developing a biomarker, and to report metrics, such as precision, reproducibility, accuracy, analytic sensitivity, limits of detection and quantification, linearity, and analytic specificity [120]. A descriptive summary of these measures is reported in Table 2.

Table 2. Principal tools used to assess analytic validation.

Features	Definition	Statistical Metric
Precision	Intra-assay agreement of a set of results among themselves. It could be expressed by coefficient of variation (CV).	$CV_{(\%)}$ = (Standard $deviation_{samples}/Mean_{samples}) \times 100$
Reproducibility	Concordance between various measurements carried out in different laboratories and experimental conditions on the same sample.	
Accuracy	Closeness of the agreement between result of a single measurement and true value obtained using a reference standard method.	
Trueness	Concordance between a series of assays and the real value of analyte concentration.	
Bias	Systematic difference of the series of measurements with true value.	$Bias_{(\%)} = (Mean_{sample} - \text{True value}) \times 100$
Limit of blank	Highest apparent analyte concentration founded by testing specimens without analyte.	$LoB = Mean_{blank} + 1.645(SD_{blank})$
Limit of detection	Average of lowest concentration of analyte which can be distinguished from a blank sample.	$LoD = LoB + 1645(SD_{samples})$
Limit of quantification	Smallest concentration of analyte with an acceptable accuracy and precision.	
Linearity	Proportionality between a set of measured values and true concentration of analyte.	
Analytic specificity	Ability to measure only and exclusively the analyte of interest.	
Analytic sensibility	Ability to measure lowest concentration of analyte.	

Clinical validity is the next important step and consists of demonstrating that biomarker measurement is associated with a clinical characteristic of interest [115]. The first steps of clinical validation are the proof of concept and prospective validation [114]. Proof of concept means to assess whether biomarker levels differ between subjects who develop the event of interest vs. non-events. This phase is essential since it allows understanding if the biomarker can play a role in the context of disease, and continuing its development is convenient. To this aim, a cross-sectional design could be sufficient [121]. Next, it is necessary, in prognostic validation, to evaluate if the biomarker is significantly associated with the event of interest, with a prospective analysis. Moreover, it is important that the magnitude of this association is not attenuated when the analysis is adjusted for traditional risk factors, such as age, gender, and proteinuria and eGFR levels in CKD patients. This step provides other useful information such as the distribution of the biomarker and, therefore, how to incorporate the biomarker levels in multivariable analyses. It is suggested to start by adding to the model the biomarker variable as a continuous variable, before applying a categorization (e.g., tertiles or quartiles) [122]. For instance, proteinuria has a skewed distribution and is often added as a log-transformed variable or restricted cubic spline in CKD prognostic models [27]. The prospective validation step is also important for selecting variables to be included in the model. This can be done by using a knowledge-driven (or a priori) method, based on the already known biological association of the variables with the outcome, or data-driven methods, which are automated tools that select a small set of variables from a larger one, in order to maximize the model fit [123]. In the case of a large number of predictors, as often happens during the development of proteomic/metabolomic classifiers, regularization or dimension reduction methods can be used [124]. The metabolomic classifier for the prediction of response to ARB treatment, which we described in Section 4, was developed by means of least absolute shrinkage and selection operator (LASSO), a regularization technique that shrinks the variables regression coefficients through a tuning parameter and retains the best predictors in the model. LASSO was also shown to work very well with small sample sizes [112]. The third phase of clinical validation is focused on the incremental value of the biomarker on the previous assessed risk models. In nephrology, what is essentially required in biomarker research is to demonstrate that a biomarker adds information, in the prediction of a defined endpoint, on top of already assessed risk factors. This process needs a hierarchical assessment, since a likelihood ratio test (LR test) should be firstly reported to determine if the biomarker remains associated with the endpoint after controlling for previously established risk factors. Next, three measures of performance should be reported: discrimination, calibration, and reclassification [125]. These three domains are important to warrant the applicability of the biomarker predictive performance to the individual patient. Discrimination refers to the ability of the model to attribute a high risk to patients who develop the outcome of interest and, accordingly, a low risk to those who do not [126]. A measure that depicts sensitivity and specificity for all possible thresholds of a biomarker is the receiver operating characteristic (ROC) curve. To evaluate discrimination, it is, thus, suggested to present the ROC derived from the model together with the area under the curve (AUC), also labeled the *c*-statistic [127]. The difference in *c*-statistic between models with and without the biomarker should also be presented. Calibration is the degree of agreement between observed and predicted outcomes. It is suggested to depict calibration graphically by plotting the mean predicted versus mean observed outcome probability for intervals (usually deciles) of risk in a predictiveness curve or by representing observed event rates versus mean predicted risk, thus creating a calibration plot, with points that should lie along a 45° line if the model is well calibrated [126]. Reclassification metrics provide useful information on the proportion (%) of patients that are reclassified in the true risk category (lower or higher risk), whether or not the new biomarker is added to a traditional risk prediction model. The most used reclassification metrics are the net reclassification improvement (NRI), the integrated discrimination index (IDI), and reclassification tables which directly depict the movement of patients between risk categories based on the risk predicted by models with and without the biomarker [127]. After showing measures of performance, it would be necessary to internally or externally validate the model. External validation implies that the risk prediction model, including the biomarker, is re-run within an external cohort of patients with similar characteristics (e.g., CKD patients) to confirm predictive accuracy in all sequences. Alternatively, several methods of internal validation, such as bootstrapping or cross-validation, can be computed [128]. The appropriateness of methodology used to develop a biomarker is a key element to obtain useful clinical results. This is particularly true if we consider that only a few prediction models in nephrology reported these measures appropriately [129]. However, this is not the only limitation. Most of the proposed biomarkers are yet to complete the sequence from discovery to clinical application, because they were developed in studies with a small sample size without validation, thus providing heterogeneous results. The ISN prompted that biomarker research would take advantage from the setting up of large, observational cohort studies and possibly a long-term follow-up in which biomarker development and validation could be strengthened and provide robust evidence for clinicians [18]. This also requires the standardization of data collection, storage, and database structure across countries, as well as a collaboration among academia, industry, and regulatory authorities in order to warrant a correct dissemination of results.

6. Biomarkers in Intervention Studies

Projecting clinical trials, which test the effect of novel pharmacological treatments on prognosis of CKD patients, is always an important challenge. In the past few decades, all nephrology communities expressed the need for clinicians to have more therapeutic tools, with each one specific for a particular etiology of CKD, in order to improve the care of patients with CKD and to deal promptly with the complexity of kidney disease, abandoning the "reductionist" approach [10,130]. The milestone of intervention studies in nephrology dates back to the years 1990–2000 when the Collaborative Study Group, the RENAAL, and the IDNT trials showed the efficacy of RAAS-i (ACEi and ARBs) in reducing CV and renal risk in patients with diabetes and CKD [76,131,132]. Since then, a number of clinical trials were carried out with an attempt to reduce the high residual risk in CKD patients, but they missed the target [133]. The reasons for this breakdown are several and include the enrolment, in clinical trials, of a large number of CKD patients with heterogeneous etiologies and the add-on strategy. The add-on strategy consists of adding a pharmacological agent to patients who are already being treated with a drug belonging to the same class. This was adopted, for example, in the Veterans Affairs Nephropathy in Diabetes (VA-NEPHRON-D) clinical trial, which tested the effect of dual RAAS blockade ACEi + ARB, or in the ALTITUDE trial, with the addition of Aliskiren, a renin inhibitor, to RAAS-i [134,135]. In these studies, the intensification of RAAS blockade did not result in further CV or renal risk protection and even increased the risk of these endpoints. Hence, a series of initiatives were started to improve clinical trial designs. The focus is indeed to move from large trials to smaller studies that enroll similar patients so that the treatment effect can be adequately measured [26]. Biomarkers play a central role in this context (Figure 2), being useful to enrich clinical trial CKD populations through at least three important ways called biomarker-based approaches: (1) by identifying patients at increased risk for developing an event (risk-based enrichment); (2) by selecting a population based on the response to a drug of interest (predictive response enrichment or adaptive enrichment); (3) by detecting subgroup of similar patients within a master trial protocol [136].

Risk-based enrichment was used in the proteomic prediction and renin angiotensin aldosterone system inhibition prevention of early diabetic nephropathy in type 2 diabetic patients with normoalbuminuria (PRIORITY) study. The PRIORITY study enrolled patients with diabetes mellitus and normal albuminuria at increased risk for developing albuminuria [137]. High or low risk was established based on urine CKD273 levels, and only high-risk patients were then randomized to receive spironolactone or placebo. Although the trials did not show a significant effect of spironolactone on preventing the development of albuminuria, high-risk patients identified with CKD273 were at increased risk of CKD progression vs. low risk patients ($p < 0.001$). PRIORITY was an innovative design, since it anticipated the treatment of albuminuria in patients who were only likely to develop albuminuria, but not yet with albuminuria. The adaptive enrichment design consists of exposing all patients to a short-term period (usually called run-in) of treatment with the drug of interest before randomization. In this case, biomarkers could inform on the response/non-response to treatment. Such a design was adopted in previous trials like the Study of Heart and Renal Protection (SHARP) study and more recently in the study of diabetic nephropathy with the endothelin receptor antagonist atrasentan (SONAR) trial [94,138]. Patients enrolled in SONAR underwent a six-month treatment period with atrasentan, and only patients who manifested a 30% reduction in albuminuria levels (measured as albumin-to-creatinine ratio) were then randomized. Hence, albuminuria worked as a biomarker for the prediction of response to treatment. Moreover, the SONAR trial included the assessment of "secondary" risk markers, such as the B-type natriuretic peptide levels. Patients who showed a significant increase in this marker during run-in were excluded from the study. This strategy allows assessing the individual response to treatment, including the effect of a drug on primary and secondary markers and, thus, to capture in a reliable manner the effect of treatment after randomization. An extension of the adaptive enrichment trial is given by the master trial protocol [139]. Master protocols can be planned to test the efficacy of multiple interventions, each targeting a subgroup of patients defined by a biomarker. Master protocols encompass umbrella, basket, and platform trials. Platform trials aroused the interest of the nephrology community [136]. The platform is an experimental cohort of patients followed periodically to assess laboratory and clinical measurements. Within the platform, multiple treatments can be started or withdrawn and, if a defined treatment shows benefits in a defined subgroup of the platform, it can be introduced in clinical practice [140]. This approach allows the acceleration of the experimental phase of drug development, to improve the application of biomarkers and to save time and financial sources. Future perspectives around the implementation of available biomarkers are depicted in Table 3.

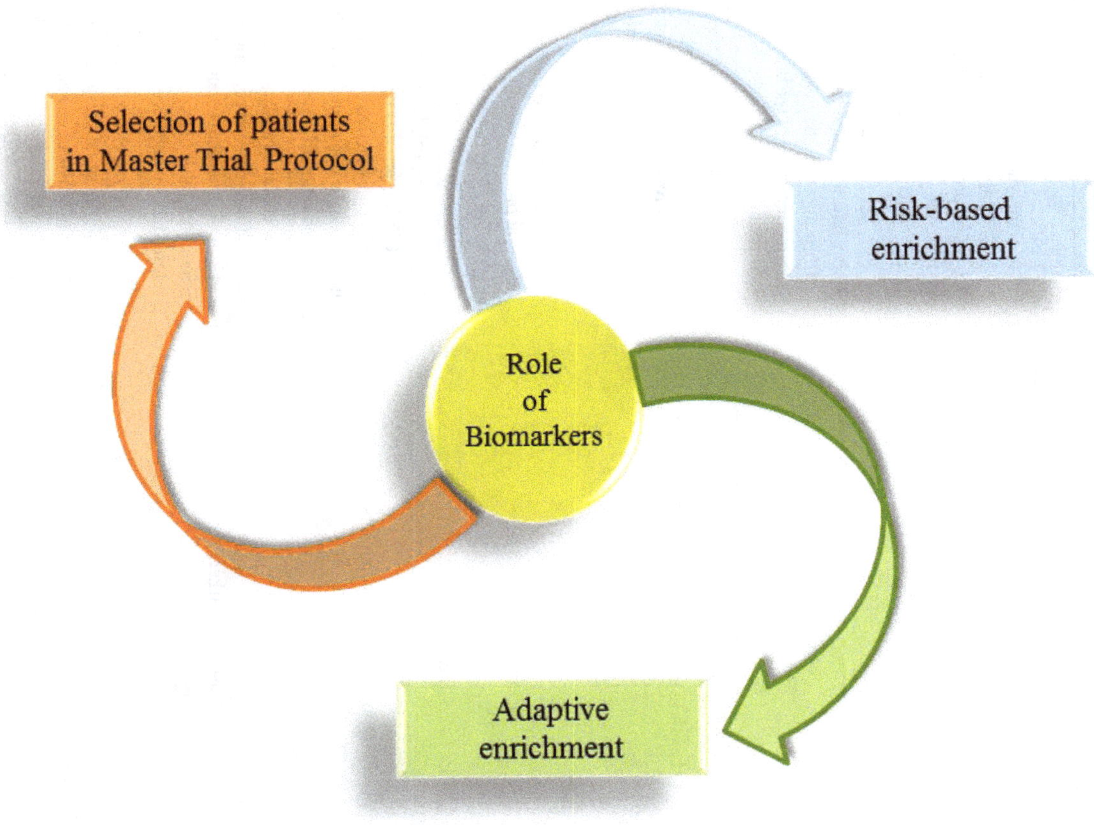

Figure 2. Biomarker-based approaches for patient selection in clinical trials.

Table 3. Validation score and future perspectives in the development of biomarkers in CKD patients.

Biomarkers	Validation Criteria	Future Perspectives
Proteinuria	Analytic validation: +/– Clinical proof of concept: + Clinical prospective validation: + Incremental value of the biomarker: + Introduction in clinical trials: +	Further studies are needed to establish (1) how this marker should be used for monitoring disease progression considering, among all factors, its variability, and (2) what are the true cut-offs for response to treatments. Inclusion of proteinuria in risk prediction models that include the presence of renal diagnoses is also needed.
$eGFR_{crea}$	Analytic validation: + Clinical proof of concept: + Clinical prospective validation: + Incremental value of the biomarker: + Introduction in clinical trials: +/–	$eGFR_{crea}$ is an important marker used to stratify risk in CKD patients. Further studies could refine the assessment of $eGFR_{crea}$ as a biomarker of response to nephroprotective treatments in clinical trials. Inclusion of $eGFR_{crea}$ in risk prediction models that include the presence of renal diagnoses is also needed.
Markers of oxidative stress, tissue remodeling, and metabolism	Analytic validation: + Clinical proof of concept: + Clinical prospective validation: +/– Incremental value of the biomarker: – Introduction in clinical trials: +/–	The prognostic role of these markers should be evaluated in larger cohort studies. Individual prognostic measures should be provided. Although pilot experimental trials showed promising results, stronger evidence in CKD patients around the changes in these markers after treatment initiation is needed.
Cardiac markers	Analytic validation: +/– Clinical proof of concept: + Clinical prospective validation: +/– Incremental value of the biomarker: +/– Introduction in clinical trials: –	Although cardiac markers levels are associated with the severity of CKD, their assessment is confounded by the coexistence of CV disease, as well as by the eGFR levels. Further studies are needed to establish the true role of these markers in CKD patients.
Filtration and urinary markers	Analytic validation: +/– Clinical proof of concept: + Clinical prospective validation: + Incremental value of the biomarker: – Introduction in clinical trials: –	The prognostic role of these markers should be evaluated in larger studies. Individual risk prediction models that include these parameters and intervention studies assessing their changes over time should be implemented.
Ultrasound markers	Analytic validation: + Clinical proof of concept: + Clinical prospective validation: + Incremental value of the biomarker: +/– Introduction in clinical trials: +/–	RRI was found to be associated with CV and renal events in CKD patients, being a promising marker. However, larger clinical trials evaluating the association between changes (treatment-induced) in RRI and clinical outcomes should be performed in the future.
Proteomics, metabolomics, and genomics	Analytic validation: + Clinical proof of concept: + Clinical prospective validation: + Incremental value of the biomarker: + Introduction in clinical trials: +/–	Omics approaches show useful prognostic and predictive information in addition to traditional risk factors. Improving the inclusion of these markers in clinical trials may inform on their clinical applicability.

+, fully present; +/–, partially present; –, absent. CKD, chronic kidney disease; eGFR, estimated glomerular filtration rate; RRI, renal resistive index; CV, cardiovascular.

7. Conclusions

CKD is a growing public health problem with high morbidity and mortality. The current classification considers the eGFR and albuminuria levels to classify patients in prognostic categories. Novel biomarkers were also developed to improve risk stratification and clinical decision-making, as well as guide CKD patient enrichment in clinical trials. Despite the great efforts made, only a few biomarkers found a large clinical application to date. More emphasis should be placed on the development process of biomarkers, which needs to be methodologically rigorous, well validated, and correctly diffused. A "real-world" assessment of biomarkers that can be performed by analyzing large databases with long-term follow-up may substantially contribute to understanding whether a definite biomarker can find clinical application. The implementation of biomarkers in CKD is highly expected in the future, since they provide information on the mechanisms of kidney disease, improve clinical practice, and, in most cases, are able to forecast both CV and renal endpoints, which represent the most frequent events in CKD patients.

Author Contributions: Conceptualization, M.P., S.R., I.G., and M.A.; methodology, M.P., S.R., P.C. and M.A.; validation, M.P., S.R., I.G., A.M., E.A., S.B., R.S., D.F., G.D.S., and M.A.; writing—original draft preparation, M.P., S.R., I.G., A.M., G.D.S., and M.A.; writing—review and editing, M.P., S.R., P.C., I.G., A.M., G.D.S., and M.A.; visualization, M.P., S.R., P.C., I.G., A.M., E.A., S.B., R.S., D.F., G.D.S., and M.A.; supervision, M.P. and M.A. All authors have read and agreed to the published version of the manuscript.

Acknowledgments: We thank all the investigators of the "Magna Graecia" University of Catanzaro and the University of Campania "L. Vanvitelli", who collaborated on the manuscript, for their insight.

References

1. FDA-NIH Biomarker Working Group. *BEST (Biomarkers, Endpoints, and other Tools) Resource*; Food and Drug Administration (US): Silver Spring, MD, USA; National Institutes of Health (US): Bethesda, MD, USA, 2020. Available online: www.ncbi.nlm.nih.gov/books/NBK326791 (accessed on 25 June 2020).
2. Pepe, M.; Janes, H. Methods for Evaluating Prediction Performance of Biomarkers and Tests. In *Risk Assessment and Evaluation of Predictions*; Lecture Notes in Statistics; Lee, M.L., Gail, M., Pfeiffer, R., Satten, G., Cai, T., Gandy, A., Eds.; Springer: New York, NY, USA, 2013; Volume 215. [CrossRef]
3. Devarajan, P.; Williams, L.M. Proteomics for biomarker discovery in acute kidney injury. *Semin. Nephrol.* **2007**, *27*, 637–651. [CrossRef] [PubMed]
4. Simon, R. Development and validation of biomarker classifiers for treatment selection. *J. Stat. Plan. Inference* **2008**, *138*, 308–320. [CrossRef] [PubMed]
5. Provenzano, M.; Coppolino, G.; De Nicola, L.; Serra, R.; Garofalo, C.; Andreucci, M.; Bolignano, D. Unraveling cardiovascular risk in renal patients: A new take on old tale. *Front. Cell Dev. Biol.* **2019**, *7*, 314. [CrossRef] [PubMed]
6. Provenzano, M.; Coppolino, G.; Faga, T.; Garofalo, C.; Serra, R.; Andreucci, M. Epidemiology of cardiovascular risk in chronic kidney disease patients: The real silent killer. *Rev. Cardiovasc. Med.* **2019**, *20*, 209–220. [CrossRef]
7. Kidney Disease Improving Global Outcomes Work Group. CVD, medication dosage, patient safety, infections, hospitalizations, and caveats for investigating complications of CKD. *Kidney Int. Suppl.* **2013**, *3*, 91–111. [CrossRef]
8. Xie, Y.; Bowe, B.; Mokdad, A.H.; Xian, H.; Yan, Y.; Li, T.; Maddukuri, G.; Tsai, C.-Y.; Floyd, T.; Al Aly, Z. Analysis of the Global Burden of Disease study highlights the global, regional, and national trends of chronic kidney disease epidemiology from 1990 to 2016. *Kidney Int.* **2018**, *94*, 567–581. [CrossRef]
9. Bikbov, B.T.; A Purcell, C.; Levey, A.S.; Smith, M.; Abdoli, A.; Abebe, M.; Adebayo, O.M.; Afarideh, M.; Agarwal, S.K.; Agudelo-Botero, M.; et al. Global, regional, and national burden of chronic kidney disease, 1990–2017: A systematic analysis for the Global Burden of Disease Study 2017. *Lancet* **2020**, *395*, 709–733. [CrossRef]

10. Hall, Y.N.; Himmelfarb, J. The CKD classification system in the precision medicine era. *Clin. J. Am. Soc. Nephrol.* **2016**, *12*, 346–348. [CrossRef]
11. Inker, L.A.; Astor, B.C.; Fox, C.H.; Isakova, T.; Lash, J.P.; Peralta, C.A.; Tamura, M.K.; Feldman, H.I. KDOQI US commentary on the 2012 KDIGO Clinical Practice Guideline for the Evaluation and Management of CKD. *Am. J. Kidney Dis.* **2014**, *63*, 713–735. [CrossRef]
12. De Nicola, L.; Provenzano, M.; Chiodini, P.; Borrelli, S.; Garofalo, C.; Pacilio, M.; Liberti, M.E.; Sagliocca, A.; Conte, G.; Minutolo, R. Independent role of underlying kidney disease on renal prognosis of patients with chronic kidney disease under nephrology care. *PLoS ONE* **2015**, *10*, e0127071. [CrossRef]
13. Haynes, R.; Staplin, N.; Emberson, J.R.; Herrington, W.G.; Tomson, C.; Agodoa, L.; Tesař, V.; Levin, A.; Lewis, D.; Reith, C.; et al. Evaluating the contribution of the cause of kidney disease to prognosis in CKD: Results from the Study of Heart and Renal Protection (SHARP). *Am. J. Kidney Dis.* **2014**, *64*, 40–48. [CrossRef] [PubMed]
14. Conte, G.; Minutolo, R.; De Nicola, L.; Hallan, S.I.; Gansevoort, R.T. Pro: Thresholds to define chronic kidney disease should not be age-dependent. *Nephrol. Dial. Transplant.* **2014**, *29*, 770–774. [CrossRef] [PubMed]
15. Glassock, R.J. Con: Thresholds to define chronic kidney disease should not be age dependent. *Nephrol. Dial. Transplant.* **2014**, *29*, 774–779. [CrossRef] [PubMed]
16. Hommos, M.S.; Glassock, R.J.; Rule, A.D. Structural and functional changes in human kidneys with healthy aging. *J. Am. Soc. Nephrol.* **2017**, *28*, 2838–2844. [CrossRef] [PubMed]
17. Levin, A.; Tonelli, M.; Bonventre, J.; Coresh, J.; Donner, J.-A.; Fogo, A.B.; Fox, C.S.; Gansevoort, R.T.; Heerspink, H.J.; Jardine, M.; et al. Global kidney health 2017 and beyond: A roadmap for closing gaps in care, research, and policy. *Lancet* **2017**, *390*, 1888–1917. [CrossRef]
18. Pena, M.J.; Stenvinkel, P.; Kretzler, M.; Adu, D.; Agarwal, S.K.; Coresh, J.; Feldman, H.I.; Fogo, A.B.; Gansevoort, R.T.; Harris, D.C.; et al. Strategies to improve monitoring disease progression, assessing cardiovascular risk, and defining prognostic biomarkers in chronic kidney disease. *Kidney Int. Suppl.* **2017**, *7*, 107–113. [CrossRef]
19. IOM (Institute of Medicine). *Evaluation of Biomarkers and Surrogate Endpoints in Chronic Disease*; The National Academies Press: Washington, DC, USA, 2010.
20. Serra, R.; Ielapi, N.; Barbetta, A.; Andreucci, M.; De Franciscis, S. Novel biomarkers for cardiovascular risk. *Biomark. Med.* **2018**, *12*, 1015–1024. [CrossRef]
21. De Nicola, L.; Provenzano, M.; Chiodini, P.; Borrelli, S.; Russo, L.; Bellasi, A.; Santoro, D.; Conte, G.; Minutolo, R. Epidemiology of low-proteinuric chronic kidney disease in renal clinics. *PLoS ONE* **2017**, *12*, e0172241. [CrossRef]
22. Minutolo, R.; Gabbai, F.B.; Chiodini, P.; Garofalo, C.; Stanzione, G.; Liberti, M.E.; Pacilio, M.; Borrelli, S.; Provenzano, M.; Conte, G.; et al. Reassessment of Ambulatory blood pressure improves renal risk stratification in nondialysis chronic kidney disease. *Hypertension* **2015**, *66*, 557–562. [CrossRef]
23. Astor, B.C.; Matsushita, K.; Gansevoort, R.T.; Van Der Velde, M.; Woodward, M.; Levey, A.S.; De Jong, P.E.; Coresh, J. Lower estimated glomerular filtration rate and higher albuminuria are associated with mortality and end-stage renal disease. A collaborative meta-analysis of kidney disease population cohorts. *Kidney Int.* **2011**, *79*, 1331–1340. [CrossRef]
24. Gansevoort, R.T.; Matsushita, K.; Van Der Velde, M.; Astor, B.C.; Woodward, M.; Levey, A.S.; De Jong, P.E.; Coresh, J. Chronic kidney disease prognosis consortium lower estimated GFR and higher albuminuria are associated with adverse kidney outcomes. A collaborative meta-analysis of general and high-risk population cohorts. *Kidney Int.* **2011**, *80*, 93–104. [CrossRef] [PubMed]
25. Matsushita, K.; Coresh, J.; Sang, Y.; Chalmers, J.P.; Fox, C.; Guallar, E.; Jafar, T.; Jassal, S.K.; Landman, G.W.; Muntner, P.; et al. Estimated glomerular filtration rate and albuminuria for prediction of cardiovascular outcomes: A collaborative meta-analysis of individual participant data. *Lancet Diabetes Endocrinol.* **2015**, *3*, 514–525. [CrossRef]
26. Tangri, N.; Stevens, L.A.; Griffith, J.; Tighiouart, H.; Djurdjev, O.; Naimark, D.M.; Levin, A.; Levey, A.S. A predictive model for progression of chronic kidney disease to kidney failure. *JAMA* **2011**, *305*, 1553–1559. [CrossRef] [PubMed]

27. Provenzano, M.; Chiodini, P.; Minutolo, R.; Zoccali, C.; Bellizzi, V.; Conte, G.; Locatelli, F.; Tripepi, G.; Del Vecchio, L.; Mallamaci, F.; et al. Reclassification of chronic kidney disease patients for end-stage renal disease risk by proteinuria indexed to estimated glomerular filtration rate: Multicentre prospective study in nephrology clinics. *Nephrol. Dial. Transplant.* **2018**, *35*. [CrossRef]
28. Schroeder, E.B.; Yang, X.; Thorp, M.L.; Arnold, B.M.; Tabano, D.; Petrik, A.F.; Smith, D.H.; Platt, R.W.; Johnson, E.S. Predicting 5-Year Risk of RRT in Stage 3 or 4 CKD: Development and external validation. *Clin. J. Am. Soc. Nephrol.* **2016**, *12*, 87–94. [CrossRef]
29. Grams, M.E.; Sang, Y.; Ballew, S.H. Predicting timing of clinical outcomes in patients with chronic kidney disease and severely decreased glomerular filtration rate. *Kidney Int.* **2018**, *94*, 1025–1026. [CrossRef]
30. Abbate, M.; Zoja, C.; Remuzzi, G. How does proteinuria cause progressive renal damage? *J. Am. Soc. Nephrol.* **2006**, *17*, 2974–2984. [CrossRef]
31. Provenzano, M.; Garofalo, C.; Chiodini, P. Ruolo della proteinuria nella ricerca clinica: Per ogni vecchia risposta, una nuova domanda [Role of proteinuria in clinical research: For each old-answer, a new key-question]. *Recenti Prog Med.* **2020**, *111*, 74–81. [CrossRef]
32. Nakano, T.; Ninomiya, T.; Sumiyoshi, S.; Fujii, H.; Doi, Y.; Hirakata, H.; Tsuruya, K.; Iida, M.; Kiyohara, Y.; Sueishi, K. Association of kidney function with coronary atherosclerosis and calcification in autopsy samples from Japanese elders: The Hisayama study. *Am. J. Kidney Dis.* **2010**, *55*, 21–30. [CrossRef]
33. Pun, P.H.; Smarz, T.R.; Honeycutt, E.F.; Shaw, L.K.; Al-Khatib, S.M.; Middleton, J.P. Chronic kidney disease is associated with increased risk of sudden cardiac death among patients with coronary artery disease. *Kidney Int.* **2009**, *76*, 652–658. [CrossRef]
34. Deo, R.; Lin, F.; Vittinghoff, E.; Tseng, Z.H.; Hulley, S.B.; Shlipak, M.G. Kidney dysfunction and sudden cardiac death among women with coronary heart disease. *Hypertension* **2008**, *51*, 1578–1582. [CrossRef] [PubMed]
35. Deo, R.; Sotoodehnia, N.; Katz, R.; Sarnak, M.J.; Fried, L.F.; Chonchol, M.; Kestenbaum, B.; Psaty, B.M.; Siscovick, D.S.; Shlipak, M.G. Cystatin C and sudden cardiac death risk in the elderly. *Circ. Cardiovasc. Qual. Outcomes* **2010**, *3*, 159–164. [CrossRef] [PubMed]
36. Meier, P.; Vogt, P.; Blanc, E. Ventricular arrhythmias and sudden cardiac death in end-stage renaldisease patients on chronic hemodialysis. *Nephron* **2001**, *87*, 199–214. [CrossRef] [PubMed]
37. Van Acker, B.A.C.; Stroomer, M.K.J.; Gosselink, M.A.H.E.; Koomen, G.C.M.; Koopman, M.G.; Arisz, L. Urinary protein excretion in normal individuals: Diurnal changes, influence of orthostasis and relationship to the renin-angiotensin system. *Contrib. Nephrol.* **1993**, *101*, 143–150.
38. Fotheringham, J.; Odudu, A.; McKane, W.; Ellam, T. Modification of the relationship between blood pressure and renal albumin permeability by impaired excretory function and diabetes. *Hypertension* **2015**, *65*, 510–516. [CrossRef]
39. Willows, J.; Odudu, A.; Logan, I.; Sheerin, N.; Tomson, C.; Ellam, T. changing protein permeability with nephron loss: Evidence for a human remnant nephron effect. *Am. J. Nephrol.* **2019**, *50*, 152–159. [CrossRef]
40. Mallamaci, F.; Tripepi, G.; D'Arrigo, G.; Borrelli, S.; Garofalo, C.; Stanzione, G.; Provenzano, M.; De Nicola, L.; Conte, G.; Minutolo, R.; et al. Blood pressure variability, mortality, and cardiovascular outcomes in CKD patients. *Clin. J. Am. Soc. Nephrol.* **2019**, *14*, 233–240. [CrossRef]
41. Zhou, T.L.; Rensma, S.P.; Van Der Heide, F.C.; Henry, R.M.; Kroon, A.A.; Houben, A.J.; Jansen, J.F.; Backes, W.H.; Berendschot, T.T.; Schouten, J.S.; et al. Blood pressure variability and microvascular dysfunction. *J. Hypertens.* **2020**, *38*. [CrossRef]
42. Xu, G.; Luo, K.; Liu, H.; Huang, T.; Fang, X.; Tu, W. The progress of inflammation and oxidative stress in patients with chronic kidney disease. *Ren. Fail.* **2014**, *37*, 45–49. [CrossRef]
43. Ismael, F.O.; Proudfoot, J.M.; Brown, B.E.; Van Reyk, D.M.; Croft, K.D.; Davies, M.J.; Hawkins, C.L. Comparative reactivity of the myeloperoxidase-derived oxidants HOCl and HOSCN with low-density lipoprotein (LDL): Implications for foam cell formation in atherosclerosis. *Arch. Biochem. Biophys.* **2015**, *573*, 40–51. [CrossRef]
44. Correa, S.; Pena-Esparragoza, J.K.; Scovner, K.M.; Waikar, S.S.; Mc Causland, F.R. Myeloperoxidase and the risk of CKD Progression, cardiovascular disease, and death in the Chronic Renal Insufficiency Cohort (CRIC) Study. *Am. J. Kidney Dis.* **2020**, *76*, 32–41. [CrossRef] [PubMed]

45. Provenzano, M.; Andreucci, M.; Garofalo, C.; Faga, T.; Michael, A.; Ielapi, N.; Grande, R.; Sapienza, P.; De Franciscis, S.; Mastroroberto, P.; et al. The association of matrix metalloproteinases with chronic kidney disease and peripheral vascular disease: A light at the end of the tunnel? *Biomolecules* **2020**, *10*, 154. [CrossRef] [PubMed]
46. Butrico, L.; Barbetta, A.; Ciranni, S.; Andreucci, M.; Mastroroberto, P.; De Franciscis, S. Role of metalloproteinases and their inhibitors in the development of abdominal aortic aneurysm: Current insights and systematic review of the literature. *Chirurgia* **2017**, *30*, 151–159. [CrossRef]
47. Lauhio, A.; Sorsa, T.; Srinivas, R.; Stenman, M.; Tervahartiala, T.; Stenman, U.-H.; Grönhagen-Riska, C.; Honkanen, E. Urinary matrix metalloproteinase -8, -9, -14 and their regulators (TRY-1, TRY-2, TATI) in patients with diabetic nephropathy. *Ann. Med.* **2008**, *40*, 312–320. [CrossRef] [PubMed]
48. Tashiro, K.; Koyanagi, I.; Ohara, I.; Ito, T.; Saitoh, A.; Horikoshi, S.; Tomino, Y. Levels of urinary matrix metalloproteinase-9 (MMP-9) and renal injuries in patients with type 2 diabetic nephropathy. *J. Clin. Lab. Anal.* **2004**, *18*, 206–210. [CrossRef]
49. Lieb, W.; Song, R.J.; Xanthakis, V.; Vasan, R.S. Association of circulating tissue inhibitor of Metalloproteinases-1 and Procollagen type III Aminoterminal peptide levels with incident heart failure and chronic kidney disease. *J. Am. Hear. Assoc.* **2019**, *8*, e011426. [CrossRef]
50. Forough, R.; Koyama, N.; Hasenstab, D.; Lea, H.; Clowes, M.; Nikkari, S.T.; Clowes, A.W. Overexpression of tissue inhibitor of matrix metalloproteinase-1 inhibits vascular smooth muscle cell functions In Vitro and In Vivo. *Circ. Res.* **1996**, *79*, 812–820. [CrossRef]
51. Newman, K.M.; Jean-Claude, J.; Li, H.; Scholes, J.V.; Ogata, Y.; Nagase, H.; Tilson, M. Cellular localization of matrix metalloproteinases in the abdominal aortic aneurysm wall. *J. Vasc. Surg.* **1994**, *20*, 814–820. [CrossRef]
52. Scialla, J.J.; Xie, H.; Rahman, M.; Anderson, A.H.; Isakova, T.; Ojo, A.; Zhang, X.; Nessel, L.; Hamano, T.; Grunwald, J.E.; et al. Fibroblast Growth Factor-23 and cardiovascular events in CKD. *J. Am. Soc. Nephrol.* **2013**, *25*, 349–360. [CrossRef]
53. Isakova, T.; Xie, H.; Yang, W.; Xie, D.; Anderson, A.H.; Scialla, J.J.; Wahl, P.; Gutiérrez, O.M.; Steigerwalt, S.; He, J.; et al. Fibroblast Growth Factor 23 and risks of mortality and end-stage renal disease in patients with chronic kidney disease. *JAMA* **2011**, *305*, 2432–2439. [CrossRef]
54. Defilippi, C.R.; De Lemos, J.A.; Christenson, R.H.; Gottdiener, J.S.; Kop, W.J.; Zhan, M.; Seliger, S. Association of serial measures of cardiac troponin T using a sensitive assay with incident heart failure and cardiovascular mortality in older adults. *JAMA* **2010**, *304*, 2494–2502. [CrossRef] [PubMed]
55. Ballew, S.H.; Matsushita, K. Cardiovascular risk prediction in CKD. *Semin. Nephrol.* **2018**, *38*, 208–216. [CrossRef] [PubMed]
56. Srisawasdi, P.; Vanavanan, S.; Charoenpanichkit, C.; Kroll, M.H. The Effect of renal dysfunction on BNP, NT-proBNP, and their ratio. *Am. J. Clin. Pathol.* **2010**, *133*, 14–23. [CrossRef] [PubMed]
57. Matsushita, K.; Ballew, S.H.; Coresh, J. Cardiovascular risk prediction in people with chronic kidney disease. *Curr. Opin. Nephrol. Hypertens.* **2016**, *25*, 518–523. [CrossRef]
58. Rangaswami, J.; Bhalla, V.; Blair, J.E.; Chang, T.I.; Costa, S.; Lentine, K.L.; Lerma, E.V.; Mezue, K.; Molitch, M.; Mullens, W.; et al. Cardiorenal syndrome: Classification, pathophysiology, diagnosis, and treatment strategies: A scientific statement from the american heart association. *Circulation* **2019**, *139*, e840–e878. [CrossRef]
59. Saunders, J.T.; Nambi, V.; De Lemos, J.A.; Chambless, L.E.; Virani, S.S.; Boerwinkle, E.; Hoogeveen, R.C.; Liu, X.; Astor, B.C.; Mosley, T.H.; et al. Cardiac troponin T measured by a highly sensitive assay predicts coronary heart disease, heart failure, and mortality in the Atherosclerosis Risk in Communities study. *Circulation* **2011**, *123*, 1367–1376. [CrossRef]
60. Agarwal, S.K.; Chambless, L.E.; Ballantyne, C.M.; Astor, B.; Bertoni, A.G.; Chang, P.P.; Folsom, A.R.; He, M.; Hoogeveen, R.C.; Ni, H.; et al. Prediction of incident heart failure in general practice: The Atherosclerosis Risk in Communities (ARIC) study. *Circ. Hear. Fail.* **2012**, *5*, 422–429. [CrossRef]
61. Matsushita, K.; Sang, Y.; Ballew, S.H.; Astor, B.C.; Hoogeveen, R.C.; Solomon, S.D.; Ballantyne, C.M.; Woodward, M.; Coresh, J. Cardiac and kidney markers for cardiovascular prediction in individuals with chronic kidney disease. *Arter. Thromb. Vasc. Boil.* **2014**, *34*, 1770–1777. [CrossRef]
62. Bansal, N.; Zelnick, L.; Shlipak, M.G.; Anderson, A.; Christenson, R.; Deo, R.; Defilippi, C.; Feldman, H.; Lash, J.; He, J.; et al. Cardiac and stress biomarkers and chronic kidney disease progression: The CRIC study. *Clin. Chem.* **2019**, *65*, 1448–1457. [CrossRef]

63. Ho, J.E.; Hwang, S.-J.; Wollert, K.C.; Larson, M.G.; Cheng, S.; Kempf, T.; Vasan, R.S.; Januzzi, J.L.; Wang, T.J.; Fox, C.S. Biomarkers of cardiovascular stress and incident chronic kidney disease. *Clin. Chem.* **2013**, *59*, 1613–1620. [CrossRef]
64. Shlipak, M.G.; Matsushita, K.; Ärnlöv, J.; Inker, L.A.; Katz, R.; Polkinghorne, K.R.; Rothenbacher, D.; Sarnak, M.J.; Astor, B.C.; Coresh, J.; et al. Cystatin C versus creatinine in determining risk based on kidney function. *N. Engl. J. Med.* **2013**, *369*, 932–943. [CrossRef] [PubMed]
65. Foster, M.C.; Coresh, J.; Hsu, C.-Y.; Xie, D.; Levey, A.S.; Nelson, R.G.; Eckfeldt, J.H.; Vasan, R.S.; Kimmel, P.L.; Schelling, J.; et al. Serum β-trace protein and β2-microglobulin as predictors of ESRD, mortality, and cardiovascular disease in adults with CKD in the Chronic Renal Insufficiency Cohort (CRIC) study. *Am. J. Kidney Dis.* **2016**, *68*, 68–76. [CrossRef] [PubMed]
66. Ix, J.H.; Katz, R.; Bansal, N.; Foster, M.; Weiner, D.E.; Tracy, R.P.; Jotwani, V.; Hughes-Austin, J.; McKay, D.; Gabbai, F.; et al. Urine fibrosis markers and risk of allograft failure in kidney transplant recipients: A Case-Cohort Ancillary Study of the FAVORIT Trial. *Am. J. Kidney Dis.* **2017**, *69*, 410–419. [CrossRef] [PubMed]
67. Puthumana, J.; Hall, I.E.; Reese, P.P.; Schroppel, B.; Weng, F.L.; Thiessen-Philbrook, H.; Doshi, M.D.; Rao, V.; Lee, C.G.; Elias, J.A.; et al. YKL-40 associates with renal recovery in deceased donor kidney transplantation. *J. Am. Soc. Nephrol.* **2017**, *28*, 661–670. [CrossRef]
68. Malhotra, R.; Katz, R.; Jotwani, V.; Ambrosius, W.T.; Raphael, K.L.; Haley, W.; Rastogi, A.; Cheung, A.K.; Freedman, B.I.; Punzi, H.; et al. Urine markers of kidney tubule cell injury and kidney function decline in SPRINT Trial participants with CKD. *Clin. J. Am. Soc. Nephrol.* **2020**, *15*, 349–358. [CrossRef] [PubMed]
69. Sun, L.; Zou, L.-X.; Chen, M.-J. Make precision medicine work for chronic kidney disease. *Med Princ. Pr.* **2016**, *26*, 101–107. [CrossRef]
70. Serra, R.; Ssempijja, L.; Provenzano, M.; Andreucci, M. Genetic biomarkers in chronic venous disease. *Biomark Med.* **2020**, *14*, 75–80. [CrossRef]
71. Serra, R.; Ielapi, N.; Barbetta, A.; Buffone, G.; Bevacqua, E.; Andreucci, M. Biomarkers for precision medicine in phlebology and wound care: A systematic review. *Acta. Phlebol.* **2017**, *18*, 52–56. [CrossRef]
72. Good, D.M.; Zürbig, P.; Argilés, A.; Bauer, H.W.; Behrens, G.; Coon, J.J.; Dakna, M.; Decramer, S.; Delles, C.; Dominiczak, A.F.; et al. Naturally occurring human urinary peptides for use in diagnosis of chronic kidney disease. *Mol. Cell. Proteom.* **2010**, *9*, 2424–2437. [CrossRef]
73. Argiles, A.; Siwy, J.; Duranton, F.; Gayrard, N.; Dakna, M.; Lundin, U.; Osaba, L.; Delles, C.; Mourad, G.; Weinberger, K.M.; et al. A new proteomics classifier assessing CKD and its prognosis. *PLoS ONE* **2013**, *8*, e62837. [CrossRef]
74. Roscioni, S.S.; De Zeeuw, D.; Hellemons, M.E.; Mischak, H.; Zürbig, P.; Bakker, S.J.L.; Gansevoort, R.T.; Reinhard, H.; Persson, F.; Lajer, M.; et al. A urinary peptide biomarker set predicts worsening of albuminuria in type 2 diabetes mellitus. *Diabetologia* **2012**, *56*, 259–267. [CrossRef] [PubMed]
75. Schanstra, J.P. Diagnosis and prediction of progression of chronic kidney disease by assessment of urinary peptides. *J. Am. Soc. Nephrol.* **2014**, *26*, 1999–2010. [CrossRef] [PubMed]
76. Kwan, B.; Fuhrer, T.; Zhang, J.; Darshi, M.; Van Espen, B.; Montemayor, D.; De Boer, I.H.; Dobre, M.; Hsu, C.-Y.; Kelly, T.N.; et al. Metabolomic markers of kidney function decline in patients with diabetes: Evidence From the Chronic Renal Insufficiency Cohort (CRIC) study. *Am. J. Kidney Dis.* **2020**. [CrossRef] [PubMed]
77. Connaughton, D.M.; Hildebrandt, F. Personalized medicine in chronic kidney disease by detection of monogenic mutations. *Nephrol. Dial. Transplant.* **2019**, *35*, 390–397. [CrossRef] [PubMed]
78. Thio, C.H.; Van Der Most, P.J.; Nolte, I.M.; Van Der Harst, P.; Bültmann, U.; Gansevoort, R.T.; Snieder, H. Evaluation of a genetic risk score based on creatinine-estimated glomerular filtration rate and its association with kidney outcomes. *Nephrol. Dial. Transplant.* **2017**, *33*, 1757–1764. [CrossRef] [PubMed]
79. Köttgen, A.; Hwang, S.-J.; Larson, M.G.; Van Eyk, J.E.; Fu, Q.; Benjamin, E.J.; Dehghan, A.; Glazer, N.L.; Kao, W.L.; Harris, T.B.; et al. Uromodulin levels associate with a common UMOD variant and risk for incident CKD. *J. Am. Soc. Nephrol.* **2009**, *21*, 337–344. [CrossRef]
80. Böger, C.A.; Gorski, M.; Li, M.; Hoffmann, M.M.; Huang, C.; Yang, Q.; Teumer, A.; Krane, V.; O'Seaghdha, C.M.; Kutalik, Z.; et al. Association of eGFR-related loci identified by GWAS with incident CKD and ESRD. *PLoS Genet.* **2011**, *7*, e1002292. [CrossRef]
81. Pays, E.; Vanhollebeke, B. Human innate immunity against African trypanosomes. *Curr. Opin. Immunol.* **2009**, *21*, 493–498. [CrossRef]

82. Parsa, A.; Kao, W.L.; Xie, D.; Astor, B.C.; Li, M.; Hsu, C.-Y.; Feldman, H.I.; Parekh, R.S.; Kusek, J.W.; Greene, T.H.; et al. APOL1 risk variants, race, and progression of chronic kidney disease. *N. Engl. J. Med.* **2013**, *369*, 2183–2196. [CrossRef]
83. Sudlow, C.; Gallacher, J.; Allen, N.; Beral, V.; Burton, P.; Danesh, J.; Downey, P.; Elliott, P.; Green, J.; Landray, M.; et al. UK Biobank: An open access resource for identifying the causes of a wide range of complex diseases of middle and old age. *PLoS Med.* **2015**, *12*, e1001779. [CrossRef]
84. Zhao, J.; Schooling, C.M. Sex-specific associations of insulin resistance with chronic kidney disease and kidney function: A bi-directional Mendelian randomisation study. *Diabetologia* **2020**, *63*, 1–10. [CrossRef]
85. Zhao, J.; Schooling, C.M. The role of testosterone in chronic kidney disease and kidney function in men and women: A bi-directional Mendelian randomization study in the UK Biobank. *BMC Med.* **2020**, *18*, 122. [CrossRef] [PubMed]
86. Casanova, F.; Tyrrell, J.; Beaumont, R.N.; Ji, Y.; Jones, S.E.; Hattersley, A.T.; Weedon, M.N.; Murray, A.; Shore, A.C.; Frayling, T.M.; et al. A genome-wide association study implicates multiple mechanisms influencing raised urinary albumin–creatinine ratio. *Hum. Mol. Genet.* **2019**, *28*, 4197–4207. [CrossRef]
87. Ledermann, J.A.; Harter, P.; Gourley, C.; Friedlander, M.; Vergote, I.; Rustin, G.; Scott, C.; Meier, W.; Shapira-Frommer, R.; Safra, T.; et al. Olaparib maintenance therapy in platinum-sensitive relapsed ovarian cancer. *N. Engl. J. Med.* **2012**, *366*, 1382–1392. [CrossRef]
88. Perco, P.; Pena, M.; Heerspink, H.J.; Mayer, G. Multimarker panels in diabetic kidney disease: The way to improved clinical trial design and clinical practice? *Kidney Int. Rep.* **2018**, *4*, 212–221. [CrossRef] [PubMed]
89. Brenner, B.M.; Cooper, M.E.; De Zeeuw, D.; Keane, W.F.; Mitch, W.E.; Parving, H.-H.; Remuzzi, G.; Snapinn, S.M.; Zhang, Z.; Shahinfar, S. Effects of losartan on renal and cardiovascular outcomes in patients with type 2 diabetes and nephropathy. *N. Engl. J. Med.* **2001**, *345*, 861–869. [CrossRef] [PubMed]
90. The GISEN Group (Gruppo Italiano di Studi Epidemiologici in Nefrologia). Randomised placebo-controlled trial of effect of ramipril on decline in glomerular filtration rate and risk of terminal renal failure in proteinuric, non-diabetic nephropathy. *Lancet* **1997**, *349*, 1857–1863. [CrossRef]
91. Heerspink, H.J.L.; Ninomiya, T.; Perkovic, V.; Woodward, M.; Zoungas, S.; Cass, A.; Cooper, M.; Grobbee, D.E.; Mancia, G.; Mogensen, C.E.; et al. Effects of a fixed combination of perindopril and indapamide in patients with type 2 diabetes and chronic kidney disease. *Eur. Hear. J.* **2010**, *31*, 2888–2896. [CrossRef]
92. Perkovic, V.; Jardine, M.J.; Neal, B.; Bompoint, S.; Heerspink, H.J.; Charytan, D.M.; Edwards, R.; Agarwal, R.; Bakris, G.; Bull, S.; et al. Canagliflozin and renal outcomes in type 2 diabetes and nephropathy. *N. Engl. J. Med.* **2019**, *380*, 2295–2306. [CrossRef]
93. Wanner, C.; E Inzucchi, S.; Lachin, J.M.; Fitchett, D.; Von Eynatten, M.; Mattheus, M.; Johansen, O.E.; Woerle, H.J.; Broedl, U.C.; Zinman, B. Empagliflozin and progression of kidney disease in type 2 diabetes. *N. Engl. J. Med.* **2016**, *375*, 323–334. [CrossRef]
94. Heerspink, H.J.L.; Parving, H.H.; Andress, D.L. SONAR Committees and Investigators. Atrasentan and renal events in patients with type 2 diabetes and chronic kidney disease (SONAR): A double-blind, randomised, placebo-controlled trial. *Lancet* **2019**, *393*, 1937–1947. [CrossRef]
95. Perkovic, V.; Ninomiya, T.; Arima, H.; Gallagher, M.; Jardine, M.; Cass, A.; Neal, B.; MacMahon, S.; Chalmers, J.P. Chronic kidney disease, cardiovascular events, and the effects of perindopril-based blood pressure lowering: Data from the PROGRESS study. *J. Am. Soc. Nephrol.* **2007**, *18*, 2766–2772. [CrossRef] [PubMed]
96. De Zeeuw, D.; Remuzzi, G.; Parving, H.-H.; Keane, W.F.; Zhang, Z.; Shahinfar, S.; Snapinn, S.; Cooper, M.E.; Mitch, W.E.; Brenner, B.M. Albuminuria, a therapeutic target for cardiovascular protection in type 2 diabetic patients with nephropathy. *Circulation* **2004**, *110*, 921–927. [CrossRef]
97. Heerspink, H.J.L.; Ninomiya, T.; Persson, F.; Brenner, B.M.; Brunel, P.; Chaturvedi, N.; Desai, A.S.; Haffner, S.M.; McMurray, J.J.; Solomon, S.D.; et al. Is a reduction in albuminuria associated with renal and cardiovascular protection? A post hoc analysis of the ALTITUDE trial. *Diabetes Obes. Metab.* **2016**, *18*, 169–177. [CrossRef] [PubMed]
98. Heerspink, H.J.L.; Gansevoort, R.T. Albuminuria is an appropriate therapeutic target in patients with CKD: The pro view. *Clin. J. Am. Soc. Nephrol.* **2015**, *10*, 1079–1088. [CrossRef]

99. Levey, A.S.; Inker, L.A.; Matsushita, K.; Greene, T.; Willis, K.; Lewis, E.; De Zeeuw, D.; Cheung, A.K.; Coresh, J. GFR decline as an end point for clinical trials in CKD: A scientific workshop sponsored by the National Kidney Foundation and the US Food and Drug Administration. *Am. J. Kidney Dis.* **2014**, *64*, 821–835. [CrossRef]
100. Heerspink, H.J.L.; Tighiouart, H.; Sang, Y.; Ballew, S.H.; Mondal, H.; Matsushita, K.; Coresh, J.; Levey, A.S.; Inker, L.A. GFR decline and subsequent risk of established kidney outcomes: A Meta-analysis of 37 Randomized Controlled Trials. *Am. J. Kidney Dis.* **2014**, *64*, 860–866. [CrossRef]
101. Heerspink, H.J.L.; Weldegiorgis, M.; Inker, L.A.; Gansevoort, R.; Parving, H.-H.; Dwyer, J.P.; Mondal, H.; Coresh, J.; Greene, T.; Levey, A.S.; et al. Estimated GFR decline as a surrogate end point for kidney failure: A post hoc analysis from the reduction of end points in non–insulin-dependent diabetes with the Angiotensin II Antagonist Losartan (RENAAL) Study and Irbesartan Diabetic Nephropathy Trial (IDNT). *Am. J. Kidney Dis.* **2014**, *63*, 244–250. [CrossRef]
102. Steinmann-Niggli, K.; Ziswiler, R.; Küng, M.; Marti, H.P. Inhibition of matrix metalloproteinases attenuates anti-Thy1.1 nephritis. *J. Am. Soc. Nephrol.* **1998**, *9*, 397–407.
103. Aggarwal, H.K.; Jain, D.; Talapatra, P.; Yadav, R.K.; Gupta, T.; Kathuria, K.L. Evaluation of role of doxycycline (a matrix metalloproteinase inhibitor) on renal functions in patients of diabetic nephropathy. *Ren. Fail.* **2010**, *32*, 941–946. [CrossRef]
104. Das, N.A.; Carpenter, A.J.; Belenchia, A.; Aroor, A.R.; Noda, M.; Siebenlist, U.; Chandrasekar, B.; Demarco, V.G. Empagliflozin reduces high glucose-induced oxidative stress and miR-21-dependent TRAF3IP2 induction and RECK suppression, and inhibits human renal proximal tubular epithelial cell migration and epithelial-to-mesenchymal transition. *Cell. Signal.* **2020**, *68*, 109506. [CrossRef] [PubMed]
105. Provenzano, M.; Rivoli, L.; Garofalo, C.; Faga, T.; Pelagi, E.; Perticone, M.; Serra, R.; Michael, A.; Comi, N.; Andreucci, M. Renal resistive index in chronic kidney disease patients: Possible determinants and risk profile. *PLoS ONE* **2020**, *15*, e0230020. [CrossRef] [PubMed]
106. Doi, Y.; Iwashima, Y.; Yoshihara, F.; Kamide, K.; Hayashi, S.-I.; Kubota, Y.; Nakamura, S.; Horio, T.; Kawano, Y. Response to renal resistive index and cardiovascular and renal outcomes in essential hypertension. *Hypertension* **2013**, *61*, e23. [CrossRef] [PubMed]
107. Sugiura, T.; Wada, A. Resistive index predicts renal prognosis in chronic kidney disease. *Nephrol. Dial. Transplant.* **2009**, *24*, 2780–2785. [CrossRef]
108. Solini, A.; Giannini, L.; Seghieri, M.; Vitolo, E.; Taddei, S.; Ghiadoni, L.; Bruno, R.M. Dapagliflozin acutely improves endothelial dysfunction, reduces aortic stiffness and renal resistive index in type 2 diabetic patients: A pilot study. *Cardiovasc. Diabetol.* **2017**, *16*, 138. [CrossRef]
109. Leoncini, G.; Martinoli, C.; Viazzi, F.; Ravera, M.; Parodi, D.; Ratto, E.; Vettoretti, S.; Tomolillo, C.; Derchi, L.E.; Deferrari, G.; et al. Changes in renal resistive index and urinary albumin excretion in hypertensive patients under long-term treatment with lisinopril or nifedipine GITS. *Nephron* **2002**, *90*, 169–173. [CrossRef]
110. Parving, H.-H.; Mauer, M.; Ritz, E. Diabetic nephropathy. In *Brenner and Rector's the Kidney*, 7th ed.; Brenner, B.M., Ed.; Boston Saunders: Cambridge, UK, 2004; pp. 1777–1818.
111. Parving, H.-H.; De Zeeuw, D.; Cooper, M.E.; Remuzzi, G.; Liu, N.; Lunceford, J.; Shahinfar, S.; Wong, P.H.; Lyle, P.A.; Rossing, P.; et al. ACE gene polymorphism and losartan treatment in type 2 diabetic patients with nephropathy. *J. Am. Soc. Nephrol.* **2008**, *19*, 771–779. [CrossRef]
112. Pena, M.J.; Heinzel, A.; Rossing, P.; Parving, H.-H.; Dallmann, G.; Rossing, K.; Andersen, S.; Mayer, B.; Heerspink, H.J.L. Serum metabolites predict response to angiotensin II receptor blockers in patients with diabetes mellitus. *J. Transl. Med.* **2016**, *14*, 203. [CrossRef]
113. Pena, M.J.; Jankowski, J.; Heinze, G.; Kohl, M.; Heinzel, A.; Bakker, S.J.; Gansevoort, R.T.; Rossing, P.; De Zeeuw, D.; Heerspink, H.J.L.; et al. Plasma proteomics classifiers improve risk prediction for renal disease in patients with hypertension or type 2 diabetes. *J. Hypertens.* **2015**, *33*, 2123–2132. [CrossRef]
114. Pencina, M.J.; Parikh, C.R.; Kimmel, P.L.; Cook, N.R.; Coresh, J.; Feldman, H.I.; Foulkes, A.S.; Gimotty, P.A.; Hsu, C.-Y.; Lemley, K.; et al. Statistical methods for building better biomarkers of chronic kidney disease. *Stat. Med.* **2019**, *38*, 1903–1917. [CrossRef]
115. McShane, L.M. Biomarker validation: Context and complexities. *J. Law Med. Ethics* **2019**, *47*, 388–392. [CrossRef]

116. Soveri, I.; Helmersson-Karlqvist, J.; Fellström, B.; Larsson, A. Day-to-day variation of the kidney proximal tubular injury markers urinary cystatin C, KIM1, and NGAL in patients with chronic kidney disease. *Ren. Fail.* **2020**, *42*, 400–404. [CrossRef] [PubMed]
117. LeDue, T.B.; Rifai, N. Preanalytic and analytic sources of variations in C-reactive protein measurement: Implications for cardiovascular disease risk assessment. *Clin. Chem.* **2003**, *49*, 1258–1271. [CrossRef] [PubMed]
118. Schinstock, C.A.; Semret, M.H.; Wagner, S.J.; Borland, T.M.; Bryant, S.C.; Kashani, K.B.; Larson, T.S.; Lieske, J.C. Urinalysis is more specific and urinary neutrophil gelatinase-associated lipocalin is more sensitive for early detection of acute kidney injury. *Nephrol. Dial. Transplant.* **2012**, *28*, 1175–1185. [CrossRef] [PubMed]
119. Jones, G.R.; Albarede, S.; Kesseler, D.; MacKenzie, F.; Mammen, J.; Pedersen, M.; Stavelin, A.; Thelen, M.; Thomas, A.; Twomey, P.J.; et al. Analytical performance specifications for external quality assessment —Definitions and descriptions. *Clin. Chem. Lab. Med.* **2017**, *55*. [CrossRef] [PubMed]
120. Jennings, L.; Van Deerlin, V.M.; Gulley, M.L. Recommended principles and practices for validating clinical molecular pathology tests. *Arch. Pathol. Lab. Med.* **2009**, *133*, 743–755. [PubMed]
121. Tripepi, G.; D'Arrigo, G.; Jager, K.J.; Stel, V.S.; Dekker, F.J.; Zoccali, C. Do we still need cross-sectional studies in Nephrology? Yes we do! *Nephrol. Dial. Transplant.* **2017**, *32*. [CrossRef]
122. Harrell, F.E., Jr.; Lee, K.L.; Mark, D.B. Multivariable prognostic models: Issues in developing models, evaluating assumptions and adequacy, and measuring and reducing errors. *Stat. Med.* **1996**, *15*, 361–387. [CrossRef]
123. Roy, J.; Shou, H.; Xie, D.; Hsu, J.Y.; Yang, W.; Anderson, A.H.; Landis, J.R.; Jepson, C.; He, J.; Liu, K.D.; et al. Statistical methods for cohort studies of CKD: Prediction modeling. *Clin. J. Am. Soc. Nephrol.* **2016**, *12*, 1010–1017. [CrossRef]
124. Tibshirani, R. Regression shrinkage and selection via the lasso. *J. R. Stat. Soc. Ser. B Stat. Methodol.* **1996**, *58*, 267–288. [CrossRef]
125. Pencina, M.J.; D'Agostino, R.B.; Vasan, R.S. Statistical methods for assessment of added usefulness of new biomarkers. *Clin. Chem. Lab. Med.* **2010**, *48*, 1703–1711. [CrossRef] [PubMed]
126. Pepe, M.S.; Kerr, K.F.; Longton, G.; Wang, Z. Testing for improvement in prediction model performance. *Stat. Med.* **2013**, *32*, 1467–1482. [CrossRef] [PubMed]
127. Pencina, M.J.; D'Agostino, R.B., Sr.; Steyerberg, E.W. Extensions of net reclassification improvement calculations to measure usefulness of new biomarkers. *Stat. Med.* **2011**, *30*, 11–21. [CrossRef]
128. Steyerberg, E.W.; Vickers, A.J.; Cook, N.R.; Gerds, T.; Gonen, M.; Obuchowski, N.; Pencina, M.J.; Kattan, M.W. Assessing the performance of prediction models. *Epidemiology* **2010**, *21*, 128–138. [CrossRef] [PubMed]
129. Tangri, N.; Kitsios, G.D.; Inker, L.A.; Griffith, J.; Naimark, D.M.; Walker, S.; Rigatto, C.; Uhlig, K.; Kent, D.M.; Levey, A.S. Risk prediction models for patients with chronic kidney disease. *Ann. Intern. Med.* **2013**, *158*, 596–603. [CrossRef]
130. Andreucci, M.; Faga, T.; Pisani, A.; Perticone, M.; Michael, A. The ischemic/nephrotoxic acute kidney injury and the use of renal biomarkers in clinical practice. *Eur. J. Intern. Med.* **2017**, *39*, 1–8. [CrossRef]
131. Lewis, E.J.; Hunsicker, L.G.; Bain, R.P.; Rohde, R.D. The Effect of angiotensin-converting-enzyme inhibition on diabetic nephropathy. *N. Engl. J. Med.* **1993**, *329*, 1456–1462. [CrossRef]
132. Lewis, E.J.; Hunsicker, L.G.; Clarke, W.R.; Berl, T.; Pohl, M.A.; Lewis, J.B.; Ritz, E.; Atkins, R.C.; Rohde, R.; Raz, I. Renoprotective effect of the angiotensin-receptor antagonist irbesartan in patients with nephropathy due to type 2 diabetes. *N. Engl. J. Med.* **2001**, *345*, 851–860. [CrossRef]
133. De Zeeuw, D.; Heerspink, H.J.L. Time for clinical decision support systems tailoring individual patient therapy to improve renal and cardiovascular outcomes in diabetes and nephropathy. *Nephrol. Dial. Transplant.* **2020**, *35*, ii38–ii42. [CrossRef]
134. Parving, H.-H.; Brenner, B.M.; McMurray, J.J.; De Zeeuw, D.; Haffner, S.M.; Solomon, S.D.; Chaturvedi, N.; Persson, F.; Desai, A.S.; Nicolaides, M.; et al. Cardiorenal end points in a trial of aliskiren for type 2 diabetes. *N. Engl. J. Med.* **2012**, *367*, 2204–2213. [CrossRef]
135. Fried, L.F.; Emanuele, N.; Zhang, J.H.; Brophy, M.; Conner, T.A.; Duckworth, W.C.; Leehey, D.J.; McCullough, P.A.; O'Connor, T.; Palevsky, P.M.; et al. Combined angiotensin inhibition for the treatment of diabetic nephropathy. *N. Engl. J. Med.* **2013**, *369*, 1892–1903. [CrossRef] [PubMed]
136. Heerspink, H.J.; List, J.; Perkovic, V. New clinical trial designs for establishing drug efficacy and safety in a precision medicine era. *Diabetes Obes. Metab.* **2018**, *20*, 14–18. [CrossRef] [PubMed]

137. Lindhardt, M.; Persson, F.; Currie, G.; Pontillo, C.; Beige, J.; Delles, C.; Von Der Leyen, H.; Mischak, H.; Navis, G.; Noutsou, M.; et al. Proteomic prediction and renin angiotensin aldosterone system inhibition prevention of early diabetic nephropathy in type 2 diabetic patients with normoalbuminuria (PRIORITY): Essential study design and rationale of a randomised clinical multicentre trial. *BMJ Open* **2016**, *6*, e010310. [CrossRef] [PubMed]

138. Baigent, C.; Landray, M.; Reith, C.; Emberson, J.R.; Wheeler, D.C.; Tomson, C.; Wanner, C.; Krane, V.; Cass, A.; Craig, J.C.; et al. The effects of lowering LDL cholesterol with simvastatin plus ezetimibe in patients with chronic kidney disease (Study of Heart and Renal Protection): A randomised placebo-controlled trial. *Lancet* **2011**, *377*, 2181–2192. [CrossRef]

139. Woodcock, J.; LaVange, L.M. Master protocols to study multiple therapies, multiple diseases, or both. *N. Engl. J. Med.* **2017**, *377*, 62–70. [CrossRef] [PubMed]

140. Berry, S.M.; Connor, J.T.; Lewis, R.J. The platform trial. *JAMA* **2015**, *313*, 1619–1620. [CrossRef]

12

Uromodulin and microRNAs in Kidney Transplantation Association with Kidney Graft Function

Špela Borštnar [1,2], Željka Večerić-Haler [1,2], Emanuela Boštjančič [3], Živa Pipan Tkalec [3], Damjan Kovač [1,2], Jelka Lindič [1,2] and Nika Kojc [3,*]

1 Department of Nephrology, University Medical Centre Ljubljana, Zaloška 7, 1000 Ljubljana, Slovenia; spela.borstnar@kclj.si (Š.B.); zeljka.veceric@gmail.com (Ž.V.-H.); damjan.kovac@kclj.si (D.K.); jelka.lindic@kclj.si (J.L.)

2 Faculty of Medicine, University of Ljubljana, Vrazov trg 2, 1000 Ljubljana, Slovenia

3 Institute of Pathology, Faculty of Medicine, University of Ljubljana, Korytkova 2, 1000 Ljubljana, Slovenia; emanuela.bostjancic@mf.uni-lj.si (E.B.); ziva.pipan-tkalec@mf.uni-lj.si (Ž.P.T.)

* Correspondence: nika.kojc@mf.uni-lj.si

Abstract: Uromodulin and microRNAs (miRNAs) have recently been investigated as potential biomarkers for kidney graft associated pathology and outcome, with a special focus on biomarkers indicating specific disease processes and kidney graft survival. The study's aim was to determine whether expression of serum uromodulin concentration and selected miRNAs might be related to renal function in kidney transplant recipients (KTRs). The uromodulin concentration and expression of six selected miRNAs (*miR-29c*, *miR-126*, *miR-146a*, *miR-150*, *miR-155*, and *miR-223*) were determined in the serum of 100 KTRs with stable graft function and chronic kidney disease of all five stages. Kidney graft function was estimated with routine parameters (creatinine, urea, cystatin C, and Chronic Kidney Disease Epidemiology Collaboration study equations) and precisely measured using chromium-51 labelled ethylenediaminetetraacetic-acid clearance. The selected miRNAs were shown to be independent of kidney graft function, indicating their potential as biomarkers of associated kidney graft disease processes. In contrast, the serum uromodulin level depended entirely on kidney graft function and thus reflected functioning tubules rather than any specific kidney graft injury. However, decreased concentrations of serum uromodulin can be observed in the early course of tubulointerstitial injury, thereby suggesting its useful role as an accurate, noninvasive biomarker of early (subclinical) kidney graft injury.

Keywords: microRNA; uromodulin; kidney graft function; biomarker; kidney transplantation

---

1. Introduction

Serum creatinine, urea, cystatin C, and estimation of glomerular filtration rate (GFR) via different equations are currently routinely used biomarkers of kidney graft function in clinical transplantation. Although they are characterized by low cost and rapid accessibility of results, these biomarkers are significantly less sensitive and specific than the aggressive and time-consuming gold standard, i.e., the measurement of GFR by an exogenous marker, such as chromium-51-ethylenediaminetetraacetic acid (^{51}CrEDTA). Many new candidate biomarkers in kidney transplantation have been proposed and tested in recent years, which address specific pathologic processes and not merely glomerular, tubular, or overall kidney graft function. Uromodulin (also known as Tamm–Horsfall's protein) is a urinary mucoprotein that is synthesized only in the thick ascending limb of Henle's loop and early distal convoluted tubules of the kidneys [1]. In addition to this classical tubular secretion, to a minor degree uromodulin also sorts to the basolateral pole of tubular epithelial cells, as shown by its presence in circulation [2]. The reduced number of tubular cells seen in chronic kidney disease (CKD) due to interstitial fibrosis/tubular atrophy (IF/TA) is paralleled by the reduced urinary and serum concentrations of uromodulin [3–5]. The potential utility of serum [4,6,7] and urine [8] uromodulin measurement in kidney transplant recipients (KTRs) has been studied, showing an association of lower serum uromodulin levels with progression to end-stage renal disease and graft failure. Although normative ranges for serum/plasma uromodulin concentration were established over 30 years ago, its characteristics have not yet been sufficiently identified as a priority in certain instances, resulting in a failure to fully implement uromodulin in clinical practice.

MicroRNAs (miRNAs) are short, endogenous non-coding ribonucleic acids (RNAs) involved in the modulation of gene expression, mainly by inhibition of messenger RNA translation [9,10]. Recent studies have indicated an association of miRNAs with pathological processes following kidney transplantation, such as T-cell or antibody-mediated rejection, delayed graft function, and IF/TA [9–11]. The diagnostic accuracy of such molecules as biomarkers is still questionable, since many of them emerge on the vascular side of the glomerular filtration barrier and can therefore reflect glomerular filtration rather than a specific disease process. We have focused on searching for miRNAs that were among the most studied in the context of fibrosis (anti-fibrotic *miR-29c*) [12], endothelial dysfunction (*miR-126*) [13–15], and immune response (*miR-146a*) [16,17], or might even be involved in more than one physiological and/or pathogenetic process, e.g., *miR-150* [18,19], *miR-155* [16,17], and *miR-223* [20–22]. Moreover, our previous pilot research on miRNA association with certain most common kidney graft pathologies, such as kidney graft rejection and the recurrence of primary glomerular disease, offered interesting insights into a possible connection of selected miRNAs with underlying kidney graft pathology. For details, see also Supplementary Table S1 and Figure S1.

In this study, we investigated the association of serum uromodulin concentration (s-Uromodulin) (which emerges on the urinary side of the filtration barrier) and selected miRNAs (which emerge on the vascular side of the glomerular filtration barrier) with standard biomarkers of kidney graft function, including measurement of ^{51}CrEDTA clearance. The study's aim was firstly to investigate whether any of the proposed biomarkers are associated with the glomerular filtration and renal function in KTRs. Based on these results, the proposed biomarkers could or could not be a reliable indicator of kidney graft associated disease processes. The possible association of reliable biomarker(s) with the course of the associated disease process and kidney graft outcome is a long-term aim of this study protocol.

2. Results

2.1. Characteristics of the Study Population

The study included 100 KTRs, all Caucasian, 55 men and 45 women. The mean age was 55 ± 11 years (range 19 to 79 years). The average time from transplantation was 10 ± 7 years (range 2 to 28 years). The cohort included in the analysis had chronic kidney disease of transplanted kidney (CKD-T) of all five stages, including patients just before starting renal replacement therapy. The data presenting parameters of GFR are shown in Figure 1.

For investigation of uromodulin, the study included also 15 patients with non-kidney diseases, all Caucasian, 7 men and 8 women. The mean age was 43 ± 13 years (range 20 to 58 years).

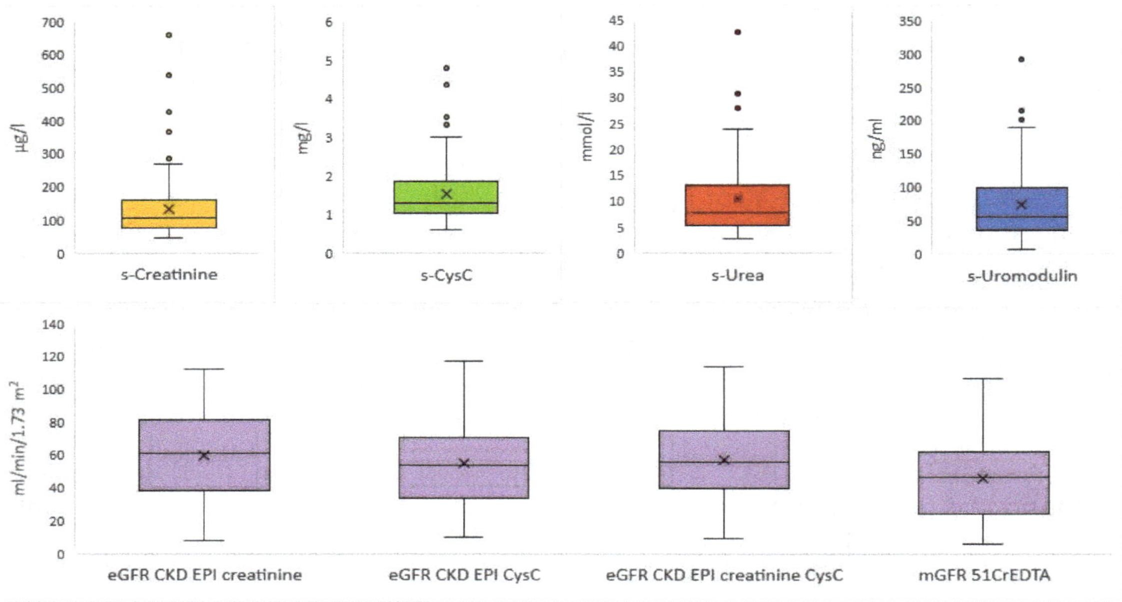

Figure 1. Boxplots for each parameter of glomerular filtration rate. Boxplots for serum creatinine concentration (s-Creatinine), serum cystatin C concentration (s-CysC), serum urea concentration (s-Urea), serum uromodulin concentration (s-Uromodulin), estimated glomerular filtration rate with Chronic Kidney Disease Epidemiology Collaboration study formula with s-Creatinine (eGFR CKD EPI creatinine), estimated glomerular filtration rate with Chronic Kidney Disease Epidemiology Collaboration study formula with s-CyC (eGFR CKD EPI CysC), estimated glomerular filtration rate with Chronic Kidney Disease Epidemiology Collaboration study formula with s-Creatinine and s-CysC (eGFR CKD EPI creatinine CysC), and measured glomerular filtration rate with Chromium-51-ethylenediaminetetraacetic acid clearance (mGFR ^{51}CrEDTA).

2.2. Relation between Kidney Function Parameters and s-Uromodulin

In the control group, the mean level of s-Uromodulin was 291 ± 71 ng/mL. S-Uromodulin levels decreased significantly in the group of KTRs ($p < 0.001$), in which the mean s-Uromodulin was 74 ± 53 ng/mL. We further analyzed s-Uromodulin in different stages of CKD-T (1–5, based on measured GFR with ^{51}CrEDTA (mGFR ^{51}CrEDTA)), in relation to the s-Uromodulin in the control group. We found that already in stage 1 of CKD-T, the s-Uromodulin significantly dropped compared to the control group ($p = 0.013$). In the other four stages (2–4), the significance of reduced s-Uromodulin compared to that in the control group was even lower ($p < 0.001$). Between CKD-T stage 1 and 2, the drop of s-Uromodulin showed borderline significance ($p = 0.067$), while s-Uromodulin was significantly lower in CKD-T stage 2 compared to CKD-T stage 3 ($p < 0.05$) and in CKD-T stage 3 compared to CKD-T stage 4 ($p < 0.05$). There were no significant differences between stages CKD-T 4 and 5 (Figure 2A).

According to receiver operating characteristics (ROC), the area under the curve (AUC) represents the probability that a randomly selected patient will have a lower or higher test result than a randomly selected control. The ROC curve of s-Uromodulin in KTRs demonstrated an AUC of 0.991 (SE-0.007) (95% Cl 0.977–1.00, $p < 0.001$) at an optimal cut-off of 191.5 ng/mL with 97% sensitivity and 100% specificity (Figure 2B).

Analyzing bivariate correlations using Spearman's correlation coefficient, s-Uromodulin was significantly associated with all parameters of kidney graft function. The highest correlation coefficient was noted for estimated glomerular filtration rate (eGFR) with Chronic Kidney Disease Epidemiology Collaboration study formula with serum creatinine concentration (s-Creatinine) and serum cystatin C concentration (s-CysC) (eGFR CKD EPI creatinine CysC) (Rho = 0.758, $p < 0.001$), followed by serum urea concentration (s-Urea) (Rho = −0.740, $p < 0.001$), eGFR with Chronic Kidney Disease Epidemiology

Collaboration study formula with s-Creatinine (eGFR CKD EPI creatinine) (Rho = −0.736, $p < 0.001$), s-CysC (Rho = −0.720, $p < 0.001$), eGFR with Chronic Kidney Disease Epidemiology Collaboration study formula with s-CysC (eGFR CKD EPI CysC) (Rho = 0.718, $p < 0.001$), s-Creatinine (Rho = −0.698, $p < 0.001$), and mGFR ^{51}CrEDTA (Rho = 0.669, $p < 0.001$) (Table 1).

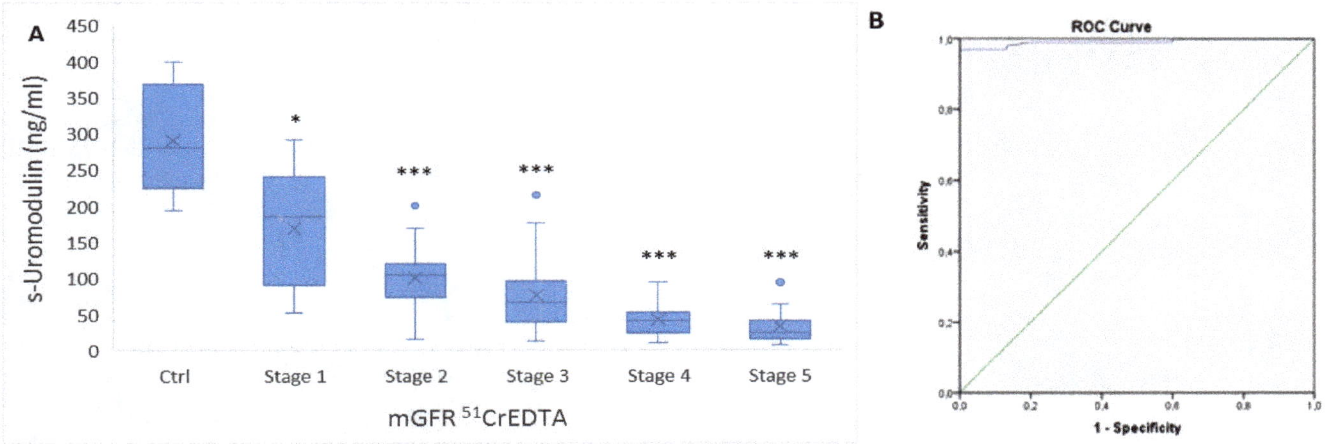

Figure 2. Uromodulin concentration in serum. (**A**) The boxplots for serum uromodulin concentration (s-Uromodulin) in chronic kidney disease of transplanted kidney (CKD-T) stages 1–5 based on measured GFR with ^{51}CrEDTA (mGFR ^{51}CrEDTA) (stage 1, $n = 5$; stage 2, $n = 21$; stage 3, $n = 43$; stage 4, $n = 17$; and stage 5, $n = 11$, with mGFR ^{51}CrEDTA not possible to perform for 3 patients) in comparison to the control group (Ctrl); (**B**) ROC curve and AUC distinguishing CKD-T from the control group without any renal diseases. Legend: * $p < 0.05$, *** $p < 0.001$ (Ctrl versus Stage 1–5).

Table 1. Bivariate correlations between serum uromodulin concentration (s-Uromodulin) and parameters of kidney graft function: serum creatinine concentration (s-Creatinine), serum cystatin C concentration (s-CysC), serum urea concentration (s-Urea), estimated glomerular filtration rate with Chronic Kidney Disease Epidemiology Collaboration study formula with s-Creatinine (eGFR CKD EPI creatinine), estimated glomerular filtration rate with Chronic Kidney Disease Epidemiology Collaboration study formula with s-CysC (eGFR CKD EPI CysC), estimated glomerular filtration rate with Chronic Kidney Disease Epidemiology Collaboration study formula with s-Creatinine and s-CysC (eGFR CKD EPI creatinine CysC) and measured GFR with Chromium-51-ethylenediaminetetraacetic acid (mGFR ^{51}CrEDTA).

Parameters of Kidney Graft Function	Spearman Correlation to s-Uromodulin	p
s-Creatinine	−0.698	<0.001
s-CysC	−0.720	<0.001
s-Urea	−0.740	<0.001
eGFR CKD EPI creatinine	0.736	<0.001
eGFR CKD EPI CysC	0.718	<0.001
eGFR CKD EPI creatinine CysC	0.758	<0.001
mGFR ^{51}CrEDTA	0.669	<0.001

2.3. *Relation between Kidney Function Parameters and Expression of Selected miRNAs*

While *miR-126*, *miR-146a*, and *miR-150* were expressed in all 100 samples of serum, *miR-29c*, *miR-155*, and *miR-223* were not expressed in 12, 8, and 8 serum samples, respectively. Using the Pearson correlation coefficient, none of the six analyzed miRNAs significantly correlated with the parameters of kidney graft function (Figure 3).

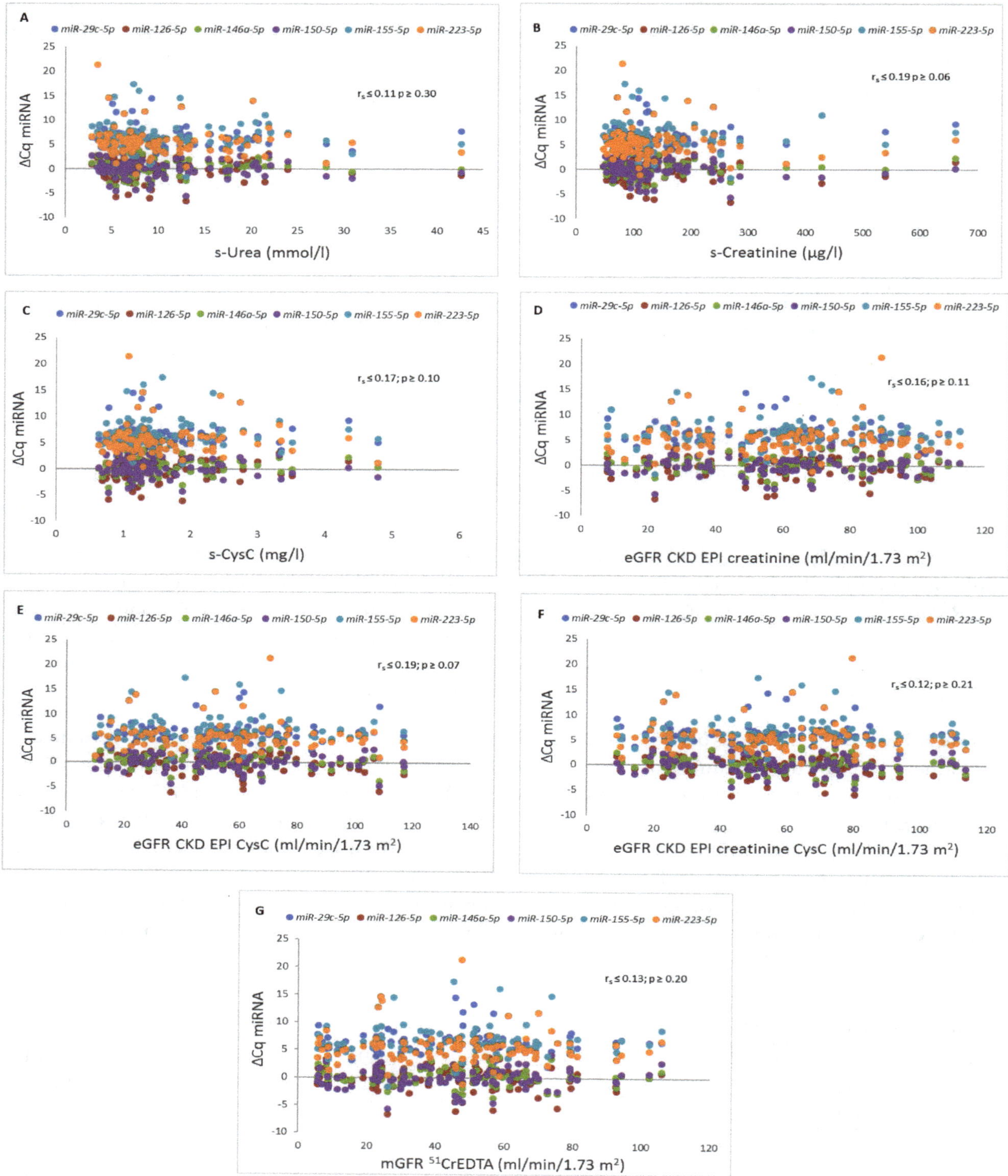

Figure 3. Correlations between different microRNAs (miRNAs) and parameters of kidney graft function. Correlation between different miRNAs and (**A**) serum urea concentration (s-Urea), (**B**) serum creatinine concentration (s-Creatinine), (**C**) serum cystatin C concentration (s-CysC), (**D**) estimated glomerular filtration rate with Chronic Kidney Disease Epidemiology Collaboration study formula with s-Creatinine (eGFR CKD EPI creatinine), (**E**) estimated glomerular filtration rate with Chronic Kidney Disease Epidemiology Collaboration study formula with s-CysC (eGFR CKD EPI CysC), (**F**) estimated glomerular filtration rate with Chronic Kidney Disease Epidemiology Collaboration study formula with s-Creatinine and s-CysC (eGFR CKD EPI creatinine CysC), (**G**) measured glomerular filtration rate with Chromium-51-ethylenediaminetetraacetic acid clearance (mGFR ^{51}CrEDTA).

3. Discussion

Although extensive scientific effort has been focused on developing biomarkers to detect kidney allograft disease processes such as rejection or IF/TA, few assays have moved from the research arena to clinical routine. The obstacle to the successful initiation of their clinical use is the still insufficiently validated specificity for renal pathology. Similar to other molecules and proteins, these biomarkers are also subject to glomerular filtration, tubular secretion, and reabsorption. Many of them, depending on the site of their production and paths of elimination, probably reflect merely kidney function and not disease. The identification of sensitive biomarkers able to reflect the subclinical steps of a pathologic process, such as rejection, is therefore of the utmost relevance to recipients of kidney transplants [23–25].

Our research confirmed previous reports showing significantly higher s-Uromodulin in healthy controls (patients without kidney disease) compared to KTRs, who in general belong to the group of CKD patients [4,5,26]. In line with the findings of other similar research in patients with kidney transplants [6], s-Uromodulin levels in our KTRs decreased stepwise from those with almost preserved graft function to the lowest values in KTRs with pre-dialysis CKD-T. We also showed in this study that s-Uromodulin correlates with all parameters of kidney graft function, the strongest association being observed for eGFR CKD EPI creatinine CysC, followed by the serum level of urea, eGFR CKD EPI creatinine, serum level of CysC, eGFR CKD EPI CysC, serum level of creatinine, and ^{51}CrEDTA. Decreased s-Uromodulin was observed in the earliest stages of CKD-T when other markers, such as serum creatinine and even the precise method of GFR determination with ^{51}CrEDTA, had still not crossed the reference range. This indicates that reabsorption of uromodulin, which is exclusively a product of tubules, is probably compromised from the earliest stages of tubulo-interstitial injury. Reduced s-Uromodulin may therefore be a more sensitive indicator of early kidney graft dysfunction not detected by serum glomerular filtration markers. In view of the simple routine of s-Uromodulin measurement and its low costs, monitoring the dynamics of s-Uromodulin concentration may serve as an accurate, noninvasive predictive biomarker of kidney graft injury and outcome.

Given that the concentration of uromodulin strongly reflects renal function, one would assume that it would never be able to act as a reliable parameter of specific kidney graft pathology. However, exceptions have already been found in the field of specificity for certain pathologies of native kidneys, such as gout [27] or Balkan nephropathy [2]. Accordingly, in the case of kidney transplantation, s-Uromodulin could be especially useful to clinicians aware of the advantages of biomarkers reflecting subclinical tubular injury. Regular s-Uromodulin checkups in KTRs could, in our opinion, become a useful tool for early detection of subclinical processes involving tubules and interstitium (such as acute tubulointerstitial rejection), or timely surveillance of IF/TA. This assumption, however, needs further exploration.

The miRNAs investigated in the present study have so far been extensively related to various physiological and pathological states of kidney graft pathology (see also Supplementary Table S1). We did not observe any association between the circulating levels of selected miRNAs (*miR-29c*, *miR-126*, *miR-146a*, *miR-150*, *miR-155*, and *miR-223*) and kidney graft function (estimated and measured by the reference method at the same time point of miRNA analysis). Previously published studies have shown that the expression of some miRNAs, such as *miR-126* or *miR-223*, is associated with renal function in an up- or downregulated manner [11,15,28]. However, many of those studies were performed with patients with CKD without kidney transplants [15] and/or focused on the functionally unstable period of delayed graft function immediately after transplantation [11,17]. The essential advantage of our analysis is that we used the reference method for GFR measurement (^{51}CrEDTA) and not only routinely used noninvasive biomarkers and/or GFR equations, but the patient cohort in this study was also larger than in most of the so far published research in the field of biomarkers in kidney transplantation [10,11,17,28].

Since selected miRNAs are independent of kidney graft function, they can be reliably used as biomarkers of various pathological processes in KTRs without adjustments to kidney function. In line with previous findings, the results of our pilot study performed on a subgroup of patients with indications of kidney graft biopsy showed a significant association with the miRNAs selected here, with histologically proven antibody-mediated kidney graft rejection and recurrence of primary glomerulonephritis. In this regard, *miR-29c* expression especially has shown potential for differentiating between these two pathologies (see also Supplementary Figure S1). Unfortunately, the sample examined was too small for reliable inference, but nevertheless pointed to the feasibility of conducting further prospective analysis with systematic serum sampling for miRNA determination and planned implementation of kidney graft biopsy, which is the long term aim of this study.

4. Materials and Methods

A prospective clinical study (NCT04413916) was conducted at the Department of Nephrology, University Medical Centre Ljubljana, Slovenia and the Institute of Pathology, Faculty of Medicine, University of Ljubljana. The study was approved by the National Medical Ethics Committee of the Republic of Slovenia (permit number 24k/06/12 approved on 15/06/2012 and 0120-625/2017/4 on 18/12/2017 (revised version number 0120-625/2017/11 on 12/12/2019)) and conducted in accordance with the Declaration of Helsinki. All patients signed informed consent.

4.1. Study Population Inclusion and Exclusion Criteria

The study included 100 kidney transplant recipients from the Slovenian Center for Kidney Transplantation. Inclusion criteria were stable graft function for more than 3 months (changes in creatinine concentration < 20%) and a time of transplantation at least two years before the study entry, since we wanted to study the expression of miRNAs in stable conditions and eliminate the influence of recent transplantation, replacement therapy, and rapid changes in renal function. The subsequent data analysis revealed unstable graft function in only one patient. Exclusion criteria were an age less than 18 years, symptomatic heart failure, malignancy, pregnancy or lactation, newly introduced drugs that may affect the function of the graft, and treatment with trimethoprim-sulfamethoxazole or cimetidine. As a control group, 15 patients with non-kidney diseases were included (nonspecific skin lesions $n = 13$, erosive stomatitis $n = 1$, and paraneoplastic dermatitis $n = 1$).

4.2. Measurement of Serum Creatinine, Serum Urea, and Cystatin C Concentration

Blood sampling was performed on the same day as the measurement of GFR ^{51}CrEDTA clearance, but before the injection of ^{51}CrEDTA. S-Creatinine was measured with the kinetic colorimetric compensated Jaffe assay (Siemens Healthcare Diagnostics Inc., Tarrytown, NY, USA) and with a calibrator traceable to primary reference material with values assigned by isotope dilution mass spectrometry [29]. S-CysC was measured using the particle-enhanced immunonephelometric method (Siemens Healthcare Diagnostics, Marburg, Germany) [30]. S-urea was determined by a Roch-Ramel enzyme reaction with urease and glutamate dehydrogenase (Siemens Healthcare Diagnostics Inc., Tarrytown, NY, USA).

4.3. eGFR

eGFR was calculated using Chronic Kidney Disease Epidemiology Collaboration study formulae with s-Creatinine (eGFR CKD EPI creatinine) and s-CysC (eGFR CKD EPI CysC) or with both s-Creatinine and s-CysC (eGFR CKD EPI creatinine CysC) [31].

4.4. Measurement of ^{51}CrEDTA Clearance

mGFR ^{51}CrEDTA was determined from a single ^{51}CrEDTA injection (activity 3 MBq) and four blood samples taken 120, 180, 240, and 300 min after intravenous application of the marker according to British Nuclear Medicine Society guidelines, using the By weight method. Samples were measured using a gamma counter (Hidex, Turku, Finland); mGFR ^{51}CrEDTA was calculated and then adjusted to the patient's body surface area (Haycock formula) and specified as mL/min/1.73 m^2 [32].

4.5. Measurement of s-Uromodulin

S-Uromodulin was assessed in 20 controls and in 100 KTRs. All serum samples were stored at −80 °C before measurements were performed. Measurements of s-Uromodulin were performed using commercial ELISA (Euroimmun, Medizinische Labordiagnostika AG, Lübeck, Germany), as described previously, based on the manufacturer's instructions [5]. Characteristics of the ELISA were as follows, given by the manufacturer: detection limit for plasma samples 2 ng/mL; mean linearity recovery 97% (83–107% at 59–397 ng/mL); intra-assay precision 1.8–3.2% (at 30–214 ng/mL); inter-assay precision 6.6–7.8% (at 35–228 ng/mL); and inter-lot precision 7.2–10.1% (at 37–227 ng/mL). Data analysis was performed using the program Analysis Software Gen5 (Gen5 2.09, BioTek).

4.6. miRNA Quantification

Total RNA isolation was performed using 200 µL of serum and a miRNeasy serum/plasma advanced kit (Qiagen, Hilden, Germany) according to the manufacturer's protocol. Elution was performed using 20 µL of RNAse-free water. The successful isolation procedure was confirmed by adding spike-ins and subsequent quantification of these spike-ins.

miRNAs *miR-29c*, *miR-126*, *miR-146a*, *miR-150*, *miR-155*, and *miR-223* were analyzed using the miRCURY LNA miRNA PCR system (Qiagen, Hilden, Germany). As the reference genes, *miR-103a-3p*, *miR-191*, and *miR-423* were used according to the manufacturer's instruction. The possibility of hemolysis was excluded by quantifying *miR-23a* and *miR-451a*. All the reagents were from Qiagen, except where otherwise indicated. qPCR was carried out using Rotor Gene Q.

For reverse transcription, a miRCURY LNA RT Kit was used in a 10 µL reaction master mix containing 2 µL of total RNA, according to the manufacturer's instructions. The resulting reverse transcription was diluted 20-fold and 3 µL was used in a 10 µL reaction master mix, according to the manufacturer's instructions. All the qPCR reactions were performed in duplicate. Prior to qPCR, RNA samples were pooled, followed by RT and qPCR as described above. Efficiency was tested for each analyzed miRNA using 10-fold dilutions and qPCR was performed in triplicate. The signal was collected at the endpoint of every cycle. Following amplification, melting curve analysis of PCR products was performed to verify the specificity and identity. Melting curves were acquired on the SYBR channel using a ramping rate of 0.7 °C/60 s for 60–95 °C.

4.7. Statistical Analysis

Correlations were analyzed using Spearman's rank correlation coefficient (Spearman's rho) or the Pearson correlation coefficient. To present relative gene expression, ΔCq was calculated for miRNA expression [33]. The *t*-test was used to calculate the difference between the expression of uromodulin between the control group and the kidney transplant group. For all statistical analyses, SPSS analytical software (IBM SPSS statistics, version 24.0, Armonk, NY, USA) was used with a cut-off point at $p < 0.05$.

5. Conclusions

In the present study, we evaluated six selected miRNAs (*miR-29c*, *miR-126*, *miR-146a*, *miR-150*, *miR-155*, and *miR-223*) and s-Uromodulin as biomarkers of kidney function in KTRs. The selected miRNAs and s-Uromodulin were compared not only with conventional GFR biomarkers (creatinine, cystatin, and estimated GFR), but also, as a novelty, with the radioisotope method, providing significant reinforcement to the credibility of the findings. To the best of our knowledge, this is the first study to compare these markers with the clinical gold standard of GFR (i.e., ^{51}CrEDTA clearance) in KTRs.

In brief, the selected miRNAs are independent of kidney graft function, indicating their potential as biomarkers of associated etiopathogenesis of kidney graft disease processes. In contrast, s-Uromodulin is dependent on all observed parameters of kidney graft function. However, s-Uromodulin reliably reflects the early stages of kidney graft disfunction, in which conventional GFR-related biomarkers, including ^{51}Cr EDTA, are still within normal limits. Since uromodulin is synthetized exclusively within tubules, though it is not a disease-specific marker, it can point to a predominantly tubular injury. Further research is needed to explore the timely expression of uromodulin and miRNAs associated with transplant pathology patterns, in order to detect kidney allograft pathology on a subclinical level, tailor response to therapy, and predict graft outcome.

Author Contributions: Conceptualization, Ž.V.-H., N.K.; methodology, Š.B., E.B., Ž.P.T., D.K.; software, Š.B., E.B., Ž.P.T.; formal analysis, Š.B., Ž.V.-H., E.B., Ž.P.T., J.L., D.K., N.K.; investigation, Š.B., Ž.V.-H., E.B., Ž.P.T., J.L., D.K., N.K.; data curation, Š.B., Ž.V.-H., E.B., Ž.P.T., J.L., D.K., N.K.; writing—original draft preparation, Š.B., E.B., Ž.P.T.; writing—review and editing, Ž.V.-H., N.K.; supervision, Ž.V.-H., N.K.; funding acquisition, Ž.V.-H., J.L., D.K., N.K. All authors have read and agreed to the published version of the manuscript.

Acknowledgments: The authors would like to thank all medical nurses from the Department of Nuclear Medicine and Center for Kidney Transplantation of the Department of Nephrology at the University Medical Center Ljubljana for their cooperation and care of our patients.

Abbreviations

CKD	chronic kidney disease
CKD-T	chronic kidney disease of transplanted kidney
^{51}CrEDTA	chromium-51-ethylenediaminetetraacetic acid
GFR	glomerular filtration rate
eGFR	estimated GFR
eGFR CKD EPI creatinine	eGFR with Chronic Kidney Disease Epidemiology Collaboration study formula with s-Creatinine
eGFR CKD EPI CysC	eGFR with Chronic Kidney Disease Epidemiology Collaboration study formula with s-CysC
eGFR CKD EPI creatinine CysC	eGFR with Chronic Kidney Disease Epidemiology Collaboration study formula with s-Creatinine and s-CysC
mGFR ^{51}CrEDTA	measured GFR with ^{51}CrEDTA
IF/TA	interstitial fibrosis/tubular atrophy
KTRs	kidney transplant recipients
miRNA	microRNA
RNA	ribonucleic acid
s-Creatinine	serum creatinine concentration
s-CysC	serum cystatin C concentration
s-Urea	serum urea concentration
s-Uromodulin	serum uromodulin concentration

References

1. Tamm, I.; Horsfall, F.L., Jr. Characterization and separation of an inhibitor of viral hemagglutination present in urine. *Proc. Soc. Exp. Biol. Med.* **1950**, *74*, 106–108. [CrossRef] [PubMed]
2. Vyletal, P.; Bleyer, A.J.; Kmoch, S. Uromodulin biology and pathophysiology—An update. *Kidney Blood Press. Res.* **2010**, *33*, 456–475. [CrossRef] [PubMed]
3. Prajczer, S.; Heidenreich, U.; Pfaller, W.; Kotanko, P.; Lhotta, K.; Jennings, P. Evidence for a role of uromodulin in chronic kidney disease progression. *Nephrol. Dial. Transplant.* **2010**, *25*, 1896–1903. [CrossRef]
4. Scherberich, J.E.; Gruber, R.; Nockher, W.A.; Christensen, E.I.; Schmitt, H.; Herbst, V.; Block, M.; Kaden, J.; Schlumberger, W. Serum uromodulin—A marker of kidney function and renal parenchymal integrity. *Nephrol. Dial. Transplant.* **2018**, *33*, 284–295. [CrossRef] [PubMed]
5. Steubl, D.; Block, M.; Herbst, V.; Nockher, W.A.; Schlumberger, W.; Satanovskij, R.; Angermann, S.; Hasenau, A.L.; Stecher, L.; Heemann, U.; et al. Plasma Uromodulin Correlates With Kidney Function and Identifies Early Stages in Chronic Kidney Disease Patients. *Medicine* **2016**, *95*, e3011. [CrossRef] [PubMed]

6. Bostom, A.; Steubl, D.; Garimella, P.S.; Franceschini, N.; Roberts, M.B.; Pasch, A.; Ix, J.H.; Tuttle, K.R.; Ivanova, A.; Shireman, T.; et al. Serum Uromodulin: A Biomarker of Long-Term Kidney Allograft Failure. *Am. J. Nephrol* **2018**, *47*, 275–282. [CrossRef]
7. Steubl, D.; Block, M.; Herbst, V.; Schlumberger, W.; Nockher, A.; Angermann, S.; Schmaderer, C.; Heemann, U.; Renders, L.; Scherberich, J. Serum uromodulin predicts graft failure in renal transplant recipients. *Biomarkers* **2017**, *22*, 171–177. [CrossRef]
8. Reznichenko, A.; van Dijk, M.C.; van der Heide, J.H.; Bakker, S.J.; Seelen, M.; Navis, G. Uromodulin in renal transplant recipients: Elevated urinary levels and bimodal association with graft failure. *Am. J. Nephrol.* **2011**, *34*, 445–451. [CrossRef]
9. Khan, Z.; Suthanthiran, M.; Muthukumar, T. MicroRNAs and Transplantation. *Clin. Lab. Med.* **2019**, *39*, 125–143. [CrossRef]
10. Wilflingseder, J.; Reindl-Schwaighofer, R.; Sunzenauer, J.; Kainz, A.; Heinzel, A.; Mayer, B.; Oberbauer, R. MicroRNAs in kidney transplantation. *Nephrol. Dial. Transplant.* **2015**, *30*, 910–917. [CrossRef]
11. Janszky, N.; Susal, C. Circulating and urinary microRNAs as possible biomarkers in kidney transplantation. *Transplant. Rev.* **2018**, *32*, 110–118. [CrossRef] [PubMed]
12. Kriegel, A.J.; Liu, Y.; Fang, Y.; Ding, X.; Liang, M. The miR-29 family: Genomics, cell biology, and relevance to renal and cardiovascular injury. *Physiol. Genomics* **2012**, *44*, 237–244. [CrossRef] [PubMed]
13. Taibi, F.; Metzinger-Le Meuth, V.; M'Baya-Moutoula, E.; Djelouat, M.; Louvet, L.; Bugnicourt, J.M.; Poirot, S.; Bengrine, A.; Chillon, J.M.; Massy, Z.A.; et al. Possible involvement of microRNAs in vascular damage in experimental chronic kidney disease. *Biochim. Biophys. Acta* **2014**, *1842*, 88–98. [CrossRef]
14. Metzinger-Le Meuth, V.; Burtey, S.; Maitrias, P.; Massy, Z.A.; Metzinger, L. microRNAs in the pathophysiology of CKD-MBD: Biomarkers and innovative drugs. *Biochim. Biophys. Acta Mol. Basis Dis.* **2017**, *1863*, 337–345. [CrossRef]
15. Fourdinier, O.; Schepers, E.; Metzinger-Le Meuth, V.; Glorieux, G.; Liabeuf, S.; Verbeke, F.; Vanholder, R.; Brigant, B.; Pletinck, A.; Diouf, M.; et al. Serum levels of miR-126 and miR-223 and outcomes in chronic kidney disease patients. *Sci. Rep.* **2019**, *9*, 4477. [CrossRef] [PubMed]
16. Testa, U.; Pelosi, E.; Castelli, G.; Labbaye, C. miR-146 and miR-155: Two Key Modulators of Immune Response and Tumor Development. *Non-Coding RNA* **2017**, *3*, 22. [CrossRef]
17. Milhoransa, P.; Montanari, C.C.; Montenegro, R.; Manfro, R.C. Micro RNA 146a-5p expression in Kidney transplant recipients with delayed graft function. *J. Bras. Nefrol.* **2019**, *41*, 242–251. [CrossRef]
18. Huang, X.L.; Zhang, L.; Li, J.P.; Wang, Y.J.; Duan, Y.; Wang, J. MicroRNA-150: A potential regulator in pathogens infection and autoimmune diseases. *Autoimmunity* **2015**, *48*, 503–510. [CrossRef]
19. De Candia, P.; Torri, A.; Pagani, M.; Abrignani, S. Serum microRNAs as Biomarkers of Human Lymphocyte Activation in Health and Disease. *Front. Immunol.* **2014**, *5*, 43. [CrossRef]
20. Yuan, X.; Berg, N.; Lee, J.W.; Le, T.T.; Neudecker, V.; Jing, N.; Eltzschig, H. MicroRNA miR-223 as regulator of innate immunity. *J. Leukoc. Biol.* **2018**, *104*, 515–524. [CrossRef]
21. Metzinger-Le Meuth, V.; Metzinger, L. miR-223 and other miRNA's evaluation in chronic kidney disease: Innovative biomarkers and therapeutic tools. *Non-Coding RNA Res.* **2019**, *4*, 30–35. [CrossRef]
22. Li, S.; Chen, H.; Ren, J.; Geng, Q.; Song, J.; Lee, C.; Cao, C.; Zhang, J.; Xu, N. MicroRNA-223 inhibits tissue factor expression in vascular endothelial cells. *Atherosclerosis* **2014**, *237*, 514–520. [CrossRef] [PubMed]
23. O'Callaghan, J.M.; Knight, S.R. Noninvasive biomarkers in monitoring kidney allograft health. *Curr. Opin. Organ. Transplant.* **2019**, *24*, 411–415. [CrossRef] [PubMed]
24. Naesens, M.; Anglicheau, D. Precision Transplant Medicine: Biomarkers to the Rescue. *J. Am. Soc. Nephrol.* **2018**, *29*, 24–34. [CrossRef] [PubMed]
25. Buron, F.; Hadj-Aissa, A.; Dubourg, L.; Morelon, E.; Steghens, J.P.; Ducher, M.; Fauvel, J.P. Estimating glomerular filtration rate in kidney transplant recipients: Performance over time of four creatinine-based formulas. *Transplantation* **2011**, *92*, 1005–1011. [CrossRef] [PubMed]
26. Fedak, D.; Kuzniewski, M.; Fugiel, A.; Wieczorek-Surdacka, E.; Przepiorkowska-Hoyer, B.; Jasik, P.; Miarka, P.; Dumnicka, P.; Kapusta, M.; Solnica, B.; et al. Serum uromodulin concentrations correlate with glomerular filtration rate in patients with chronic kidney disease. *Pol. Arch. Med. Wewn.* **2016**, *126*, 995–1004. [CrossRef]
27. Gibson, T. Hyperuricemia, gout and the kidney. *Curr. Opin. Rheumatol.* **2012**, *24*, 127–131. [CrossRef]
28. Millan, O.; Budde, K.; Sommerer, C.; Aliart, I.; Rissling, O.; Bardaji, B.; Matz, M.; Zeier, M.; Silva, I.; Guirado, L.; et al. Urinary miR-155-5p and CXCL10 as prognostic and predictive biomarkers of rejection,

graft outcome and treatment response in kidney transplantation. *Br. J. Clin. Pharmacol.* **2017**, *83*, 2636–2650. [CrossRef]
29. Delanaye, P.; Mariat, C. The applicability of eGFR equations to different populations. *Nat. Rev. Nephrol.* **2013**, *9*, 513–522. [CrossRef]
30. Inker, L.A.; Eckfeldt, J.; Levey, A.S.; Leiendecker-Foster, C.; Rynders, G.; Manzi, J.; Waheed, S.; Coresh, J. Expressing the CKD-EPI (Chronic Kidney Disease Epidemiology Collaboration) cystatin C equations for estimating GFR with standardized serum cystatin C values. *Am. J. Kidney Dis.* **2011**, *58*, 682–684. [CrossRef]
31. Levin, A.; Stevens, P.E.; Bilous, R.W.; Coresh, J.; De Francisco, A.L.M.; De Jong, P.E.; Griffith, K.E.; Hemmelgarn, B.R.; Iseki, K.; Lamb, E.J.; et al. Kidney disease: Improving Global Outcomes (KDIGO) CKD Work Group. KDIGO 2012 Clinical Practice Guideline for the Evaluation and Management of Chronic Kidney Disease. *Kidney Int. Suppl.* **2013**, *3*, 1–150.
32. Blaufox, M.D.; Aurell, M.; Bubeck, B.; Fommei, E.; Piepsz, A.; Russell, C.; Taylor, A.; Thomsen, H.S.; Volterrani, D. Report of the Radionuclides in Nephrourology Committee on renal clearance. *J. Nucl. Med.* **1996**, *37*, 1883–1890. [PubMed]
33. Latham, G.J. Normalization of microRNA quantitative RT-PCR data in reduced scale experimental designs. *Methods Mol. Biol.* **2010**, *667*, 19–31. [PubMed]

13

Role of the Furosemide Stress Test in Renal Injury Prognosis

Armando Coca [1], Carmen Aller [1], Jimmy Reinaldo Sánchez [1], Ana Lucía Valencia [1], Elena Bustamante-Munguira [2,†] and Juan Bustamante-Munguira [3,*,†]

1 Department of Nephrology, Hospital Clinico Universitario de Valladolid, 47003 Valladolid, Spain; a.coca.rojo@gmail.com (A.C.); mcaller@saludcastillayleon.es (C.A.); jreinaldo@salud.castillayleon.es (J.R.S.); avalenciape@saludcastillayleon.es (A.L.V.)

2 Department of Intensive Care Medicine, Hospital Clinico Universitario de Valladolid, 47003 Valladolid, Spain; ebustamante@saludcastillayleon.es

3 Department of Cardiac Surgery, Hospital Clinico Universitario de Valladolid, 47003 Valladolid, Spain

* Correspondence: jbustamantemunguira@gmail.com

† These authors contributed equally to this work.

Abstract: Risk stratification and accurate patient prognosis are pending issues in the management of patients with kidney disease. The furosemide stress test (FST) has been proposed as a low-cost, fast, safe, and easy-to-perform test to assess tubular integrity, especially when compared to novel plasma and urinary biomarkers. However, the findings regarding its clinical use published so far provide insufficient evidence to recommend the generalized application of the test in daily clinical routine. Dosage, timing, and clinical outcomes of the FST proposed thus far have been significantly different, which further accentuates the need for standardization in the application of the test in order to facilitate the comparison of results between series. This review will summarize published research regarding the usefulness of the FST in different settings, providing the reader some insights about the possible implications of FST in clinical decision-making in patients with kidney disease and the challenges that research will have to address in the near future before widely applying the FST.

Keywords: acute kidney injury; renal biomarkers; furosemide stress test; functional assessment

1. Introduction

Acute kidney injury (AKI) is an intricate clinical syndrome defined by a sudden decrease of kidney function, the accumulation of nitrogen waste products such as urea, electrolyte, and acid-base disturbances and volume overload [1]. The incidence of such complication has been increasing in recent years, affecting 20% of adult and 33% of pediatric patients during hospital admission, especially among subjects with predisposing factors, such as advanced age, diabetes, cardiovascular disease, chronic kidney disease (CKD), or those exposed to nephrotoxins or to cardio-pulmonary bypass. Patients developing AKI have increased morbidity and worse surviving rates than those with normal renal function. In addition, it increases ICU and in-hospital stay, risk of infection, and hospitalization costs. AKI associates a pooled mortality rate of 23.9% in adults and 13.8% in children, rates that increase with higher degrees of severity [1–3].

Diagnosis of AKI should comprise several steps, including a thoughtful clinical evaluation, physical examination, consideration of alternative diagnoses, and laboratory data. An abrupt increase of serum creatinine (≥0.3 mg/dL) is still the laboratory finding most closely associated to AKI [4–6]. Creatinine is an uncharged 113 Da molecule formed in muscles from creatine, freely filtered at the glomerulus and completely eliminated through the kidney in healthy subjects [7]. Although serum creatinine fulfills most requisites of an ideal filtration marker, it is far from being perfect. In healthy individuals approximately 15% of urinary creatinine is secreted in the proximal tubule, a percentage that can be increased in CKD patients [8]. Additionally, as a product of muscular catabolism, serum creatinine is not an adequate marker of kidney function in subjects with extremely high or low muscle mass such as the elderly or children [9]. Certain drugs (i.e., trimethoprim, cimetidine) can also interfere with tubular secretion of creatinine, producing an increase of serum creatinine levels without real kidney function loss [10,11]. Finally, there is a 48–72 h delay between actual kidney injury and the rise of serum creatinine, which limits early diagnosis and initiation of the appropriate therapeutic measures [12].

Several possible solutions have been developed to overcome this issue. Equations that estimate glomerular filtration rate (eGFR) take into account individual characteristics such as age, gender, weight, or ethnicity to better estimate renal function [13,14]. However, serum creatinine-derived eGFR equations should not be used in the AKI setting due high biases and unacceptably poor performance [15]. Moreover, GFR is not a constant parameter; it changes throughout the day and it is modified by protein consumption and other processes [16].

The development of proteomic technology has triggered extensive research in novel protein indicators that may help characterize AKI mechanisms, improve risk stratification, and facilitate clinical decision making and treatment response monitoring [17]. As a result, multiple potential markers have been discovered in recent years, such as kidney injury molecule-1 (KIM-1) [18,19], neutrophil gelatinase-associated lipocalin (NGAL) [20,21], cystatin C [22], N-acetyl-β-D-glucosaminidase (NAG) [23,24], or liver fatty-acid binding protein (L-FABP) [25,26]. However, despite intensive research effort, none of the discovered biomarkers have managed to replace serum creatinine in clinical practice. Timing of sample procurement, differences in urine concentration and flow, inconsistency among laboratory assays, or higher price are some of the barriers that routine application of novel renal biomarkers must overcome [27]. Additional validation studies that may associate biomarker levels to patient-centered clinical outcomes such as dialysis or death are needed [28].

2. Kidney Tubular Stress Test Assessment

Human organ systems have developed the capability to increase their workload in stressful situations. The analysis of this reserve capacity is a useful tool to uncover subclinical disease [16]. Reserve capacity tests are widely applied to study other pathologies, such as coronary artery disease (dobutamine stress echocardiography or exercise electrocardiogram tests). The kidney reserve capacity is built upon two main components, glomerular and tubular (Figure 1). The degree of injury of each component in AKI or CKD can present great variability and be completely independent. Therefore, testing both components could help describe the underlying pathophysiological process with much greater accuracy.

Glomerular reserve testing has been described in detail, but is sparingly used in day-to-day clinical practice. In brief, GFR, which is commonly used as a surrogate of kidney function, depends on age, sex, weight, or diet and presents great fluctuation among individuals. In healthy subjects, a protein load of 1–1.2 g/kg can induce a considerable increase of GFR above its baseline in 60–120 min. The difference between baseline and maximum GFR is considered the renal glomerular function reserve and is directly associated with stress-associated nephron recruitment and increased renal blood flow [16]. However, the lack of large cohort studies that may help describe the population variability of renal glomerular function reserve is an important limitation of this test.

The study of tubular reserve capacity is a relatively new diagnostic tool whose clinical application holds great potential [16,29]. The tubules and tubulointerstitium occupy a significant portion of the kidney and are responsible for a wide variety of functions, such as water and electrolyte handling, secretion of endogenous and exogenous acids, and protein catabolism. Tubular epithelial cells (TECs) regulate tubulointerstitial inflammation and are key mediators of tissue repair and fibrosis processes due to their capability to release cytokines, chemokines, and reactive-oxygen species [16,30]. Damaged TECs facilitate tubulointerstitial inflammation due to their capability to modulate the immune response through the formation of several proinflammatory cytokines such as interleukin-6, interleukin-34, or tumor necrosis factor alpha [30,31]. The consequent macrophage infiltration and neutrophil recruitment can aggravate tubular cell injury and perpetuate the pro-inflammatory response to AKI [32,33]. Furthermore, TECs can endure adaptative changes after kidney injury and modify their structure and phenotype, increasing the production of profibrotic factors that stimulate fibroblast proliferation, tubular cell de-differentiation, and epithelial–mesenchymal transition such as connective tissue growth factor, tubular growth factor beta, or renin-angiotensin components [34–36]. The epithelial–mesenchymal transition of TECs is a potential key point in the progression of renal fibrosis. This phenomenon involves the replacement of epithelial-type markers, such as E-cadherin or cytokeratin, for mesenchymal-type markers such as vimentin, fibronectin, or type I collagen [30,37].

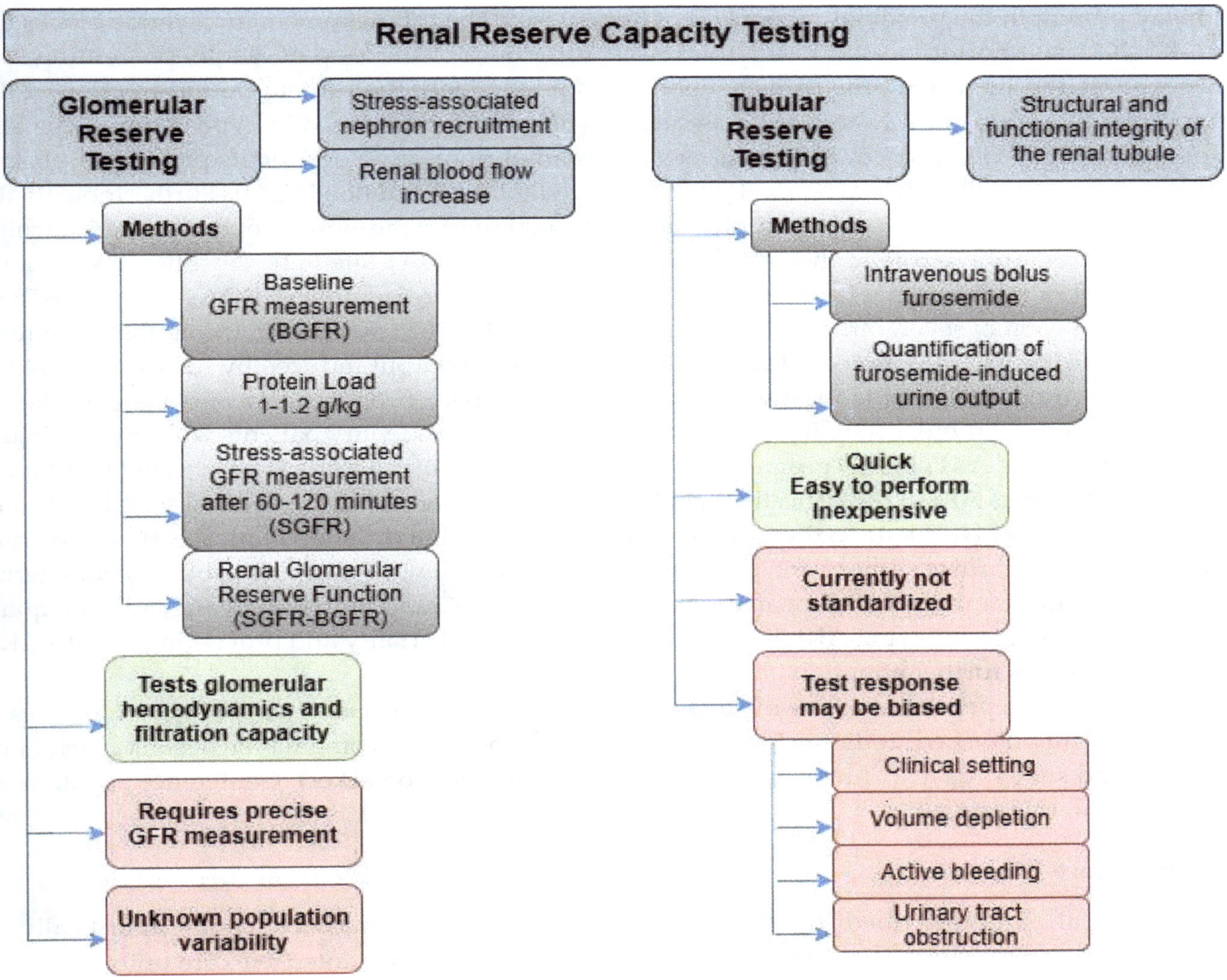

Figure 1. Renal reserve capacity testing.

Recent studies have also described the role of incomplete healing of tubulointerstitial damage as a possible link between AKI and CKD. Although TECs have several repair mechanisms to facilitate full recovery after injury, the repair process can be halted in an intermediate phase, inducing cell atrophy and fibrosis [38]. Mitochondria also play a significant part in AKI associated cell death. The use of SS-31, a drug with mitochondria-protecting effects, has been shown to diminish the development of ischemic damage and interstitial fibrosis in the kidney [39]. Additionally, disturbances of TEC energy-producing pathways, fundamentally fatty acid oxidation, can induce cell death, fibrogenesis, and inflammation [40].

The main tool to assess tubular function is to study tubular secretion of an endogenous or exogenous substance, such as creatinine or furosemide. Salt or acid loading can be used to analyze the efficiency of the tubule to eliminate sodium or acid, while water deprivation or the administration of desmopressin would serve as tests of the concentrating capabilities of the tubule [16].

3. Furosemide Stress Test

Furosemide is a short-acting loop diuretic frequently used to treat hypertension, acute or chronic heart failure, or cirrhosis-associated volume overload [41]. This drug can also be used for diagnostic purposes, which constitutes the fundamental bases of the furosemide stress test (FST). The FST is based on the pharmacokinetic properties of furosemide and is aimed to assess the functional integrity of the renal tubule. The drug is strongly bound to plasma proteins and reaches the proximal tubule lumen through active secretion using the human organic acid transporter (hOAT) pathway present in the proximal tubule [42]. After entering the tubule lumen, furosemide blocks the Na^+-K^+-$2Cl^-$ symporter located in the thick ascending limb of the loop of Henle, preventing Na^+ reabsorption and increasing the urinary volume excreted. Only the protein-bound fraction of the drug is pharmacodynamically active and as such its effect could be reduced in hypoalbuminemia [42]. In patients with CKD, furosemide produces a lower amount of urine despite its prolonged plasma half-life, due to diminished renal blood flow and reduced tubular secretion [42,43]. Furthermore, in the AKI setting, the accumulation of uremic organic acids could reduce the amount of furosemide reaching the lumen of the tubule due to increased competition at the hOAT site [42]. Additional structural modifications of the proximal tubule during AKI, including upregulation of hOAT1 and hOAT3 or reduced expression of several transporters, such as the Na^+-K^+-$2Cl^-$ symporter, the epithelial sodium channel or the Na^+/K^+ ATPase could further modify the urine output induced by furosemide [44,45].

In this setting, furosemide-induced urinary output has been proposed as a surrogate marker of the integrity of renal tubular function which could help clinicians identify patients with tubular injury and at higher risk of AKI or CKD progression. The clinical utility of the FST has been tested in different backgrounds such as AKI in the critically ill, kidney transplantation, or CKD prognosis (Table S1) since its inception in 1973 [46]. Due to the growing relevance of AKI in different clinical settings, such as those undergoing cardiac surgery, the potential application of the FST as a tool to better characterize the degree of tubular injury, achieve an earlier diagnosis of AKI and help initiate the most adequate treatment aimed at minimizing AKI-associated morbidity and mortality and preventing AKI-to-CKD transition deserves further attention.

To perform the present review, we searched the PubMed, Web of Science, and Scopus databases to identify relevant published studies in English. Search terms included a combination of subject headings, abstracts, and keywords (e.g., furosemide stress test, furosemide biomarker). Conference papers were excluded from this review.

4. Critical Care

Baek et al., first described in 1973 the application of a furosemide challenge in critically ill, postoperative patients [46]. The study included 38 patients admitted to intensive care units without a past history of CKD. A subset of 15 adequately hydrated patients without diagnosis of AKI and a free water clearance between +15 and -15 received a furosemide bolus dose ranging from 80 to 400 mg. The inability to produce an adequate response to the furosemide challenge was assumed by the authors as a predictor of imminent AKI in this set of patients.

In 2013, Chawla et al., developed a standardized version of the FST [47]. The authors studied two cohorts of 23 and 54 critically ill patients, respectively. All recruited subjects suffered stage I or II AKI according to the Acute Kidney Injury Network (AKIN) classification [5]. Dosing of furosemide was standardized: loop diuretic naïve patients received an intravenous dose of 1 mg/kg while those previously treated with loop diuretics were administered a dose of 1.5 mg/kg. Urine output during the 6 h after furosemide administration was replaced with either saline or Ringers lactate in a 1:1 ratio. The main outcome of the study was the progression to AKIN stage III within 14 days after furosemide administration. The FST was fairly safe, with no adverse events or episodes of hypotension considered attributable to it. A 2-h urine output cutoff of 200 cc showed the best combination of sensitivity (87.1%) and specificity (84.1%) and was a robust predictor of progression to AKIN stage III. The area under the receiver operator characteristic curves (AUC) for the complete urine output over the first 2 h after the FST to predict the primary outcome was 0.87. Nonetheless, the authors highlight that, for the test to be applied, patients should be euvolemic and any obstruction to urinary flow should have been resolved before the administration of the FST.

A secondary analysis of the same cohort was published in 2017 [48]. In this study, Koyner et al., compared the predictive capacity of FST with that of eight plasma and urinary biomarkers such as NGAL, KIM-1, interleukin-18, uromodulin, tissue inhibitor of metalloproteinases (TIMP-2), IGF-binding protein-7 (IGFBP-7), or albumin-to-creatinine ratio. The 2-h urine output after FST outperformed all studied urinary biomarkers when predicting progression to AKIN stage III with an AUC of 0.87. Furthermore, the FST outperformed most urinary biomarkers when predicting the need of renal replacement therapy (RRT) (AUC: 0.86) or a composite outcome of patient death or progression to AKIN stage III (AUC: 0.81). The combined use of FST and urinary biomarkers to predict outcomes did not significantly improve the performance of FST as a predictor when used alone. Authors concluded that FST was a promising tool that may help clinicians to improve risk stratification in patients with early stages of AKI.

Another approach to test the predictive capacity of the FST was used by van der Voort et al. [49]. In this study, urinary production was measured during a 4-h period after termination of continuous renal replacement therapy (CRRT) in a sample of critically ill patients with AKI. After this period, a subset of patients received either furosemide 0.5 mg/kg/h or placebo with a 4-h urine output repeated measurement after 24 h. In this study, both spontaneous urinary production after CRRT cessation and furosemide-induced urine output were significantly higher in those subjects with immediate recovery of renal function. The AUC for the total urinary output over the first 4 h after the FST to predict in-hospital renal recovery was 0.79. The authors postulated that the FST could be used as a potential predictor to assess renal function recovery after CRRT.

In 2018, Matsuura et al., retrospectively analyzed 95 patients admitted to an intensive care unit and who were treated with bolus furosemide [50]. Authors excluded those patients with AKI stage 3 according to the Kidney Disease: Improving Global Outcomes (KDIGO) AKI classification and those who received a continuous intravenous furosemide infusion. The final sample included 95 subjects with either no AKI or AKI stage 1 or 2. Furosemide responsiveness was defined as the urine output (ml) produced in 2 h divided by the dose of furosemide administered (mg). Urinary biomarkers such as plasma NGAL and urinary L-FABP and NAG were also determined. Main outcomes were progression to AKI stage 3 and a combined outcome of progression to AKI stage 3 or patient death. Furosemide responsiveness was significantly higher among non-progressors, with an AUC for the combined outcome of 0.88, which was higher than that of plasma NGAL (0.81), urinary L-FABP (0.62), or urinary NAG (0.53). Furthermore, the efficacy of furosemide responsiveness was tested in a group of 51 patients with plasma NGAL levels >142 ng/mL at the time of furosemide administration. In this subset, furosemide responsiveness presented an AUC of 0.88 to predict the composite outcome AKI stage 3 progression or patient death.

An alternative clinical use for the FST was tested by Lumlertgul et al., in a prospective, multicenter, randomized controlled trial [51]. In this study, investigators used the FST as an initial triage strategy to identify patients for randomization to different RRT initiation times. Those subjects with poor response after the FST were randomized to either early or standard RRT initiation. Although in this study FST was not assessed as a predictor of clinical outcomes, the test proved to be a safe and effective tool to stratify AKI patients at high risk for RRT.

Recently, Rewa et al., prospectively analyzed the predictive power of FST in a sample of 92 critically ill patients with AKIN stage I or II, recruited from five intensive care units [52]. Patients with evidence of volume depletion, active bleeding, or obstructive uropathy were excluded from the analysis. The dose of intravenous bolus furosemide administered was that proposed by Chawla et al.,: 1 mg/kg for loop diuretic naïve patients and 1.5 mg/kg for those previously treated with loop diuretics. The primary outcome was progression to AKIN stage III within 30 days of FST administration. FST-induced urine output was a significant predictor of the primary outcome, with an AUC of 0.87. However, the FST failed to predict in-hospital patient survival. Moreover, in a multivariate logistic regression model that included the Acute Physiology and Chronic Health Evaluation (APACHE II) score, baseline urine output or serum creatinine at the time of FST, only FST-induced urine output and sex were significant predictors of AKI progression. Authors also registered adverse events that occurred after FST; 9.8% of patients suffered an episode of clinically significant hypotension and 5.4% developed hypokalemia or hypomagenesemia, with no life-threatening events recorded. Authors concluded that FST was a safe and effective predictive tool in patients with mild to moderate AKI.

Sakhuja et al., examined if FST could be used to detect AKI stage 3 patients at risk of needing RRT [53]. Due to the retrospective nature of this study, the furosemide dose was not standardized, but only subjects that received at least 1 mg/kg of intravenous bolus furosemide or its equivalent dose of intravenous bumetanide were included. Patients that had previously received loop diuretics before the FST were excluded from this analysis. Primary and secondary outcomes for Sakhuja et al., were defined as the need for urgent dialysis within 24 or 72 h after the FST. A total of 687 patients were included in the final sample. Dialysis had to be administered to 162 patients (23.6%) during the first 24 h after FST. The 6-h urinary production after FST had only modest discriminative power to predict need of dialysis within the next 24 h, but, according to authors, its application could be useful to evaluate the need for dialysis in critically ill patients with AKI stage 3.

Finally, the usefulness of furosemide response as a predictor of AKI has also been tested in the pediatric critical care setting. Borasino et al., retrospectively examined a sample of 90 infants and neonates younger than 90 days old who received at least one dose of furosemide in the first 24 h after cardiopulmonary bypass surgery [54]. Average furosemide dose was 1.1 ± 0.3 mg/kg. The primary endpoint of the study was the development of cardiac surgery-associated AKI, defined as the doubling of serum creatinine within 72 h of index surgery or a urinary output <0.5 mL/kg/h on average in a 24 h period over the first 72 h after index surgery. Response to furosemide predicted cardiac surgery-associated AKI in this setting, with an AUC of 0.69. Additionally, furosemide response predicted peritoneal dialysis initiation and fluid overload.

5. Kidney Transplantation

There is a paucity of literature regarding the application of FST outside of the intensive care setting. The FST has been tested as a predictive tool after kidney transplantation with different approaches regarding timing of administration and furosemide dosage. McMahon et al. [55] published in 2018 a single-center retrospective analysis of a random sample of 200 deceased-donor kidney transplant recipients who received an intraoperative bolus of 100 mg furosemide. Urinary production was measured 2 and 6 h after furosemide administration. The primary outcome was the development of delayed graft function, defined as the need of dialysis within 7 days of transplantation. Authors included as secondary outcomes safety endpoints such as incidence of hypotension or hypokalemia during the first 24 h after the bolus, graft loss, rejection, death with functioning graft or length of hospital stay. Subjects who developed delayed graft function presented a significantly lower urine output 2 and 6 h after FST. A 6-h urinary output <600 mL (which defined FST non-responders) presented an AUC of 0.85 for the development of DGF. Regarding safety-related outcomes, no episodes of hypotension (defined as mean arterial pressure <60 mmHg) or change in plasma potassium levels were observed in the sample. Although FST non-responders showed longer length of in-hospital stay, the rates of graft loss or death were similar between both groups.

The usefulness of FST after kidney transplantation was also studied by Udomkarnjananun et al. [56]. The authors prospectively studied a sample of 59 adult deceased-donor kidney transplant recipients without hypoalbuminemia or surgical complications that required reoperation during the first 24 h after transplantation. Dry weight adjustment was used to ensure euvolemia prior to transplantation.

An intravenous bolus dose of 1.5 mg/kg furosemide was administered 3 h after allograft reperfusion. Urinary production was registered for 6 h after the bolus. Each mL of urine produced during the first 24 h was replaced by 1 mL of saline to avoid volume depletion. The primary outcome was incidence of DGF, using the same definition applied by McMahon et al. Mean cumulative urine volume was significantly lower in those who developed DGF compared to that of non-DGF patients. A 4-h cumulative urine output <350 mL presented the highest accuracy to predict DGF with an AUC of 0.94. The FST was the only significant predictor of DGF in multivariate logistic regression analysis. Moreover, FST was the most accurate predictor of DGF when compared to urinary NGAL, resistive index of renal arteries measured by ultrasonography or effective renal plasma flow measured by 99mTc-MAG3 renography.

These two single-center studies show that FST could improve risk stratification in the early post-transplant period, promptly detecting patients with higher risk of DGF who could benefit from an early initiation of therapeutic interventions. FST was a more accurate predictor of DGF than oliguria (defined as a daily urinary production <400 mL) [55], ultrasonography, 99mTc-MAG3 renography or novel biomarkers such as urinary NGAL. The test was also safe and well tolerated, in line with published results in critically ill patients.

However, although these studies provide an interesting starting point for the application of FST as a predictive tool after kidney transplantation they also suffer significant limitations: both were small sized, single-center studies, limiting external validity of results. The analysis by McMahon et al., was a retrospective review, which means exposure or outcome assessment could not be controlled. Furthermore, furosemide dosage had different timing and dosage in both studies. The possibility of volume depletion after transplant surgery and/or obstructive uropathy due to urinary elimination of blood clots, complications which are commonly associated to active bleeding, were not adequately addressed in these studies. Therefore, additional prospective multi-center studies should be planned to analyze if FST could improve risk stratification and patient management after kidney transplantation.

6. Other Clinical Settings (CKD)

As previously stated, most research regarding the use of FST is centered in the AKI setting. However, Rivero et al. [57] have recently published a prospective study regarding the usefulness of FST as a tool to assess interstitial fibrosis in a sample of CKD patients. To that end, the authors included adult subjects admitted for a kidney biopsy, including transplant recipients. Hypovolemic or subjects with hemodynamic instability were excluded from the study. A standardized dose of 1 mg/kg furosemide, or 1.5 mg/kg furosemide if exposed to loop diuretics during the seven days prior to FST was administered. Fluid therapy was dispensed according to post-FST urine output to avoid furosemide-induced volume depletion. A nephropathologist assessed kidney interstitial fibrosis percentage using morphometry and classified patients in one of three categories: <25%, 26–50% and >50%. Subjects with >50% interstitial fibrosis had a significantly lower urine output after FST, with an inverse correlation between FST response and degree of fibrosis. FST could thus be a potential tool to non-invasively assess interstitial fibrosis, offering a complementary instrument to eGFR and proteinuria to evaluate prognosis and disease progression in CKD patients.

7. Current Limitations and Future Challenges

The FST is a safe, non-invasive, easy to perform, low-cost tool to evaluate the severity of tubular injury which has shown promising initial results in different clinical contexts. Its capacity as a predictive tool could facilitate risk stratification and clinical decision-making in areas as disparate as AKI, kidney transplantation, or CKD. However, there is still a long way to go before the FST can be included in diagnostic and treatment algorithms. Most published clinical research to date is based on small-sized, single center pilot or feasibility studies. Several studies are based on retrospective analysis of patients who received a furosemide bolus, which makes the task of controlling possible sources of bias extremely difficult. Moreover, doses and timing of furosemide administration are highly variable, even in studies framed within the same clinical setting. Standardization of dosage, such as that proposed by Chawla et al. [47] should help to homogenize the FST in order to facilitate comparison of results between studies.

Additionally, some of the published studies solely rely on AUC values to define the predictive capacity of the test. It has been pointed that such statistic may not be the most adequate choice to assess models that predict risk or stratify individuals into risk categories, a setting in which calibration may play a significant role [58]. In these instances, actual or absolute predicted risk, which is not captured by the AUC, could be of outmost interest. Therefore, when comparing models for risk prediction, a combined analysis including global model fit and analysis of calibration and discrimination would be recommended.

8. Conclusions

In summary, tubular stress test assessment using the FST is a rediscovered and promising new tool to stratify risk in different kidney diseases. Multi-center, prospective studies with large enough sample sizes, applying standardized furosemide dosage and timing and comparing the FST to other novel plasma and urinary biomarkers are necessary to adequately validate results and define the possible clinical applications of the test.

Author Contributions: Development of the idea: A.C. and J.B.-M. Writing—Review and Editing: C.A., J.R.S. and A.L.V. Supervision: A.C., E.B.-M. and J.B.-M. All authors have read and agreed to the published version of the manuscript.

Abbreviations

AKI	acute kidney injury
AKIN	acute kidney injury network
AUC	area under the curve
CKD	chronic kidney disease
CRRT	continuous renal replacement therapy
DGF	delayed graft function
FEM	furosemide excreted mass
FR	furosemide response
FST	furosemide stress test
IL-18	interleukin 18
KIM-1	kidney injury molecule 1
L-FABP	L-type fatty acid binding protein
MC	multi-center
NA	not applicable
NGAL	neutrophil gelatinase-associated lipocalin
P	prospective
R	retrospective
RRT	renal replacement therapy
SC	single-center
TIMP-2	tissue inhibitor of metalloproteinases 2
UO	urine output

References

1. Hoste, E.; Kellum, J.A.; Selby, N.M.; Zarbock, A.; Palevsky, P.M.; Bagshaw, S.M.; Goldstein, S.L.; Cerdá, J.; Chawla, L.S. Global epidemiology and outcomes of acute kidney injury. *Nat. Rev. Nephrol.* **2018**, *14*, 607–625. [CrossRef] [PubMed]

2. Jorge-Monjas, P.; Bustamante-Munguira, J.; Lorenzo, M.; Heredia-Rodríguez, M.; Fierro, I.; Gómez-Sánchez, E.; Hernandez, A.; Álvarez, F.J.; Bermejo-Martin, J.F.; Gómez-Pesquera, E.; et al. Predicting cardiac surgery–associated acute kidney injury: The CRATE score. *J. Crit. Care* **2016**, *31*, 130–138. [CrossRef] [PubMed]
3. Gameiro, J.; Agapito, F.J.; Jorge, S.; Lopes, J.A. Acute kidney injury definition and diagnosis: A narrative review. *J. Clin. Med.* **2018**, *7*, 307. [CrossRef]
4. Bellomo, R.; Ronco, C.; Kellum, J.A.; Mehta, R.L.; Palevsky, P.; Acute Dialysis Quality Initiative Workgroup. Acute renal failure—Definition, outcome measures, animal models, fluid therapy and information technology needs: The Second International Consensus Conference of the Acute Dialysis Quality Initiative (ADQI) Group. *Crit. Care* **2004**, *8*, R204–R212. [CrossRef] [PubMed]
5. Mehta, R.L.; Kellum, J.A.; Shah, S.V.; Molitoris, B.A.; Ronco, C.; Warnock, D.G.; Levin, A. Acute kidney injury network: Report of an initiative to improve outcomes in acute kidney injury. *Crit. Care* **2007**, *11*, R31. [CrossRef]
6. Kellum, J.A.; Lameire, N.; Aspelin, P.; Barsoum, R.S.; Burdmann, E.A.; Goldstein, S.L.; Herzog, C.A.; Joannidis, M.; Kribben, A.; Levey, A.S.; et al. Kidney disease: Improving global outcomes (KDIGO) acute kidney injury work group. KDIGO clinical practice guideline for acute kidney injury. *Kidney Int. Suppl.* **2012**, *2*, 1–138.
7. Thongprayoon, C.; Cheungpasitporn, W.; Kashani, K.B. Serum creatinine level, a surrogate of muscle mass, predicts mortality in critically ill patients. *J. Thorac. Dis.* **2016**, *8*, E305–E311. [CrossRef]
8. Delanaye, P.; Cavalier, E.; Pottel, H. Serum creatinine: Not so simple! *Nephron* **2017**, *136*, 302–308. [CrossRef]
9. Baxmann, A.C.; Ahmed, M.S.; Marques, N.C.; Menon, V.B.; Pereira, A.B.; Kirsztajn, G.M.; Heilberg, I.P. Influence of muscle mass and physical activity on serum and urinary creatinine and serum cystatin C. *Clin. J. Am. Soc. Nephrol.* **2008**, *3*, 348–354. [CrossRef]
10. Delanaye, P.; Mariat, C.; Cavalier, E.; Maillard, N.; Krzesinski, J.-M.; White, C.A. Trimethoprim, creatinine and creatinine-based equations. *Nephron* **2011**, *119*, 187–194. [CrossRef]
11. Van Acker, B.; Koopman, M.; Arisz, L.; Koomen, G.; de Waart, D. Creatinine clearance during cimetidine administration for measurement of glomerular filtration rate. *Lancet* **1992**, *340*, 1326–1329. [CrossRef]
12. Parikh, C.R.; Mishra, J.; Thiessen-Philbrook, H.; Dursun, B.; Ma, Q.; Kelly, C.; Dent, C.; Devarajan, P.; Edelstein, C. Urinary IL-18 is an early predictive biomarker of acute kidney injury after cardiac surgery. *Kidney Int.* **2006**, *70*, 199–203. [CrossRef] [PubMed]
13. Levey, A.S.; Bosch, J.P.; Lewis, J.B.; Rogers, N.; Greene, T.; Roth, D. A more accurate method to estimate glomerular filtration rate from serum creatinine: A new prediction equation. *Ann. Intern. Med.* **1999**, *130*, 461–470. [CrossRef] [PubMed]
14. Levey, A.S.; Stevens, L.A.; Schmid, C.H.; Zhang, Y.L.; Castro, A.F., III; Feldman, H.I.; Kusek, J.W.; Eggers, P.; Van Lente, F.; Greene, T.; et al. A new equation to estimate glomerular filtration rate. *Ann. Intern. Med.* **2009**, *150*, 604–612. [CrossRef] [PubMed]
15. Bragadottir, G.; Redfors, B.; Ricksten, S.-E. Assessing glomerular filtration rate (GFR) in critically ill patients with acute kidney injury - true GFR versus urinary creatinine clearance and estimating equations. *Crit. Care* **2013**, *17*, R108. [CrossRef]
16. Chawla, L.S.; Ronco, C. Renal stress testing in the assessment of kidney disease. *Kidney Int. Rep.* **2016**, *1*, 57–63. [CrossRef]
17. Siew, E.D.; Ware, L.B.; Ikizler, T.A. Biological markers of acute kidney injury. *J. Am. Soc. Nephrol.* **2011**, *22*, 810–820. [CrossRef]
18. Ichimura, T.; Bonventre, J.V.; Bailly, V.; Wei, H.; Hession, C.A.; Cate, R.L.; Sanicola, M. Kidney Injury Molecule-1 (KIM-1), a putative epithelial cell adhesion molecule containing a novel immunoglobulin domain, is up-regulated in renal cells after injury. *J. Biol. Chem.* **1998**, *273*, 4135–4142. [CrossRef]
19. Tanase, D.M.; Gosav, E.M.; Radu, S.; Costea, C.; Ciocoiu, M.; Carauleanu, A.; Lacatusu, C.; Maranduca, M.; Floria, M.; Rezus, C. The predictive role of the biomarker Kidney Molecule-1 (KIM-1) in Acute Kidney Injury (AKI) cisplatin-induced nephrotoxicity. *Int. J. Mol. Sci.* **2019**, *20*, 5238. [CrossRef]
20. Fan, H.; Zhao, Y.; Sun, M.; Zhu, J.H. Urinary neutrophil gelatinase-associated lipocalin, kidney injury molecule-1, N-acetyl-beta-D-glucosaminidase levels and mortality risk in septic patients with acute kidney injury. *Arch. Med. Sci.* **2018**, *14*, 1381–1386. [CrossRef]

21. Murray, P.T.; Wettersten, N.; Van Veldhuisen, D.J.; Mueller, C.; Filippatos, G.; Nowak, R.; Hogan, C.; Kontos, M.C.; Cannon, C.M.; Müeller, G.A.; et al. Utility of urine neutrophil gelatinase-associated lipocalin for worsening renal function during hospitalization for acute heart failure: Primary findings of the urine N-gal acute kidney injury N-gal evaluation of symptomatic heart failure study (AKINESIS). *J. Card. Fail.* **2019**, *25*, 654–665. [CrossRef]
22. Park, M.Y.; Lee, Y.W.; Choi, S.J.; Kim, J.K.; Hwang, S. Urinary cystatin C levels as a diagnostic and prognostic biomarker in patients with acute kidney injury. *Nephrology* **2013**, *18*, 256–262. [CrossRef] [PubMed]
23. Westhuyzen, J.; Endre, Z.H.; Reece, G.; Reith, D.M.; Saltissi, D.; Morgan, T.J. Measurement of tubular enzymuria facilitates early detection of acute renal impairment in the intensive care unit. *Nephrol. Dial. Transplant.* **2003**, *18*, 543–551. [CrossRef] [PubMed]
24. Heise, D.; Rentsch, K.; Braeuer, A.; Friedrich, M.; Quintel, M. Comparison of urinary neutrophil glucosaminidase-associated lipocalin, cystatin C, and ?1-microglobulin for early detection of acute renal injury after cardiac surgery. *Eur. J. Cardio-Thorac. Surg.* **2011**, *39*, 38–43. [CrossRef] [PubMed]
25. Yanishi, M.; Kinoshita, H.; Mishima, T.; Taniguchi, H.; Yoshida, K.; Komai, Y.; Yasuda, K.; Watanabe, M.; Sugi, M.; Matsuda, T. Urinary l-type fatty acid-binding protein is a predictor of early renal function after partial nephrectomy. *Ren. Fail.* **2016**, *39*, 7–12. [CrossRef] [PubMed]
26. Doi, K.; Noiri, E.; Sugaya, T. Urinary L-type fatty acid-binding protein as a new renal biomarker in critical care. *Curr. Opin. Crit. Care* **2010**, *16*, 545–549. [CrossRef]
27. Tang, K.W.A.; Toh, Q.C.; Teo, B.W. Normalisation of urinary biomarkers to creatinine for clinical practice and research—When and why. *Singap. Med. J.* **2015**, *56*, 7–10. [CrossRef]
28. Parikh, C.R.; Mansour, S.G. Perspective on clinical application of biomarkers in AKI. *J. Am. Soc. Nephrol.* **2017**, *28*, 1677–1685. [CrossRef]
29. McMahon, B.A.; Koyner, J.L. Risk stratification for acute kidney injury: Are biomarkers enough? *Adv. Chronic Kidney Dis.* **2016**, *23*, 167–178. [CrossRef]
30. Liu, B.-C.; Tang, T.-T.; Lv, L.-L.; Lan, H.-Y. Renal tubule injury: A driving force toward chronic kidney disease. *Kidney Int.* **2018**, *93*, 568–579. [CrossRef]
31. Yard, B.A.; Daha, M.R.; Kooymans-Couthino, M.; Bruijn, J.A.; Paape, M.E.; Schrama, E.; Van Es, L.A.; Van Der Woude, F.J. IL-1α stimulated TNFα production by cultured human proximal tubular epithelial cells. *Kidney Int.* **1992**, *42*, 383–389. [CrossRef] [PubMed]
32. Baek, J.-H.; Zeng, R.; Weinmann-Menke, J.; Valerius, M.T.; Wada, Y.; Ajay, A.K.; Colonna, M.; Kelley, V.R. IL-34 mediates acute kidney injury and worsens subsequent chronic kidney disease. *J. Clin. Investig.* **2015**, *125*, 3198–3214. [CrossRef] [PubMed]
33. Disteldorf, E.M.; Krebs, C.; Paust, H.-J.; Turner, J.-E.; Nouailles, G.; Tittel, A.; Meyer-Schwesinger, C.; Stege, G.; Brix, S.R.; Velden, J.; et al. CXCL5 Drives neutrophil recruitment in TH17-Mediated GN. *J. Am. Soc. Nephrol.* **2014**, *26*, 55–66. [CrossRef] [PubMed]
34. Geng, H.; Lan, R.; Singha, P.K.; Gilchrist, A.; Weinreb, P.H.; Violette, S.M.; Weinberg, J.M.; Saikumar, P.; Venkatachalam, M.A. Lysophosphatidic acid increases proximal tubule cell secretion of profibrotic cytokines PDGF-B and CTGF through LPA2- and Galphaq-mediated Rho and alphavbeta6 integrin-dependent activation of TGF-beta. *Am. J. Pathol.* **2012**, *181*, 1236–1249. [CrossRef]
35. Meng, X.M.; Tang, P.M.; Li, J.; Lan, H.Y. TGF-beta/Smad signaling in renal fibrosis. *Front. Physiol.* **2015**, *6*, 82. [CrossRef]
36. Zhou, Y.; Xiong, M.; Fang, L.; Jiang, L.; Wen, P.; Dai, C.; Zhang, C.Y.; Yang, J. miR-21–containing microvesicles from injured tubular epithelial cells promote tubular phenotype transition by targeting PTEN protein. *Am. J. Pathol.* **2013**, *183*, 1183–1196. [CrossRef]
37. Strutz, F. EMT and proteinuria as progression factors. *Kidney Int.* **2009**, *75*, 475–481. [CrossRef]
38. Cosentino, C.C.; Skrypnyk, N.I.; Brilli, L.L.; Chiba, T.; Novitskaya, T.; Woods, C.; West, J.; Korotchenko, V.N.; McDermott, L.; Day, B.W.; et al. Histone deacetylase inhibitor enhances recovery after AKI. *J. Am. Soc. Nephrol.* **2013**, *24*, 943–953. [CrossRef]
39. Liu, S.; Soong, Y.; Seshan, S.V.; Szeto, H.H. Novel cardiolipin therapeutic protects endothelial mitochondria during renal ischemia and mitigates microvascular rarefaction, inflammation, and fibrosis. *Am. J. Physiol. Physiol.* **2014**, *306*, F970–F980. [CrossRef]

40. Kang, H.M.; Ahn, S.H.; Choi, P.; Ko, Y.A.; Han, S.H.; Chinga, F.; Park, A.S.; Tao, J.; Sharma, K.; Pullman, J.; et al. Defective fatty acid oxidation in renal tubular epithelial cells has a key role in kidney fibrosis development. *Nat. Med.* **2015**, *21*, 37–46. [CrossRef]
41. Ponto, L.L.; Schoenwald, R.D. Furosemide (frusemide). A pharmacokinetic/pharmacodynamic review (Part II). *Clin. Pharmacokinet.* **1990**, *18*, 460–471. [PubMed]
42. Mariano, F.; Mella, A.; Vincenti, M.; Biancone, L. Furosemide as a functional marker of acute kidney injury in ICU patients: A new role for an old drug. *J. Nephrol.* **2019**, *32*, 883–893. [CrossRef] [PubMed]
43. Brown, C.B.; Ogg, C.S.; Cameron, J.S. High dose frusemide in acute renal failure: A controlled trial. *Clin. Nephrol.* **1981**, *15*, 90–96.
44. Schmidt, C.; Hocherl, K.; Schweda, F.; Kurtz, A.; Bucher, M. Regulation of renal sodium transporters during severe inflammation. *J. Am. Soc. Nephrol.* **2007**, *18*, 1072–1083. [CrossRef] [PubMed]
45. Kunin, M.; Holtzman, E.J.; Melnikov, S.; Dinour, D. Urinary organic anion transporter protein profiles in AKI. *Nephrol. Dial. Transplant.* **2011**, *27*, 1387–1395. [CrossRef] [PubMed]
46. Baek, S.M.; Brown, R.S.; Shoemaker, W.C. Early prediction of acute renal failure and recovery. *Crit. Care Med.* **1973**, *1*, 179. [CrossRef]
47. Chawla, L.S.; Davison, D.; Brasha-Mitchell, E.; Koyner, J.L.; Arthur, J.; Shaw, A.; Tumlin, J.; Trevino, S.A.; Kimmel, P.L.; Seneff, M.G. Development and standardization of a furosemide stress test to predict the severity of acute kidney injury. *Crit. Care* **2013**, *17*, R207. [CrossRef]
48. Koyner, J.L.; Davison, D.L.; Brasha-Mitchell, E.; Chalikonda, D.M.; Arthur, J.; Shaw, A.; Tumlin, J.A.; Trevino, S.A.; Bennett, M.R.; Kimmel, P.L.; et al. Furosemide stress test and biomarkers for the prediction of aki severity. *J. Am. Soc. Nephrol.* **2015**, *26*, 2023–2031. [CrossRef]
49. Van der Voort, P.H.J.; Boerma, E.C.; Pickkers, P. The furosemide stress test to predict renal function after continuous renal replacement therapy. *Crit. Care* **2014**, *18*, 429. [CrossRef]
50. Matsuura, R.; Komaru, Y.; Miyamoto, Y.; Yoshida, T.; Yoshimoto, K.; Isshiki, R.; Mayumi, K.; Yamashita, T.; Hamasaki, Y.; Nangaku, M.; et al. Response to different furosemide doses predicts AKI progression in ICU patients with elevated plasma NGAL levels. *Ann. Intensiv. Care* **2018**, *8*, 8. [CrossRef]
51. Lumlertgul, N.; Peerapornratana, S.; Trakarnvanich, T.; Pongsittisak, W.; Surasit, K.; Chuasuwan, A.; Tankee, P.; Tiranathanagul, K.; Praditpornsilpa, K.; Tungsanga, K.; et al. Early versus standard initiation of renal replacement therapy in furosemide stress test non-responsive acute kidney injury patients (the FST trial). *Crit. Care* **2018**, *22*, 101. [CrossRef] [PubMed]
52. Rewa, O.G.; Bagshaw, S.; Wang, X.; Wald, R.; Smith, O.; Shapiro, J.; McMahon, B.; Liu, K.; Trevino, S.; Chawla, L.; et al. The furosemide stress test for prediction of worsening acute kidney injury in critically ill patients: A multicenter, prospective, observational study. *J. Crit. Care* **2019**, *52*, 109–114. [CrossRef] [PubMed]
53. Sakhuja, A.; Bandak, G.; Barreto, E.F.; Vallabhajosyula, S.; Jentzer, J.; Albright, R.; Kashani, K.B. Role of loop diuretic challenge in stage 3 acute kidney injury. *Mayo Clin. Proc.* **2019**, *94*, 1509–1515. [CrossRef] [PubMed]
54. Borasino, S.; Wall, K.M.; Crawford, J.H.; Hock, K.M.; Cleveland, D.C.; Rahman, F.; Martin, K.D.; Alten, J.A. Furosemide response predicts acute kidney injury after cardiac surgery in infants and neonates. *Pediatr. Crit. Care Med.* **2018**, *19*, 310–317. [CrossRef]
55. McMahon, B.A.; Koyner, J.L.; Novick, T.; Menez, S.; Moran, R.A.; Lonze, B.E.; Desai, N.; Alasfar, S.; Borja, M.; Merritt, W.T.; et al. The prognostic value of the furosemide stress test in predicting delayed graft function following deceased donor kidney transplantation. *Biomarkers* **2017**, *23*, 61–69. [CrossRef]
56. Udomkarnjananun, S.; Townamchai, N.; Iampenkhae, K.; Petchlorlian, A.; Srisawat, N.; Katavetin, P.; Sutherasan, M.; Santingamkun, A.; Praditpornsilpa, K.; Eiam-Ong, S.; et al. Furosemide stress test as a predicting biomarker for delayed graft function in kidney transplantation. *Nephron* **2019**, *141*, 236–248. [CrossRef]
57. Rivero, J.; Rodríguez, F.; Soto, V.; Macedo, E.; Chawla, L.S.; Mehta, R.L.; Vaingankar, S.; Garimella, P.S.; Garza, C.; Madero, M. Furosemide stress test and interstitial fibrosis in kidney biopsies in chronic kidney disease. *BMC Nephrol.* **2020**, *21*, 1–9. [CrossRef]
58. Cook, N.R. Use and misuse of the receiver operating characteristic curve in risk prediction. *Circulation* **2007**, *115*, 928–935. [CrossRef]

14

Differential Urinary Proteome Analysis for Predicting Prognosis in Type 2 Diabetes Patients with and without Renal Dysfunction

Hee-Sung Ahn [1,†], Jong Ho Kim [2,†], Hwangkyo Jeong [3], Jiyoung Yu [1], Jeonghun Yeom [4], Sang Heon Song [2], Sang Soo Kim [2], In Joo Kim [2,*] and Kyunggon Kim [1,3,5,6,*]

1 Asan Institute for Life Sciences, Asan Medical Center, Seoul 05505, Korea; zaulim3@gmail.com (H.-S.A.); yujiyoung202@gmail.com (J.Y.)
2 Department of Internal Medicine and Biomedical Research Institute, Pusan National University Hospital, Busan 49241, Korea; bedaya@hanmail.net (J.H.K.); shsong0209@gmail.com (S.H.S.); drsskim7@gmail.com (S.S.K.)
3 Department of Biomedical Sciences, University of Ulsan College of Medicine, Seoul 05505, Korea; hkyo723@naver.com
4 Convergence Medicine Research Center, Asan Institute for Life Sciences, Seoul 05505, Korea; nature8309@gmail.com
5 Clinical Proteomics Core Laboratory, Convergence Medicine Research Center, Asan Medical Center, Seoul 05505, Korea
6 Bio-Medical Institute of Technology, Asan Medical Center, Seoul 05505, Korea
* Correspondence: injkim@pusan.ac.kr (I.J.K.); kkkon1@amc.seoul.kr (K.K.)
† These authors contributed equally to this work.

Abstract: Renal dysfunction, a major complication of type 2 diabetes, can be predicted from estimated glomerular filtration rate (eGFR) and protein markers such as albumin concentration. Urinary protein biomarkers may be used to monitor or predict patient status. Urine samples were selected from patients enrolled in the retrospective diabetic kidney disease (DKD) study, including 35 with good and 19 with poor prognosis. After removal of albumin and immunoglobulin, the remaining proteins were reduced, alkylated, digested, and analyzed qualitatively and quantitatively with a nano LC-MS platform. Each protein was identified, and its concentration normalized to that of creatinine. A prognostic model of DKD was formulated based on the adjusted quantities of each protein in the two groups. Of 1296 proteins identified in the 54 urine samples, 66 were differentially abundant in the two groups (area under the curve (AUC): p-value < 0.05), but none showed significantly better performance than albumin. To improve the predictive power by multivariate analysis, five proteins (ACP2, CTSA, GM2A, MUC1, and SPARCL1) were selected as significant by an AUC-based random forest method. The application of two classifiers—support vector machine and random forest—showed that the multivariate model performed better than univariate analysis of mucin-1 (AUC: 0.935 vs. 0.791) and albumin (AUC: 1.0 vs. 0.722). The urinary proteome can reflect kidney function directly and can predict the prognosis of patients with chronic kidney dysfunction. Classification based on five urinary proteins may better predict the prognosis of DKD patients than urinary albumin concentration or eGFR.

Keywords: urine; diabetic kidney disease; kidney function; proteomics; mass spectrometry; statistical clinical model; machine learning

1. Introduction

About 30% of people with diabetes develop diabetic kidney disease (DKD), and the spread of diabetes is increasing worldwide [1,2]. Complications of type 2 diabetes (T2D) mainly cause end-stage renal disease, which is related to high heart disease incidence and mortality [2,3]. Early detection and screening of patients at risk for DKD is important, which may reduce the global burden of T2D.

Because the kidneys filter waste from blood and discharge it as urine, urine can directly reflect kidney function. Unlike plasma, urine can be easily collected non-invasively, with proteins in urine being stable and not vulnerable to sudden degradation [4]. Albuminuria and estimated glomerular filtration rate (eGFR), have been generally used to assess kidney function [2,5]. However, albuminuria is only evaluated after glomerular damage has occurred, and sometimes kidney disease develops before the outbreak of albuminuria [6,7]. Better markers are required to help delay progression to DKD.

Multiple-biomarker approaches based on proteomics, including urinary proteomics, may overcome the limitations of markers diagnostic for DKD [4,8]. This study was designed to identify a urinary multi-protein panel that could predict progression to DKD in patients with T2D.

2. Results

2.1. Baseline Characteristics of Clinical Samples Used in the Study

Table 1 summarizes the baseline characteristics of patients in the poor and good prognosis groups. All factors did not differ significantly in the two groups, including sex, age, body mass index (BMI), duration of follow-up, systolic blood pressure (SBP), glycated hemoglobin concentration (HbA1c), lipid profile, percent with diabetic retinopathy, and the percentages treated with RAS inhibitors, anti-hypertensive agents, and lipid-lowering agents (Bonferroni corrected p-value $> 0.05/17 = 0.0029$; Table S1).

Table 1. Baseline characteristics of the patients with type 2 diabetes (T2D) with and without renal outcomes.

Variable	With Renal Outcome	Without Renal Outcome
Sex, n (%)		
Male	8 (42.1)	11 (31.4)
Female	11 (57.9)	24 (68.6)
Age at diagnosis of diabetic kidney disease, mean ± SD (years)	54.58 ± 11.66	58.66 ± 9.19
BMI, mean ± SD (kg/m^2)	22.64 ± 3.46	23.81 ± 3.00
Duration of follow-up, mean ± SD (years)	4.80 ± 1.96	4.73 ± 1.94
SBP, mean ± SD (mmHg)	126.58 ± 15.70	125.97 ± 12.07
LDL cholesterol, mean ± SD (mg/dL)	104.89 ± 41.00	99.83 ± 32.32
HDL cholesterol, mean ± SD (mg/dL)	48.42 ± 7.50	52.51 ± 11.51
Triglycerides, mean ± SD (mg/dL)	145.74 ± 99.80	154.57 ± 128.88
eGFR after 1 years, mean ± SD (mL/min/1.73 m^2)	91.52 ± 17.57	88.33 ± 15.46
HbA1c, mean ± SD (%)	8.34 ± 2.09	7.16 ± 1.36
ACR, mean ± SD (mg/g)	213.66 ± 446.75	126.11 ± 419.70
NAPCR, mean ± SD (mg/g)	178.18 ± 209.30	154.76 ± 299.68
PCR, mean ± SD (mg/g)	391.84 ± 652.79	280.87 ± 711.04
Diabetic retinopathy, n (%)	9 (47.37)	11 (31.43)
RAS inhibitor, n (%)	6 (31.58)	15 (42.86)
Anti-hypertensive agent, n (%)	5 (26.32)	12 (34.29)
Lipid-lowering agent, n (%)	10 (52.63)	20 (57.14)

Abbreviations: BMI, body mass index; SBP, systolic blood pressure; LDL, low-density lipoprotein; HDL, high-density lipoprotein; eGFR, estimated glomerular filtration rate; HbA1c, glycated hemoglobin; ACR, urine albumin-to-creatinine ratio; NAPCR, urine nonalbumin protein-to-creatinine ratio; PCR, urine protein-to-creatinine ratio.

2.2. Urinary Proteome Analysis for Identification and Label-Free Quantitation

The workflow of data processes contained identified and quantified urinary proteins indicative of disease status, as well as significant proteins to build the clinical models (Figure 1A). Liquid chromatography–mass spectrometry (LC-MS) analysis of the 54 urine samples identified 1296 proteins (Table S2). Of these proteins, 1244 were quantified, and their quantities were adjusted relative to the concentration of creatinine [9,10]. Sample-to-sample variation was subsequently fixed by the amount of proteins, leading to the selection of six endogenous normalization proteins that showed stable abundance in all LC-MS analyses. A boxplot of protein abundances in the 54 samples, composed of 35 patients in good-prognostic group (GPG) and 19 patients in poor-prognostic group (PPG), is depicted in Figure 1B. The normalized abundance of 68 proteins significantly correlated with their immunoassay [11] determined concentrations in urine, with a Pearson's coefficient of 0.502 (permutation p-value < 0.001; Figure 1C).

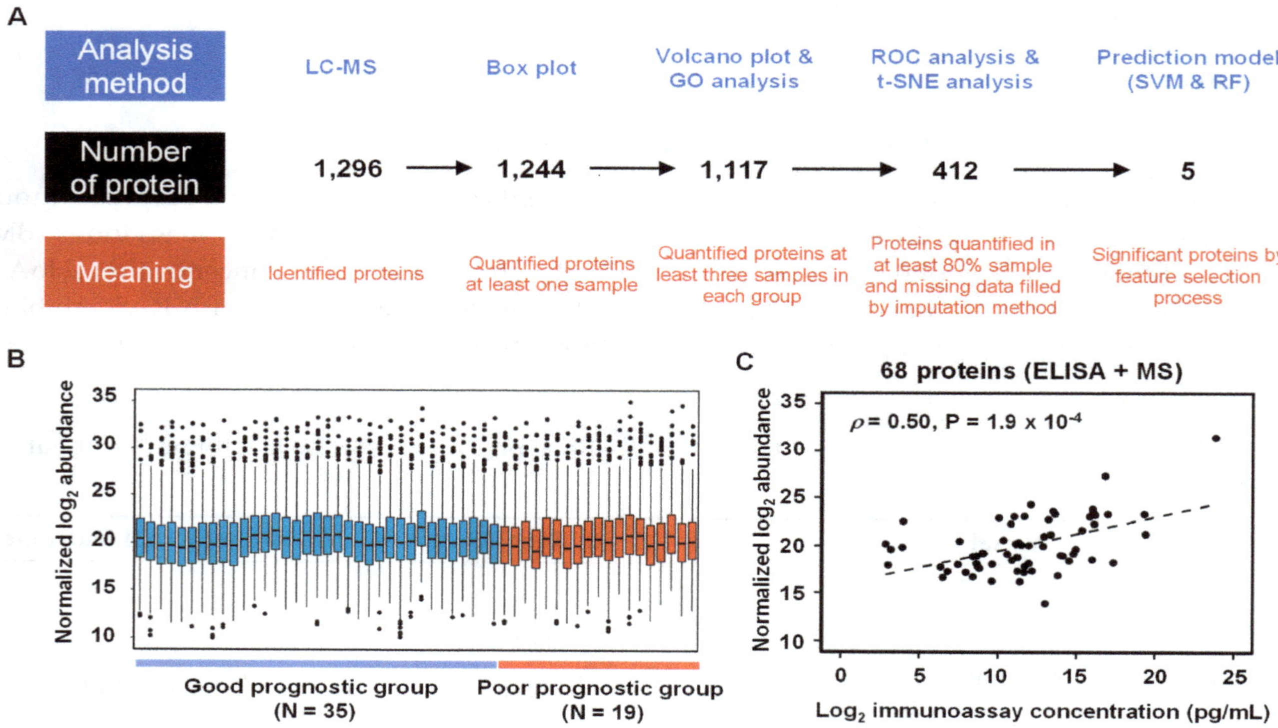

Figure 1. (**A**) Analysis workflow of urinary proteins in the 54 diabetic kidney disease (DKD) patients. The analysis method is written in the upper part, the number of proteins in the middle, and the meaning of the protein in the bottom part. (**B**) Boxplots of normalized urinary protein abundances in the 54 samples (35 patients in good-prognostic group and 19 patients in poor-prognostic group) measured by LC-MS analysis. (**C**) Scatter plot of 68 urine proteins between normalized log2 abundance and log2 immunoassays concentration (Pearson correlation coefficient (ρ): 0.5 and p-value: 1.9×10^{-4}).

2.3. Functional Annotation of Differential Protein Expression in the PPG and GPG Groups

To find the differential abundant proteins (DAPs) from among the 1117 proteins, fold-changes and p-values were calculated by Mann–Whitney U tests of the two groups. A volcano plot showing log2-fold-changes against minus $\log_{10}$ p-values identified 46 proteins as being upregulated in the PPG and 54 proteins in the GPG ($|\log_2$ fold-change$| > 0.5$; p-value < 0.05; Figure 2 and Table S3). These differentially expressed proteins included the six previously described candidate urinary biomarkers (APOE, CO3, COF1, NID1, OSTP-5, and PODXL) of glomerular or tubular injury [11].

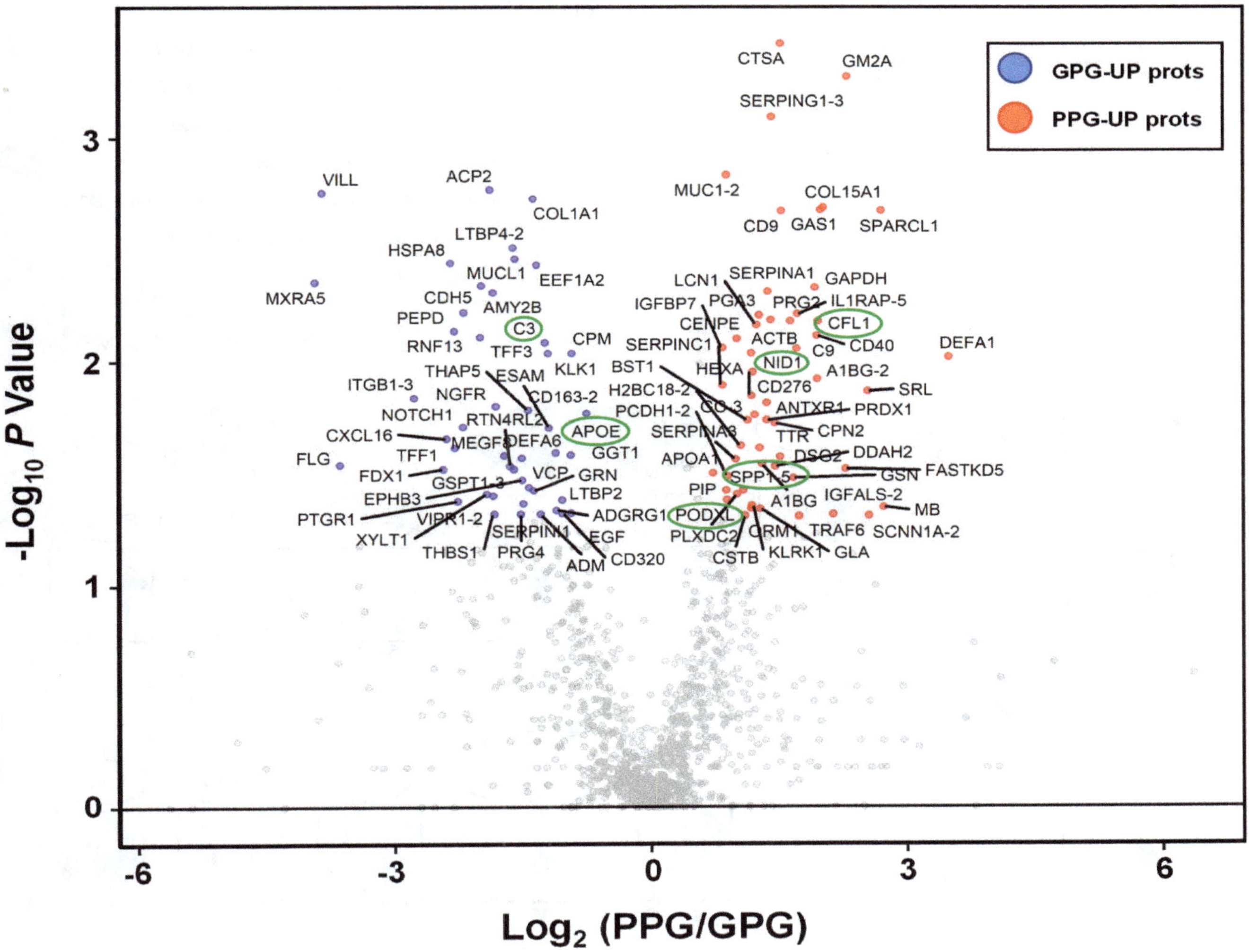

Figure 2. Volcano plot of urinary proteomic data. Volcano plots are depicted with the fold change of each protein abundance and the p value was calculated by performing a Mann–Whitney U-test. The averages of the urinary proteomic abundance data of good prognostic group (N = 35) were compared with the averages of the data for poor prognostic group (N = 19). Red circles show 54 urinary proteins that have significant increases in PPG. Blue circles show 46 urinary proteins which have significant decreases in PPG. Gray circles are urinary proteins without statistical meaning. Green circles are previously released as urinary protein markers for glomerular injury or tubular injury.

To determine whether urinary DAPs were associated with specific biological processes, up- and downregulated proteins in the PPG were subjected to gene ontology (GO) enrichment analysis. To integrate the three domains of GO and easily visualize the relationship between terms, ClueGO tools were applied with default settings (kappa score 0.4 and group merger of 50% of genes) to functionally organize the GO term networks [12].

Downregulated proteins in PPG were significantly enriched with an FDR < 0.01 (Figure 3A,B). Biological processes associated with these proteins included negative regulation of lipid localization, collagen catabolic process, positive regulation of neural precursor cell proliferation, and neuron projection regeneration. Resulting analysis of molecular function indicated that transforming growth factor beta binding and cargo receptor activity were annotated. The networks between proteins and functional GO terms showed that three proteins were negative regulators of lipid transport, as well as being associated with another GO term (Figure 3C). These included APOE, which is involved in neuron projection regeneration; THBS1, which is involved in transforming growth factor beta binding; and EGF, which is involved in positive regulation of neural precursor cell proliferation.

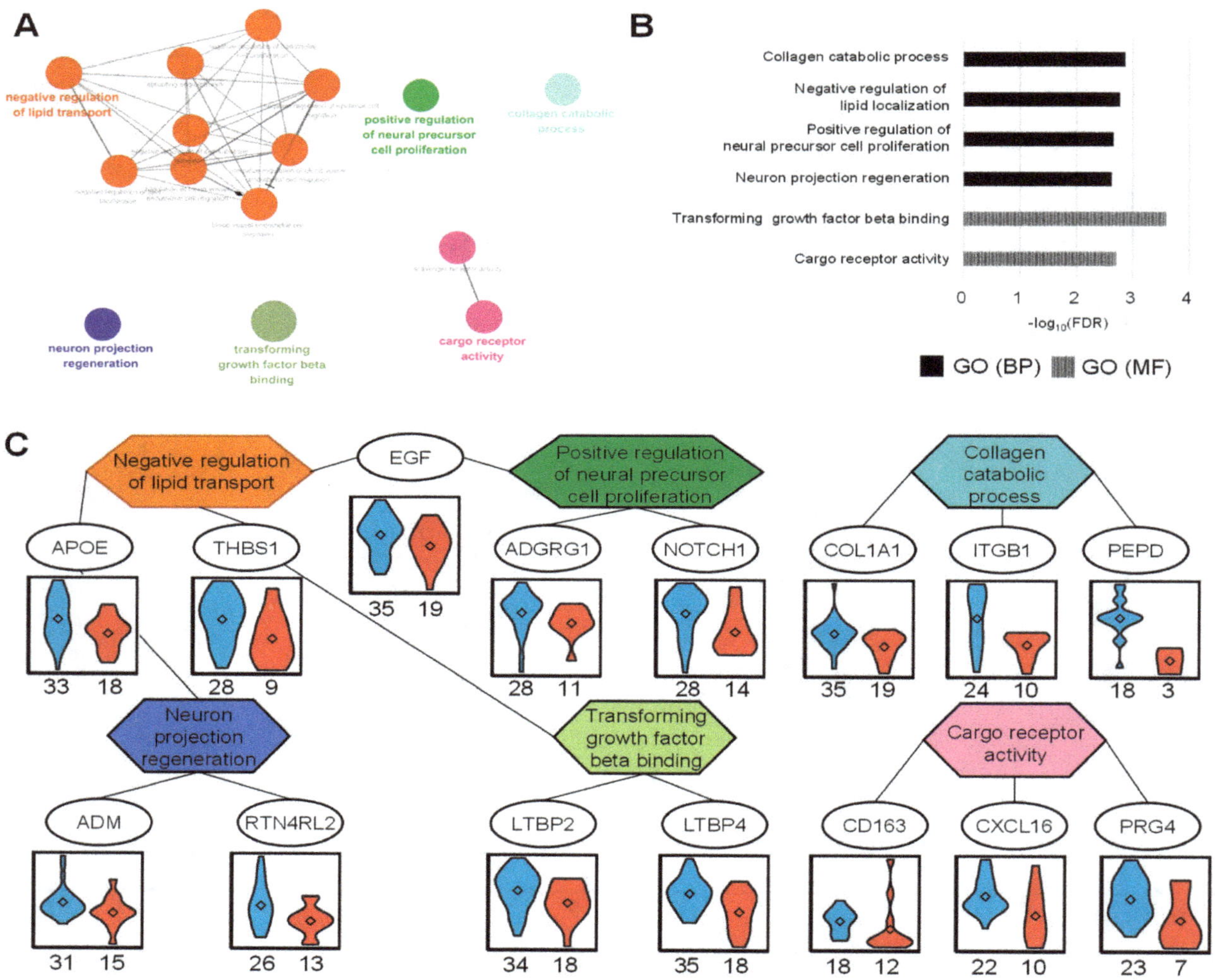

Figure 3. Up-regulated proteome in good prognosis group (GPG) and gene ontology (GO) analysis. (**A**) Functional GO network displaying grouping of GO terms enriched in GPG up-regulated proteins. (**B**) Enriched GO terms in biological process and molecular function. (**C**) The network between GO terms and corresponding proteins represents the relationship between GO terms via the proteins. The abundances of each protein represent the violin plots in two groups. The numbers listed below represent the measured numbers for each group.

Upregulated proteins in PPG were identified in enriched functional GO groups with an FDR < 0.01 (Figure 4A,B). Biological processes associated with these proteins included platelet degranulation, retina homeostasis, and heterotypic cell–cell adhesion. The molecular functional processes related with these proteins contained collagen binding. These urinary proteins were located in the lysosomal lumen and blood microparticles. The networks between proteins and functional GO terms indicated that the proteins in blood microparticles were functionally involved in platelet degranulation (Figure 4C). Platelets in patients with CKD are deficient in reactivity [13]. Leukocytes adhere to and destroy damaged kidney cell walls in patients with CKD [14], accompanied by bone marrow-derived kidney fibrosis, which is highly associated with cell–cell adhesion [15]. CKD is also associated with retinal abnormalities [16] and the possible destruction of retinal homeostasis, as confirmed in this study.

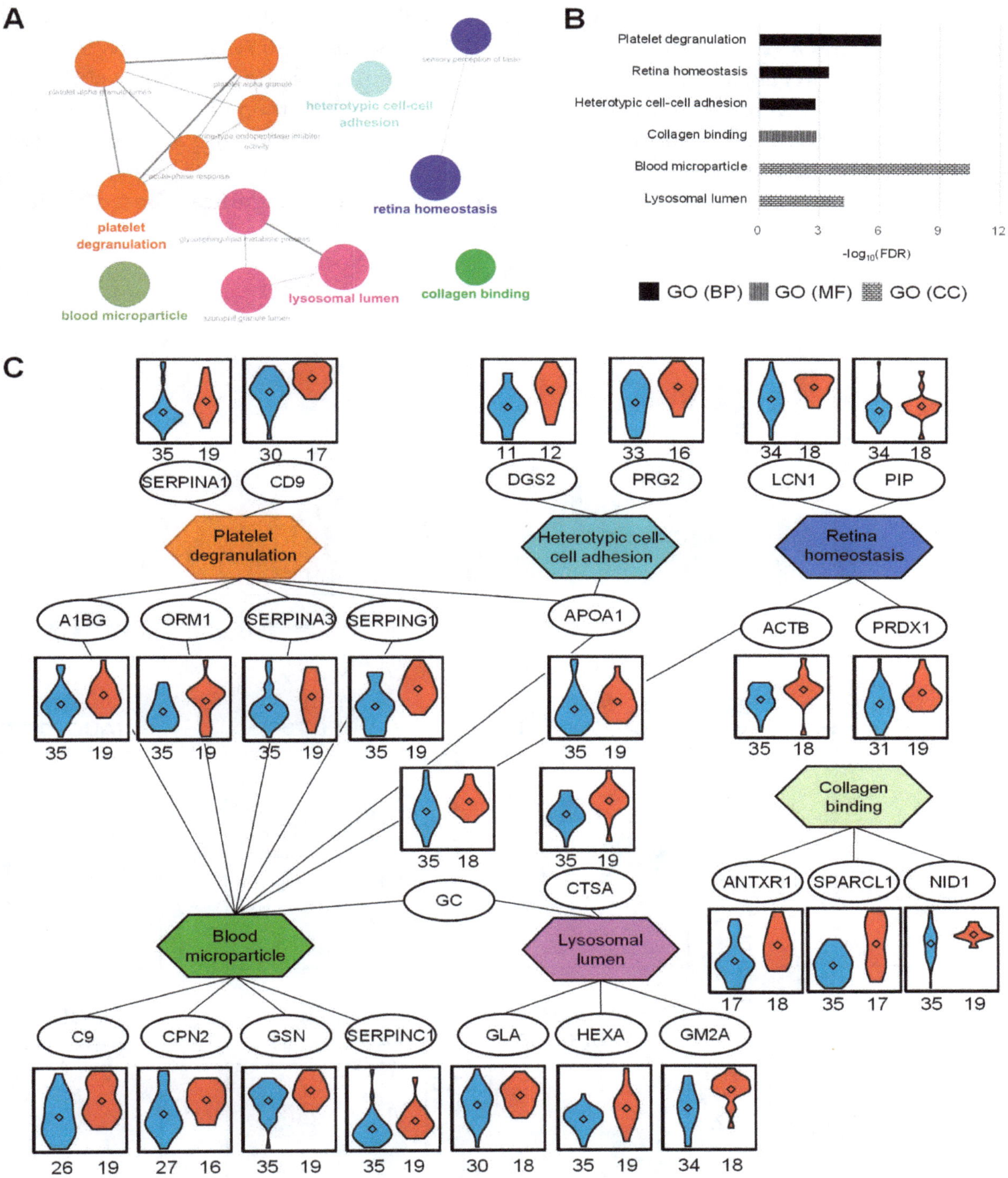

Figure 4. Up-regulated proteome in poor-prognostic group (PPG) and GO analysis. (**A**) Functional GO network displaying grouping of GO terms enriched in PPG up-regulated proteins. (**B**) Enriched GO terms in biological process, molecular function, and cellular component. (**C**) The network between GO terms and their contained proteins represents the relationship between GO terms via the proteins. The abundance of proteins represents the violin plots in two sample groups. The numbers listed below represent the measured numbers for each group.

2.4. Univariate ROC Analysis for Predicting Renal Outcome

To ensure statistical reliability, this study focused on 412 proteins quantified in more than 80% of urine samples [17], with missing values filled by local least squares imputation [18] (Table S4). To confirm that quantified urinary proteins could act as individual biomarkers, univariate receiver operating characteristic (ROC) analysis was performed in samples from the PPG and GPG, with the resulting histogram of AUC values shown in Figure 5. The AUC values of MUC1, CTSA, ACP2, SERPING1, AMY2B, GM2A, and COL1A1 were 0.791, 0.786, 0.773, 0.771, 0.768, 0.759, and 0.753, respectively. ACP2, AMY2B, and COL1A1 were significantly more abundant, whereas MUC1, CTSA, SERPING1, and GM2A were significantly less abundant, in the GPG than in the PPG (p-value < 0.05 each). The 66 urinary proteins showed significance with AUCs of 0.5 (p-value < 0.05; Table S5). Clinically, urinary albumin is a common marker of DKD [2,5]. The AUCs of 18 proteins were higher than that of albumin (0.722), but the differences were not statistically significant based on likelihood ratio tests.

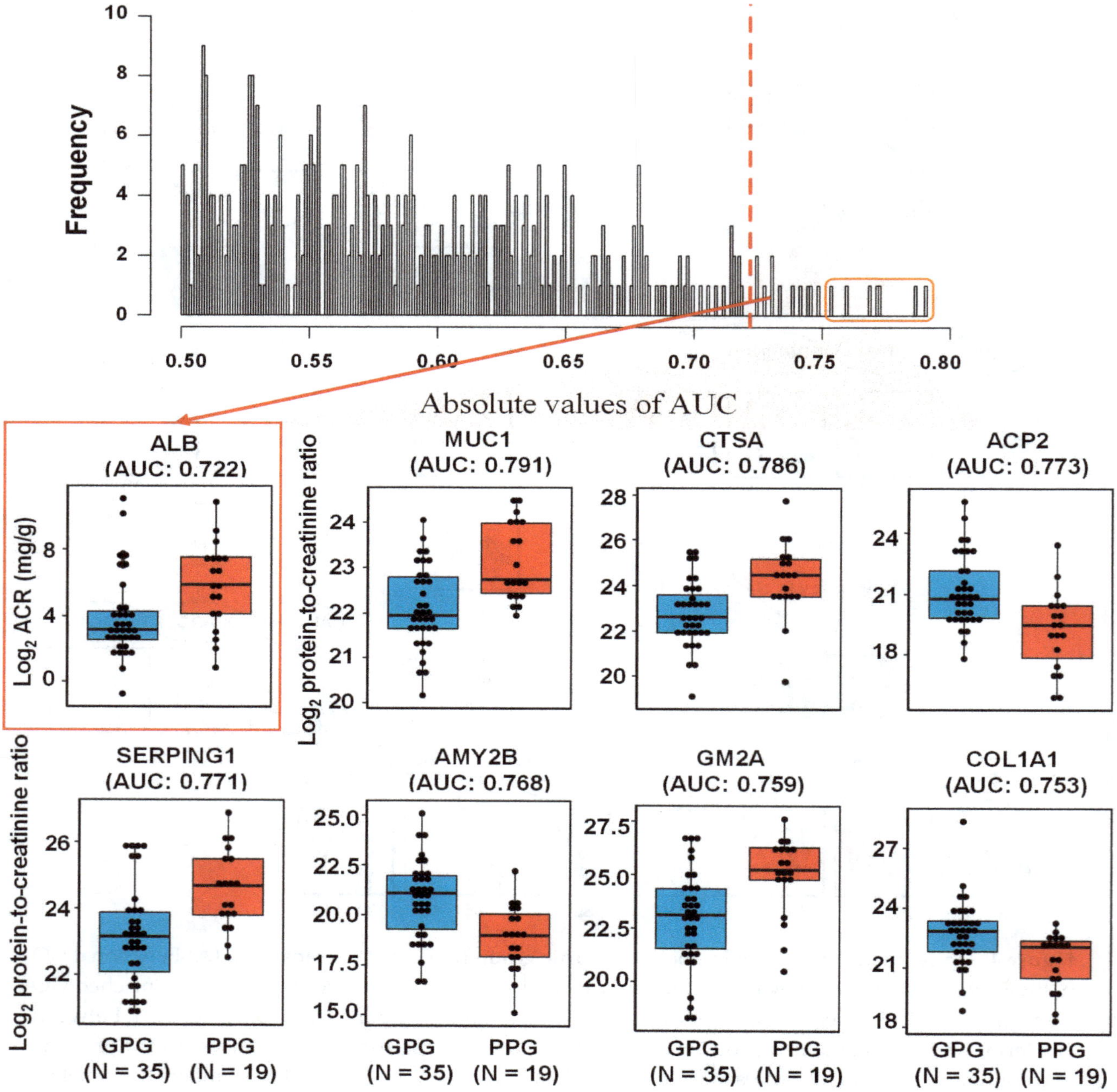

Figure 5. Histogram of area under the ROC curves (AUC) of 412 urinary proteins and ACR. Top seven proteins (MUC1, CTSA, ACP2, SERPING1, AMY2B, GM2A, and COL1A1) and ACR are represented with box plots.

2.5. Multivariate Analysis for Predicting Renal Outcome

To improve predictive performance and find a meaningful combination of proteins that could distinguish patients who were and were not at risk of disease progression, two classifiers of the 412 proteins were generated, one based on random forest (RF) [19] and the other on support vector machine (SVM) [20]. Both the RF and SVM methods selected five proteins (ACP2, CTSA, GM2A, MUC1, and SPARCL1) by an AUC-based RF backward-elimination process [21], according to a >0.3 importance of selection (Table 2). These variables were used to establish a RF model by generating 20,000 decision trees, and a linear SVM model by three repeated iterations of 10-fold cross-validation. Evaluation of the performance of these classifiers showed that the AUC values for RF and SVM were 1.000 and 0.935, respectively (Figure 6A). The nominal binary results of RF and SVM models were transformed in disease prediction scores, which ranged from 0 to 1 (Figure 6B and Table S6). The two classifiers differed significantly from albumin-to-creatinine ratio (likelihood ratio test: p-value < 0.05). These five proteins were located in extracellular exosomes, vesicles, or organelles, with three (ACP2, CTSA, and GM2A) located in the lysosomal lumen, MUC1 placed in plasma membrane, and SPARCL1 interacted with collagen in extracellular matrix.

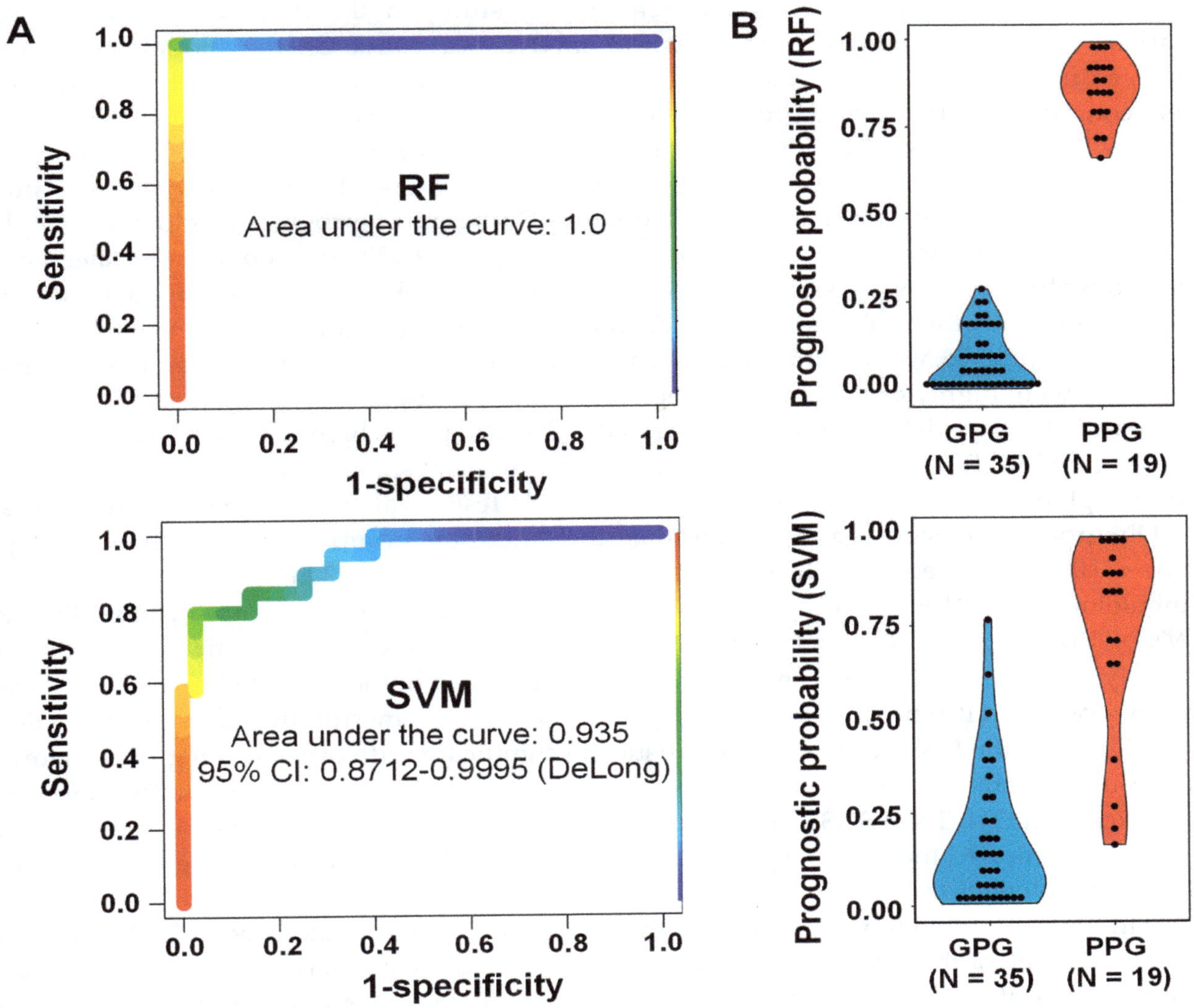

Figure 6. ROC curves of RF and SVM classifiers for five selected proteins (ACP2, CTSA, GM2A, MUC1 and SPARCL1). Performance of the two classifiers in the set of 54 samples, 35 from patients with good prognosis and 19 from patients with poor prognosis. (**A**) Areas under the curve (AUC) for the RF (1.0) and SVM (0.935) classifiers. (**B**) Clinical indices (0–1) of the two classifiers.

Table 2. AUC-based RF backward-elimination process-based selected feature proteins.

Uniprot Accession No.	Gene Name	Importance	Prob. Select	Selection	Univariate AUC
P10619	*CTSA*	0.422	0.700	Y	0.737
Q14515	*SPARCL1*	0.378	0.583	Y	0.659
P17900	*GM2A*	0.373	0.613	Y	0.726
P15941-2	*MUC1*	0.332	0.543	Y	0.791
P11117	*ACP2*	0.312	0.563	Y	0.718
P19961	*AMY2B*	0.299	0.510	N	0.779
P00734	*F2*	0.296	0.483	N	0.694
P06865	*HEXA*	0.274	0.466	N	0.651
P05155-3	*SERPING1*	0.275	0.377	N	0.771
P11142	*HSPA8*	0.238	0.330	N	0.734
P10451	*SPP1*	0.228	0.323	N	0.680

Probability of selection for each variable.

2.6. External Validation of Clinical Models in Public Studies

Since we were unable to find a benchmarking study in the discovery of urine protein biomarkers that could validate our statistical model, we validated the models with mRNA expression in the kidney, an organ that undoubtedly affects urine samples. The SVM and RF models consisting of five urine proteins were applied to four publicly available GEO datasets (GSE99339 [22], GSE47185 [23], GSE30122 [24], and GSE96804 [25,26]) without model adjustment. In the first GSE99339 dataset, mRNA expression in the renal glomerulus of 187 patients was studied, and the 11 disease groups are diabetic nephropathy (DN), rapidly progressive glomerulonephritis (RPGN), tumor nephrectomies (TN), hypertensive nephropathy (HT), IgA nephropathy, membranous glomerulonephritis (MGN), systemic lupus erythematosus (SLE), thin membrane disease (TMD), focal and segmental glomerulosclerosis (FSGS), focal and segmental glomerulosclerosis and minimal change disease (FSGS&MCD), and minimal change disease (MCD). The two classifiers' prognostic probabilities were highly correlated with each other in 187 samples ($\rho = 0.817$, Pearson correlation coefficient). In both models, the highest value in the DN group was higher than the other ten disease groups (Figure 7A). RF prediction values in the DN group were significantly higher than other eight groups except for RPGN and HT group (Mann-Whitney U Test: p-value < 0.05). SVM prediction values in the DN group were significantly higher than the other nine groups excluding the RPGN group (p-value < 0.05). In the second GSE99339 data set, there are a total of 223 kidney glomerulus ($N = 122$) and tubulointerstitia ($N = 101$) mRNA expression levels. The eight disease groups include DN, RPGN, TN, MGN, TMD, FSGS, FSGS&MCD, and MCD. The two classifiers' prognostic probabilities were also highly correlated in 223 samples ($r = 0.637$). The tendency of the predicted values was different depending on the cell type of the kidney (Figure 7B). In the glomeruli, the two model predictions are the highest in the DN group and are statistically significant with other seven groups. However, in the tubulointerstitium, the SVM model prediction values in DN were significant with four other groups except RPGN, TN, FSGS&MCD, and RF model prediction values in DN is only significant with MCD. It indicated that the five urine proteins are more closely related to the glomeruli than the kidney tubulointerstitium.

Meanwhile, we tried to verify whether the prognostic models could predict DKD. In the third GSE30122 data set, of the total of 69 samples, 26 of the 35 kidney glomerulus were normal obtained from living allograft donors, 9 of which were DKD, 34 of which were renal tubulus, of which 24 were normal and 10 were DKD. The results of the RF model in the glomeruli statistically were divided the normal and disease groups (p-value < 0.05), but the SVM model were not (p-value > 0.05; Figure 7C). The results of the both models in the tubulus statistically were not divided the normal and disease groups (p-value > 0.05). In the fourth GSE30122 dataset, 20 kidney glomerulus out of a total of 62 samples were glomerulus from the non-neoplastic part of tumor nephrectomies and 41 of them were from DN. The results of the both models statistically were not divided the normal and disease groups (p-value > 0.05; Figure 7D). It indicated that models for predicting kidney prognosis with urine protein markers in diabetics are difficult to distinguish DKD from normal groups by mRNA expression level in kidney.

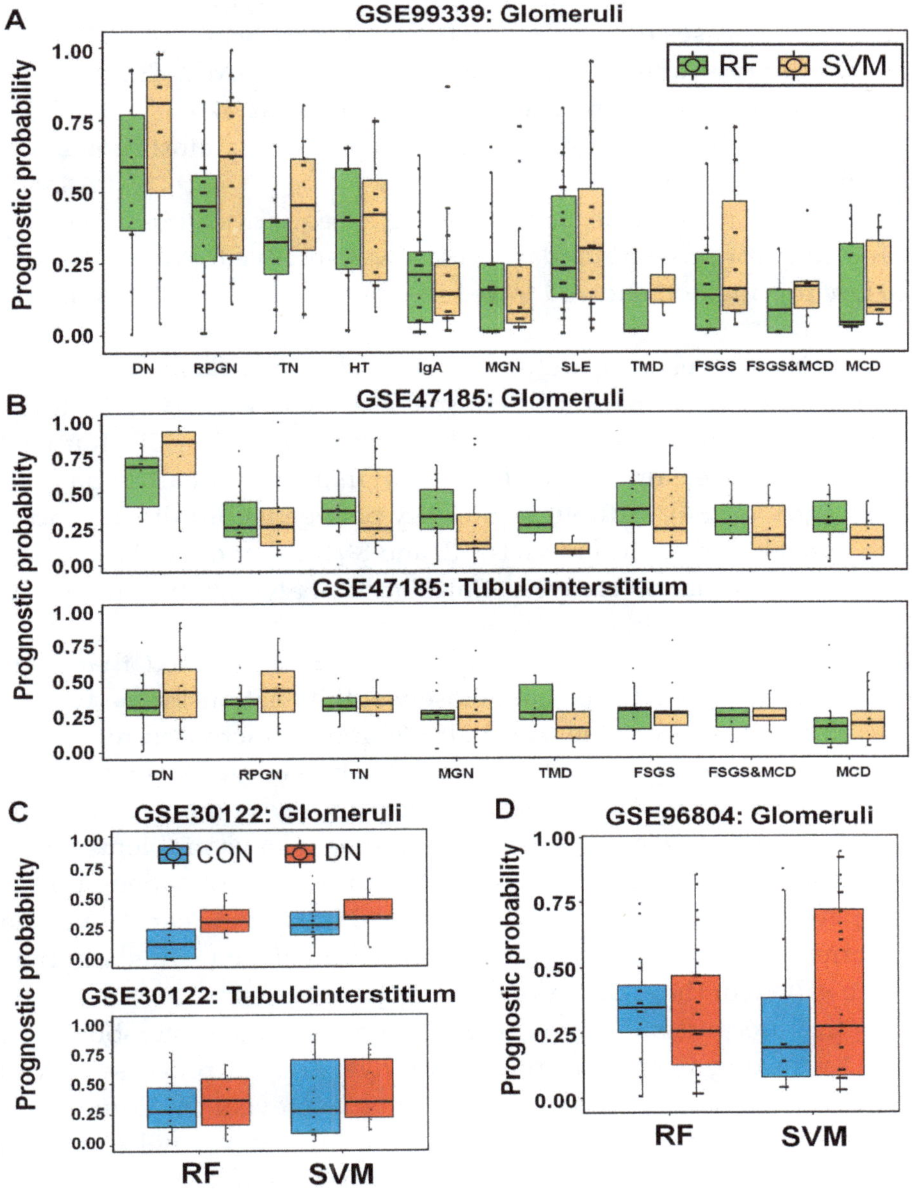

Figure 7. External validation of RF and SVM clinical models in public four GEO datasets (GSE99339, GSE47185, GSE30122 and GSE96804). (**A**) In the GSE99339 dataset, boxplot of the prognostic probabilities of the two classifiers in 11 disease groups including DN (N = 14), RPGN (N = 23), TN (N = 14), HT (N = 15), IgA nephropathy (N = 26), MGN (N = 21), SLE (N = 30), TMD (N = 3), FSGS (N = 22), FSGS&MCD (N = 6), and MCD (N = 13). (**B**) In the GSE30122 data set, the prognostic indexes of the two classifiers in the eight disease groups in the renal glomeruli with DN (N = 14), RPGN, (N = 23), TN (N = 17), MGN (N = 21), TMD (N = 3), FSGS (N = 23), FSGS&MCD (N = 6), and MCD (N = 15) and in the renal tubulointerstitia with DN (N = 18), RPGN (N = 21), TN (N = 6), MGN (N = 18), TMD (N = 6), FSGS (N = 13), FSGS&MCD (N = 4), and MCD (N = 15). (**C**) In the GSE30122 data set, the prediction values of the two classifiers in the control and disease groups in renal glomerulus (N = 26; control and N = 9; disease) and in renal tubulus (N = 24; control and N = 10; disease). (**D**) In the GSE30122 data set, the prediction probabilities of the two classifiers in the control (N = 20) and disease (N = 41) groups in renal glomeruli.

3. Discussion

Urine-based approaches for measuring internal biomolecules can be normalized. Ideally, urine should be collected for 24 h and urinary biomolecules measured. Because this method is practically difficult, urinary proteins in random spot samples were calibrated relative to creatinine concentrations [9]. Prolonged storage of urine samples for studying proteins is important because of the activity of urinary proteases depending on the temperature and pH [27]. In this retrospective study, urine samples were stored at −80 °C for 7–8 years before LC-MS/MS measurements. In general, it is known that it is stable without urine preservatives stored at −70 or −80 °C, and urine samples stored for more than 2.3 years have no significant change in not only most proteins including albumin but also metabolites including creatinine [28–31].

Proteins were extracted from urine samples using an equal volume-based approach similar to ELISA [32]. This procedure for protein standardization was suitable for downstream analysis. Urinary proteins normalized by this method showed lower sample-to-sample variation and higher correlation with immunoassay results.

Albuminuria is primarily used to detect DKD in clinical practice [2,5]. Because glomeruli filter blood, albumin is a good biomarker of chronic kidney disease (CKD) caused by glomerular abnormalities but is insufficient to determine subsequent prognosis [5]. Rather than this, it was determined that finding and measuring specific protein markers that affect pathological function is more clinically meaningful [33,34]. Although causality between albuminuria and prognostic values from the five-protein panel-based clinical models (RF and SVM) cannot be clarified in this retrospective study, it can be inferred by correlation analysis. Correlation analysis between two classifiers and ACR in the 54 enrolled patients reveals a little of bit correlation but no significance ($r = 0.086$; p-value > 0.05; SVM and $r = 0.094$; p-value > 0.05; RF). Therefore, it was confirmed that there was no causal relationship as well as a correlation. To consider closely at the relationship between them, we divided the three classes based on the ACR value (normal; <30 mg/g, microalbuminuria; 30–300 mg/g and macroalbuminuria; >300 mg/g) and plotted the predicted values of the SVM model according to the two prognostic groups (Figure S1). In T2D patients with normal range and microalbuminuria, SVM results were almost separated between two groups. Rather, it seems to have problems with predictive power in patients with macroalbuminuria. It means that SVM results did not depend on the development of albuminuria in T2D patients and showed the possibility to predict the earlier disease stage before the development of albuminuria. Moreover, the predicted value of RF results accurately separates two prognostic groups regardless of the ACR value.

As a rule, diabetics are persistently exposed to miscellaneous metabolic and hemodynamic risks [35], with DKD resulting from multiple pathophysiological processes. Multiple-biomarker approaches using proteomics and metabolomics may better reveal the complicated disease status thought to be associated with the onset of DKD [4,8]. CKD273, a panel consisting of 273 urinary peptides currently undergoing Phase 3 testing, was a high performance urine peptidomic classifier for CKD diagnosis [36]. Moreover, this classifier was recently validated as a predictor of the development of microalbuminuria in normoalbuminuric with diabetic patients [37]. These 273 intact peptides were derived from 30 independent proteins, 24 of which were quantified in this study. CKD273, which includes cleaved collagenase peptides and SERPINA1 peptides, is a good prognostic marker, showing that the concentrations of cleaved collagenase peptides decrease and those of SERPINA1 peptides increase in the urine of patients with CKD [38,39]. The present study showed a similar pattern of abundance in the urine of PPG patients despite artificial digestion. Our approach, based on protein concentrations in urine samples, could better explain the pathological pathway associated with DKD than the peptidome approach. Indicators of kidney dysfunction include increased blood particles in urine; lysosomal dysfunction in glomerular cells [40], which is related to the autophagy-lysosome pathway [41] abnormal heterotypic cell–cell adhesion among glomerular, tubular, and immune cell compartments, collagenase, and binding proteins (driven by rapid changes in glycolipids) [42] and platelet activation [43].

Our clinical models consist of five selected proteins, four proteins (CTSA, MUC1, GM2A, and SPARCL1) are high in PPG and other one protein (ACP2) is low in PPG. Cystatin A (CTSA), in the same protein family as cystatin C that can measure kidney function [44–46], has been found in our urinary biomarker discovery study. Muc1 is a multifaceted tumor protein, and its relationship with the kidney has recently been highlighted [47] and has been identified as a mutant that causes mendelian disorder medullary cystic kidney disease type 1 [48]. In a meta-analysis study of rat glomerular transcriptome profiling, it was confirmed that GM2A was highly expressed in various diabetic kidney disease rat [49]. Through the mouse kidney injury model experiment, SPARCL1 showed that mRNA expression was not changed in the acute phase, but the expression level was high in the fibrosis of the kidney [50], and it inhibited the movement and invasion of renal cell carcinoma [51]. Lastly, ACP 2, one of the lysosomal enzymes, is a protein used in peptiduria [52] or lysosomal enzymuria [53] that measures kidney disease in diabetic patients. Through the external kidney mRNA published studies, these urine biomarkers we found confirmed differential expression in kidney tissue with DKD.

This study had several limitations. First, the patient population in this study was homogeneous and of small sample size. These results require further validation in a multiethnic cohort including larger numbers of patients to assess applicability to a wider population with T2D, a study currently in progress. Second, DKD was clinically diagnosed in the absence of renal biopsies. Third, it is unclear which organ is derived from the urinary protein signatures. More research is needed to determine whether urinary protein signatures are biomarkers of tubular damage in pathological conditions with a glomerular protein load.

4. Materials and Methods

4.1. Patients and Urine Samples

Urine samples were collected from 54 outpatients with T2D and eGFR $\geq$ 60 mL/min/1.72 m^2 who were enrolled in the DKD study at Pusan National University Hospital, South Korea, from February 2010 to January 2011 and who met previously described inclusion and exclusion criteria [54]. After one year, patients were followed-up with until September 2017. Patients were managed according to standard guidelines, including treatment with RAS inhibitors, and eGFR was measured at least twice during a follow-up period $\geq$12 months. Renal function decline was defined as an eGFR < 60 mL/min/1.72 m^2, annual eGFR reduction > 3 mL/min/1.72 m^2, or CKD progression, defined as a reduction in GFR category, accompanied by a $\geq$ 25% deterioration in eGFR from baseline. The patients were divided into two groups—19 with renal outcomes (poor prognosis group (PPG)) and 35 without renal outcomes (good prognosis group (GPG)). The protocols and consent procedures were approved by the Institutional Review Board of Pusan National University Hospital (approval No. 2013033). Total proteinuria and albuminuria, as well as creatinine concentrations, were measured in random spot urine samples [55].

4.2. Measurements of Nephrology Parameters

eGFR was calculated using the equation eGFR = 141 $\times$ min (serum creatinine/kappa, 1) alpha $\times$ max (serum creatinine/kappa, 1) $-$ 1.209 $\times$ 0.993 $\times$ age $\times$ sex $\times$ race. For females, sex = 1.018; alpha = $-$0.329; and kappa = 0.7; for males, sex = 1; alpha = $-$0.411; and kappa = 0.9. Renal outcomes were chronic kidney disease (CKD) progression based on guidelines of the International Society of Nephrology; accelerated eGFR decline, defined as an annual eGFR reduction > 3 mL/min/1.72 m^2; or the development of CKD stage $\geq$ 3. CKD stages 1, 2, 3a, 3b, 4, and 5 were defined as eGFRs of $\geq$ 90, 60–89, 45–59, 30–44, 15–29, and < 15 mL/min/1.73 m^2, respectively, and CKD progression was defined as a decline in eGFR category accompanied by a $\geq$ 25% deterioration in eGFR from baseline [56].

4.3. Urinary Protein Sample Preparation

Urine samples were centrifuged at 13,000 rpm for 30 min to remove debris, and 300 µL of each supernatant was mixed with 100 µL High Select™ HSA/Immunoglobulin Depletion Resin (Cat. No:

A36368, Thermo Fisher Scientific, Waltham, MA, USA) and incubated for 1 h at 4 °C to remove albumin and immunoglobulin. Following centrifugation at 13,000 rpm for 10 min, the supernatant was dried using a speed vac with a cold trap (CentriVap Cold Traps, Labconco, Kansas City, MO, USA).

4.4. Enzymatic Digestion in-Solution

Each dried urine sample was dissolved in 100 µL of 8 M urea, reduced with 20 mM dithiothreitol in 50 mM NH_4HCO_3 for 60 min at 25 °C, and alkylated with 40 mM iodoacetamide in 50 mM NH4HCO3 for 60 min in the dark. Urea concentration was diluted to less than 1.0 M. Each urine sample was incubated overnight at 37 °C with 12.5 µg sequencing grade modified trypsin/LysC (Promega, Madison, WI, USA) in 50 mM NH4HCO3 buffer (pH 7.8), followed by quenching with 10uL of 5% formic acid and lyophilization with a cold trap. The samples were re-suspended in 0.1% formic acid, desalted using C18 ZipTips (Millipore, Burlington, MA, USA), and dried for LC-MS analysis.

4.5. Nano-LC-ESI-MS/MS Analysis

Digested peptides were separated using a Dionex UltiMate 3000 RSLCnano system (Thermo Fisher Scientific, Waltham, MA, USA). Tryptic peptides from the bead column were reconstituted in 100 µL of 0.1% formic acid and separated on an Acclaim™ Pepmap 100 C18 column (500 mm × 75 µm i.d., 3 µm, 100 Å) equipped with a C18 Pepmap trap column (20 mm × 100 µm i.d., 5 µm, 100 Å; Thermo Fisher Scientific, Waltham, MA, USA) over 200 min (250 nL/min) using a 0–48% acetonitrile gradient in 0.1% formic acid and 5% DMSO for 150 min at 50 °C. The LC was coupled to a Q Exactive™ Plus Hybrid Quadrupole-Orbitrap™ mass spectrometer with a nano-ESI source. Mass spectra were acquired in a data-dependent mode with an automatic switch between a full scan and 10 data-dependent MS/MS scans. The target value for the full scan MS spectra, selected from a 350 to 1800 *m/z*, was 3,000,000 with a maximum injection time of 50 ms and a resolution of 70,000 at *m/z* 400. The selected ions were fragmented by higher-energy collisional dissociation in the following parameters: 2 Da precursor ion isolation window and 27% normalized collision energy. The ion target value for MS/MS was set to 1,000,000 with a maximum injection time of 100 ms and a resolution of 17,500 at *m/z* 400. Repeated peptides were dynamically excluded for 20 s. All MS data were measured once per sample and have been deposited in the PRIDE archive (www.ebi.ac.uk/pride/archive/projects/PXD016571) [57] under Project 1-20191129-77373 12.

4.6. Database Searching and Label-Free Quantitation

The SwissProt human database (May 2017) was searched for acquired MS/MS spectra using SequestHT on Proteome discoverer (version 2.2, Thermo Fisher Scientific, USA) [58]. The search parameters were set as default including cysteine carbamidomethylation as a fixed modification, and N-terminal acetylation and methionine oxidation as variable modifications with two miscleavages. Peptides were identified based on a search with an initial mass deviation of the precursor ion of up to 10 ppm, with the allowed fragment mass deviation set to 20 ppm. When assigning proteins to peptides, both unique and razor peptides were used. Label-free quantitation (LFQ) was performed using peak intensity for unique peptides of each protein.

4.7. Normalization of Protein Abundance

To correct for sampling variations resulting from random spot urine collection, the raw LFQ values for each protein were divided by the amounts of total protein and creatinine in each sample, followed by normalization of the corrected LFQ values by endogenous proteins without spike-in standards [59]. To identify endogenous urinary proteins for normalization, the 112 initial completely quantified proteins were considered, with six selected based on the following criteria: (1) quantified in all 54 samples; (2) corrected LFQ values did not differ significantly in the poor and good prognosis groups by the Mann–Whitney U Test (p-value > 0.05); and (3) had nearly persistent urine concentrations throughout the sample as top-ranked by NormFinder stability value [60].

The corrected LFQ values of the six selected normalization proteins in each sample were divided by their median value in all samples. The median of these six ratios was defined as the normalization scaling factor (NSF) for that sample. For example, NSF for sample s can be determined using the equation:

$$NSF_s = median\left(\frac{N_{1,s}}{\hat{N}_1}, \frac{N_{2,s}}{\hat{N}_2}, \cdots, \frac{N_{6,s}}{\hat{N}_6}\right) \quad (1)$$

where $N_{i,\,s}$ is the corrected LFQ value of normalization protein i in sample s and $\hat{N}_i$ is the median corrected LFQ value of normalization protein i in all samples. Except for the six normalization proteins in a sample, the normalized LFQ value of each protein was calculated by dividing its corrected LFQ value by NSF.

$$LF\check{Q}_{j,s} = \frac{LFQ_{j,\,s}}{NSF_s} \quad (2)$$

where $LF\check{Q}_{j,s}$ is the normalized LFQ of urinary protein j in sample s and $LFQ_{j,s}$ is the corrected LFQ of the corresponding protein [61].

4.8. *Differential Data Analysis by Filling Missing Data*

For clinical utility, the LFQ data were filtered to <20% of quantified proteins in each sample group to analyze the differential urinary proteins in these groups, with the missing data filled by the local least squared imputation method at the normalized abundance [18].

4.9. *GO Analysis*

Differential abundant proteins (DAPs) in the poor and good prognosis groups were analyzed using the ClueGO (version 2.5.1) [12] plugin for Cytoscape (version 3.6.1) [62]. To group GO terms, the kappa score was set at 0.4 and the number of overlapping genes to combine groups was set at 50%.

4.10. *Statistical Clinical Model Generation Based on Feature Selection*

The process of feature selection was to find the best subset for classifying two disease progression groups out of 412 proteins. There are two steps. In the first step, 50,000 decision trees containing eight variables were randomly generated 50,000 trees and had AUC values. Based on the AUCs values, the optimal number of proteins were determined by out-of-bag error estimation and the value is 11. Second, through the 100 iterations with three-fold cross-validation for from the selected 11 optimal variables, the probability and importance that each variable was included in the model was calculated. We selected five proteins (>0.3 importance). Prior to model building, centering and scaling were performed as preprocessing on the data. In the clinical models, SVM model with linear kernel was generated by a 10 repeated three-fold cross validation method (parameter C = 0.1052) and The RF model was made by a three-fold cross validation method repeated 100 times with 1000 trees, mtry = 5 and nodesize = 5.

4.11. *Mining Public Microarray Data*

We downloaded the mRNA expression data (series accession number: GSE99339, GSE47185, GSE30122, and GSE96804) in the Gene Expression Omnibus database [63]. Then, using GEO2R interactive web tool, five identifiers matching the five selected genes according to the platform record and their expression values were extracted.

4.12. *Statistical Analysis*

Data were analyzed using RStudio (version 1.1.456) including R (version 3.6.0). Statistical R software packages included ggplot2 for drawing box, scattering, volcano and violin plots, permcor for calculating permutation-based *p*-values for Pearson correlation [64], pcaMethods for missing value estimation [65], pROC for univariate ROC analysis [66], ROCR for multivariate ROC analysis,

AUCRF for feature selection [21], caret for building statistical classifiers [67], randomForest for building a RF classifier, and e1071 for building a SVM classifier.

5. Conclusions

These results suggest that measurement of urinary proteome was more promising than albuminuria alone for predicting renal outcomes in patients with type 2 diabetes. A panel of five proteins had the potential for use as a biomarker in clinical practice.

Supplementary Materials:
4236/s1. Figure S1. Prognostic probability of 54 patients by RF and SVM classifier divided into three groups by albumin-to-creatinine ratio.; Table S1. Demographic and clinical characteristics of the 54 patients with type 2 diabetes.; Table S2. Search result of MS/MS spectra of protein sequences obtained from the 54 urine samples in the Human Swissprot proteome database using the SequestHT search engine.; Table S3. Results of volcano plot analysis.; Table S4. Normalized abundance of 412 urinary proteins in the 54 patients with type 2 diabetes.; Table S5. Univariate receiver operating curve analysis of the areas under the curves of 412 urinary proteins.; Table S6. Prognostic probability by RF and SVM classifier of 54 patients.

Author Contributions: Conceptualization, J.H.K., S.H.S., S.S.K., I.J.K., and K.K.; methodology, H.J.; formal analysis, H.-S.A.; investigation, J.Y. (Jiyoung Yu); data curation, H.-S.A., S.S.K., and I.J.K.; writing—original draft preparation, H.-S.A. and K.K.; writing—review and editing, J.H.K., J.Y. (Jiyoung Yu), J.Y. (Jeonghun Yeom), S.H.S., S.S.K., and I.J.K; visualization, H.-S.A.; supervision, I.J.K and K.K.; funding acquisition, J.H.K. All authors have read and agreed to the published version of the manuscript.

Acknowledgments: The authors thank the Department of Biostatistics, Clinical Trial Center, Biomedical Research Institute, Pusan National University Hospital.

Abbreviations

T2D	Type 2 diabetes
eGFR	Estimated glomerular filtration rate
DKD	Diabetic kidney disease
BMI	Body mass index
SBP	Systolic blood pressure
HbA1c	Glycated hemoglobin concentration
LDL	Low-density lipoprotein
HDL	High-density lipoprotein
ACR	Albumin-to-creatinine ratio
NAPCR	Nonalbumin protein-to-creatinine ratio
PCR	Urine protein-to-creatinine ratio
GPG	Good-prognostic group
PPG	Poor-prognostic group
LC-MS	Liquid chromatography–mass spectrometry
DAP	Differential abundant protein
GO	Gene ontology
FDR	False discovery rate
ROC	Receiver operating characteristic
AUC	Area under the receiver operating characteristic curve
RF	Random forest
SVM	Support vector machine
ELISA	Enzyme-linked immunosorbent assay
CKD	Chronic kidney disease
MS/MS	Tandem mass spectrometry
LFQ	Label-free quantitation
NSF	Normalization scaling factor

DN	Diabetic nephropathy
FSGS	Focal and segmental glomerulosclerosis
FSGS&MCD	Focal and segmental glomerulosclerosis and minimal change disease
HT	Hypertensive nephropathy
MCD	Minimal change disease
MGN	Membranous glomerulonephritis
RPGN	Rapidly progressive glomerulonephritis
SLE	Systemic lupus erythematosus
TMD	Thin membrane disease
TN	Tumor nephrectomies

References

1. Ahn, J.H.; Yu, J.H.; Ko, S.H.; Kwon, H.S.; Kim, D.J.; Kim, J.H.; Kim, C.S.; Song, K.H.; Won, J.C.; Lim, S.; et al. Prevalence and determinants of diabetic nephropathy in Korea: Korea national health and nutrition examination survey. *Diabetes Metab. J.* **2014**, *38*, 109–119. [CrossRef]
2. Tuttle, K.R.; Bakris, G.L.; Bilous, R.W.; Chiang, J.L.; de Boer, I.H.; Goldstein-Fuchs, J.; Hirsch, I.B.; Kalantar-Zadeh, K.; Narva, A.S.; Navaneethan, S.D.; et al. Diabetic kidney disease: A report from an ADA Consensus Conference. *Diabetes Care* **2014**, *37*, 2864–2883. [CrossRef] [PubMed]
3. Collins, A.J.; Foley, R.N.; Chavers, B.; Gilbertson, D.; Herzog, C.; Johansen, K.; Kasiske, B.; Kutner, N.; Liu, J.; St Peter, W.; et al. United States Renal Data System 2011 Annual Data Report: Atlas of chronic kidney disease & end-stage renal disease in the United States. *Am. J. Kidney Dis.* **2012**, *59*, A7. [CrossRef] [PubMed]
4. Currie, G.; Delles, C. Urinary Proteomics for Diagnosis and Monitoring of Diabetic Nephropathy. *Curr. Diabetes Rep.* **2016**, *16*, 104. [CrossRef] [PubMed]
5. KDIGO Working Group. KDIGO clinical practice guideline for the evaluation and management of chronic kidney disease. Chapter 2: Definition, identification, and prediction of CKD progression. *Kidney Int. Suppl.* **2013**, *3*, 63–72. [CrossRef]
6. Barratt, J.; Topham, P. Urine proteomics: The present and future of measuring urinary protein components in disease. *CMAJ* **2007**, *177*, 361–368. [CrossRef] [PubMed]
7. Retnakaran, R.; Cull, C.A.; Thorne, K.I.; Adler, A.I.; Holman, R.R.; Group, U.S. Risk factors for renal dysfunction in type 2 diabetes: U.K. Prospective Diabetes Study 74. *Diabetes* **2006**, *55*, 1832–1839. [CrossRef] [PubMed]
8. Kamijo-Ikemori, A.; Sugaya, T.; Kimura, K. Novel urinary biomarkers in early diabetic kidney disease. *Curr. Diabetes Rep.* **2014**, *14*, 513. [CrossRef]
9. Abitbol, C.; Zilleruelo, G.; Freundlich, M.; Strauss, J. Quantitation of proteinuria with urinary protein/creatinine ratios and random testing with dipsticks in nephrotic children. *J. Pediatr.* **1990**, *116*, 243–247. [CrossRef]
10. Lemann, J., Jr.; Doumas, B.T. Proteinuria in health and disease assessed by measuring the urinary protein/creatinine ratio. *Clin. Chem.* **1987**, *33*, 297–299. [CrossRef]
11. Zhao, M.; Li, M.; Yang, Y.; Guo, Z.; Sun, Y.; Shao, C.; Li, M.; Sun, W.; Gao, Y. A comprehensive analysis and annotation of human normal urinary proteome. *Sci. Rep.* **2017**, *7*, 3024. [CrossRef] [PubMed]
12. Bindea, G.; Mlecnik, B.; Hackl, H.; Charoentong, P.; Tosolini, M.; Kirilovsky, A.; Fridman, W.H.; Pages, F.; Trajanoski, Z.; Galon, J. ClueGO: A Cytoscape plug-in to decipher functionally grouped gene ontology and pathway annotation networks. *Bioinformatics* **2009**, *25*, 1091–1093. [CrossRef] [PubMed]
13. Van Bladel, E.R.; de Jager, R.L.; Walter, D.; Cornelissen, L.; Gaillard, C.A.; Boven, L.A.; Roest, M.; Fijnheer, R. Platelets of patients with chronic kidney disease demonstrate deficient platelet reactivity in vitro. *BMC Nephrol.* **2012**, *13*, 127. [CrossRef] [PubMed]
14. Prozialeck, W.C.; Edwards, J.R. Cell adhesion molecules in chemically-induced renal injury. *Pharmacol. Ther.* **2007**, *114*, 74–93. [CrossRef]
15. Yan, J.; Zhang, Z.; Jia, L.; Wang, Y. Role of Bone Marrow-Derived Fibroblasts in Renal Fibrosis. *Front. Physiol.* **2016**, *7*, 61. [CrossRef]

16. Deva, R.; Alias, M.A.; Colville, D.; Tow, F.K.; Ooi, Q.L.; Chew, S.; Mohamad, N.; Hutchinson, A.; Koukouras, I.; Power, D.A.; et al. Vision-threatening retinal abnormalities in chronic kidney disease stages 3 to 5. *Clin. J. Am. Soc. Nephrol.* **2011**, *6*, 1866–1871. [CrossRef]
17. Dziura, J.D.; Post, L.A.; Zhao, Q.; Fu, Z.; Peduzzi, P. Strategies for dealing with missing data in clinical trials: From design to analysis. *Yale J. Biol. Med.* **2013**, *86*, 343–358.
18. Karpievitch, Y.V.; Dabney, A.R.; Smith, R.D. Normalization and missing value imputation for label-free LC-MS analysis. *BMC Bioinform.* **2012**, *13* (Suppl. 16), S5. [CrossRef]
19. Breiman, L. Random forests. *Mach Learn* **2001**, *45*, 5–32. [CrossRef]
20. Cortes, C.; Vapnik, V. Support-Vector Networks. *Mach. Learn.* **1995**, *20*, 273–297. [CrossRef]
21. Calle, M.L.; Urrea, V.; Boulesteix, A.L.; Malats, N. AUC-RF: A new strategy for genomic profiling with random forest. *Hum. Hered.* **2011**, *72*, 121–132. [CrossRef] [PubMed]
22. Shved, N.; Warsow, G.; Eichinger, F.; Hoogewijs, D.; Brandt, S.; Wild, P.; Kretzler, M.; Cohen, C.D.; Lindenmeyer, M.T. Transcriptome-based network analysis reveals renal cell type-specific dysregulation of hypoxia-associated transcripts. *Sci. Rep.* **2017**, *7*, 8576. [CrossRef] [PubMed]
23. Ju, W.; Greene, C.S.; Eichinger, F.; Nair, V.; Hodgin, J.B.; Bitzer, M.; Lee, Y.S.; Zhu, Q.; Kehata, M.; Li, M.; et al. Defining cell-type specificity at the transcriptional level in human disease. *Genome Res.* **2013**, *23*, 1862–1873. [CrossRef] [PubMed]
24. Woroniecka, K.I.; Park, A.S.; Mohtat, D.; Thomas, D.B.; Pullman, J.M.; Susztak, K. Transcriptome analysis of human diabetic kidney disease. *Diabetes* **2011**, *60*, 2354–2369. [CrossRef] [PubMed]
25. Shi, J.S.; Qiu, D.D.; Le, W.B.; Wang, H.; Li, S.; Lu, Y.H.; Jiang, S. Identification of Transcription Regulatory Relationships in Diabetic Nephropathy. *Chin. Med. J.* **2018**, *131*, 2886–2890. [CrossRef] [PubMed]
26. Pan, Y.; Jiang, S.; Hou, Q.; Qiu, D.; Shi, J.; Wang, L.; Chen, Z.; Zhang, M.; Duan, A.; Qin, W.; et al. Dissection of Glomerular Transcriptional Profile in Patients With Diabetic Nephropathy: SRGAP2a Protects Podocyte Structure and Function. *Diabetes* **2018**, *67*, 717–730. [CrossRef]
27. Kania, K.; Byrnes, E.A.; Beilby, J.P.; Webb, S.A.; Strong, K.J. Urinary proteases degrade albumin: Implications for measurement of albuminuria in stored samples. *Ann. Clin. Biochem.* **2010**, *47*, 151–157. [CrossRef]
28. Parekh, R.S.; Kao, W.H.; Meoni, L.A.; Ipp, E.; Kimmel, P.L.; La Page, J.; Fondran, C.; Knowler, W.C.; Klag, M.J.; Family Investigation of Nephropathy and Diabetes; et al. Reliability of urinary albumin, total protein, and creatinine assays after prolonged storage: The Family Investigation of Nephropathy and Diabetes. *Clin. J. Am. Soc. Nephrol.* **2007**, *2*, 1156–1162. [CrossRef]
29. Chapman, D.P.; Gooding, K.M.; McDonald, T.J.; Shore, A.C. Stability of urinary albumin and creatinine after 12 months storage at −20 degrees C and −80 degrees C. *Pract. Lab. Med.* **2019**, *15*, e00120. [CrossRef]
30. Herrington, W.; Illingworth, N.; Staplin, N.; Kumar, A.; Storey, B.; Hrusecka, R.; Judge, P.; Mahmood, M.; Parish, S.; Landray, M.; et al. Effect of Processing Delay and Storage Conditions on Urine Albumin-to-Creatinine Ratio. *Clin. J. Am. Soc. Nephrol.* **2016**, *11*, 1794–1801. [CrossRef]
31. Klasen, I.S.; Reichert, L.J.; de Kat Angelino, C.M.; Wetzels, J.F. Quantitative determination of low and high molecular weight proteins in human urine: Influence of temperature and storage time. *Clin. Chem.* **1999**, *45*, 430–432. [CrossRef] [PubMed]
32. Voller, A.; Bartlett, A.; Bidwell, D.E. Enzyme immunoassays with special reference to ELISA techniques. *J. Clin. Pathol.* **1978**, *31*, 507–520. [CrossRef] [PubMed]
33. Frantzi, M.; Bhat, A.; Latosinska, A. Clinical proteomic biomarkers: Relevant issues on study design & technical considerations in biomarker development. *Clin. Transl. Med.* **2014**, *3*, 7. [CrossRef] [PubMed]
34. Borrebaeck, C.A. Precision diagnostics: Moving towards protein biomarker signatures of clinical utility in cancer. *Nat. Rev. Cancer* **2017**, *17*, 199–204. [CrossRef]
35. Thomas, M.C.; Burns, W.C.; Cooper, M.E. Tubular changes in early diabetic nephropathy. *Adv. Chronic Kidney Dis.* **2005**, *12*, 177–186. [CrossRef]
36. Good, D.M.; Zurbig, P.; Argiles, A.; Bauer, H.W.; Behrens, G.; Coon, J.J.; Dakna, M.; Decramer, S.; Delles, C.; Dominiczak, A.F.; et al. Naturally occurring human urinary peptides for use in diagnosis of chronic kidney disease. *Mol. Cell. Proteomics* **2010**, *9*, 2424–2437. [CrossRef]
37. Lindhardt, M.; Persson, F.; Zurbig, P.; Stalmach, A.; Mischak, H.; de Zeeuw, D.; Lambers Heerspink, H.; Klein, R.; Orchard, T.; Porta, M.; et al. Urinary proteomics predict onset of microalbuminuria in normoalbuminuric type 2 diabetic patients, a sub-study of the DIRECT-Protect 2 study. *Nephrol. Dial. Transplant.* **2017**, *32*, 1866–1873. [CrossRef]

38. Rodriguez-Ortiz, M.E.; Pontillo, C.; Rodriguez, M.; Zurbig, P.; Mischak, H.; Ortiz, A. Novel Urinary Biomarkers For Improved Prediction Of Progressive Egfr Loss In Early Chronic Kidney Disease Stages And In High Risk Individuals Without Chronic Kidney Disease. *Sci. Rep.* **2018**, *8*, 15940. [CrossRef]
39. Pontillo, C.; Mischak, H. Urinary peptide-based classifier CKD273: Towards clinical application in chronic kidney disease. *Clin. Kidney J.* **2017**, *10*, 192–201. [CrossRef] [PubMed]
40. Surendran, K.; Vitiello, S.P.; Pearce, D.A. Lysosome dysfunction in the pathogenesis of kidney diseases. *Pediatr. Nephrol.* **2014**, *29*, 2253–2261. [CrossRef] [PubMed]
41. Liu, W.J.; Shen, T.T.; Chen, R.H.; Wu, H.L.; Wang, Y.J.; Deng, J.K.; Chen, Q.H.; Pan, Q.; Huang Fu, C.M.; Tao, J.L.; et al. Autophagy-Lysosome Pathway in Renal Tubular Epithelial Cells Is Disrupted by Advanced Glycation End Products in Diabetic Nephropathy. *J. Biol. Chem.* **2015**, *290*, 20499–20510. [CrossRef]
42. Rops, A.L.; van der Vlag, J.; Lensen, J.F.; Wijnhoven, T.J.; van den Heuvel, L.P.; van Kuppevelt, T.H.; Berden, J.H. Heparan sulfate proteoglycans in glomerular inflammation. *Kidney Int.* **2004**, *65*, 768–785. [CrossRef] [PubMed]
43. Landray, M.J.; Wheeler, D.C.; Lip, G.Y.; Newman, D.J.; Blann, A.D.; McGlynn, F.J.; Ball, S.; Townend, J.N.; Baigent, C. Inflammation, endothelial dysfunction, and platelet activation in patients with chronic kidney disease: The chronic renal impairment in Birmingham (CRIB) study. *Am. J. Kidney Dis.* **2004**, *43*, 244–253. [CrossRef] [PubMed]
44. Shlipak, M.G.; Matsushita, K.; Arnlov, J.; Inker, L.A.; Katz, R.; Polkinghorne, K.R.; Rothenbacher, D.; Sarnak, M.J.; Astor, B.C.; Coresh, J.; et al. Cystatin C versus creatinine in determining risk based on kidney function. *N. Engl. J. Med.* **2013**, *369*, 932–943. [CrossRef]
45. Inker, L.A.; Schmid, C.H.; Tighiouart, H.; Eckfeldt, J.H.; Feldman, H.I.; Greene, T.; Kusek, J.W.; Manzi, J.; Van Lente, F.; Zhang, Y.L.; et al. Estimating glomerular filtration rate from serum creatinine and cystatin C. *N. Engl. J. Med.* **2012**, *367*, 20–29. [CrossRef] [PubMed]
46. Ingelfinger, J.R.; Marsden, P.A. Estimated GFR and risk of death–is cystatin C useful? *N. Engl. J. Med.* **2013**, *369*, 974–975. [CrossRef] [PubMed]
47. Al-Bataineh, M.M.; Sutton, T.A.; Hughey, R.P. Novel roles for mucin 1 in the kidney. *Curr. Opin. Nephrol. Hypertens.* **2017**, *26*, 384–391. [CrossRef]
48. Kirby, A.; Gnirke, A.; Jaffe, D.B.; Baresova, V.; Pochet, N.; Blumenstiel, B.; Ye, C.; Aird, D.; Stevens, C.; Robinson, J.T.; et al. Mutations causing medullary cystic kidney disease type 1 lie in a large VNTR in MUC1 missed by massively parallel sequencing. *Nat. Genet.* **2013**, *45*, 299–303. [CrossRef]
49. Tryggvason, S.H.; Guo, J.; Nukui, M.; Norlin, J.; Haraldsson, B.; Jornvall, H.; Tryggvason, K.; He, L. A meta-analysis of expression signatures in glomerular disease. *Kidney Int.* **2013**, *84*, 591–599. [CrossRef]
50. Feng, D.; Ngov, C.; Henley, N.; Boufaied, N.; Gerarduzzi, C. Characterization of Matricellular Protein Expression Signatures in Mechanistically Diverse Mouse Models of Kidney Injury. *Sci. Rep.* **2019**, *9*, 16736. [CrossRef]
51. Ye, H.; Wang, W.G.; Cao, J.; Hu, X.C. SPARCL1 suppresses cell migration and invasion in renal cell carcinoma. *Mol. Med. Rep.* **2017**, *16*, 7784–7790. [CrossRef] [PubMed]
52. Gudehithlu, K.P.; Hart, P.D.; Vernik, J.; Sethupathi, P.; Dunea, G.; Arruda, J.A.L.; Singh, A.K. Peptiduria: A potential early predictor of diabetic kidney disease. *Clin. Exp. Nephrol.* **2019**, *23*, 56–64. [CrossRef]
53. Gatsing, D.; Garba, I.H.; Adoga, G.I. The use of lysosomal enzymuria in the early detection and monitoring of the progression of diabetic nephropathy. *Indian J. Clin. Biochem.* **2006**, *21*, 42–48. [CrossRef]
54. Kim, S.S.; Song, S.H.; Kim, I.J.; Yang, J.Y.; Lee, J.G.; Kwak, I.S.; Kim, Y.K. Clinical implication of urinary tubular markers in the early stage of nephropathy with type 2 diabetic patients. *Diabetes Res. Clin. Pract.* **2012**, *97*, 251–257. [CrossRef] [PubMed]
55. Lane, C.; Brown, M.; Dunsmuir, W.; Kelly, J.; Mangos, G. Can spot urine protein/creatinine ratio replace 24 h urine protein in usual clinical nephrology? *Nephrology* **2006**, *11*, 245–249. [CrossRef] [PubMed]
56. Summary of Recommendation Statements. *Kidney Int* **2013**, *3*, 5–14. [CrossRef] [PubMed]
57. Deutsch, E.W.; Bandeira, N.; Sharma, V.; Perez-Riverol, Y.; Carver, J.J.; Kundu, D.J.; Garcia-Seisdedos, D.; Jarnuczak, A.F.; Hewapathirana, S.; Pullman, B.S.; et al. The ProteomeXchange consortium in 2020: Enabling 'big data' approaches in proteomics. *Nucleic Acids Res.* **2019**. [CrossRef] [PubMed]
58. The UniProt Consortium. UniProt: The universal protein knowledgebase. *Nucleic Acids Res.* **2017**, *45*, D158–D169. [CrossRef]

59. Wisniewski, J.R.; Hein, M.Y.; Cox, J.; Mann, M. A "proteomic ruler" for protein copy number and concentration estimation without spike-in standards. *Mol. Cell. Proteomics* **2014**, *13*, 3497–3506. [CrossRef]
60. Andersen, C.L.; Jensen, J.L.; Orntoft, T.F. Normalization of real-time quantitative reverse transcription-PCR data: A model-based variance estimation approach to identify genes suited for normalization, applied to bladder and colon cancer data sets. *Cancer Res.* **2004**, *64*, 5245–5250. [CrossRef] [PubMed]
61. Ahn, H.S.; Sohn, T.S.; Kim, M.J.; Cho, B.K.; Kim, S.M.; Kim, S.T.; Yi, E.C.; Lee, C. SEPROGADIC—Serum protein-based gastric cancer prediction model for prognosis and selection of proper adjuvant therapy. *Sci. Rep.* **2018**, *8*, 16892. [CrossRef] [PubMed]
62. Saito, R.; Smoot, M.E.; Ono, K.; Ruscheinski, J.; Wang, P.L.; Lotia, S.; Pico, A.R.; Bader, G.D.; Ideker, T. A travel guide to Cytoscape plugins. *Nat. Methods* **2012**, *9*, 1069–1076. [CrossRef] [PubMed]
63. Barrett, T.; Edgar, R. Gene expression omnibus: Microarray data storage, submission, retrieval, and analysis. *Methods Enzymol.* **2006**, *411*, 352–369. [CrossRef] [PubMed]
64. Legendre, P. Comparison of permutation methods for the partial correlation and partial Mantel tests. *J Stat Comput. Sim.* **2000**, *67*, 37–73. [CrossRef]
65. Stacklies, W.; Redestig, H.; Scholz, M.; Walther, D.; Selbig, J. pcaMethods–a bioconductor package providing PCA methods for incomplete data. *Bioinformatics* **2007**, *23*, 1164–1167. [CrossRef]
66. Robin, X.; Turck, N.; Hainard, A.; Tiberti, N.; Lisacek, F.; Sanchez, J.C.; Muller, M. pROC: An open-source package for R and S+ to analyze and compare ROC curves. *BMC Bioinformatics* **2011**, *12*, 77. [CrossRef]
67. Kuhn, M. Building Predictive Models in R Using the caret Package. *J. Stat. Softw* **2008**, *28*, 1–26. [CrossRef]

15

Urinary Biomarkers for Diagnosis and Prediction of Acute Kidney Allograft Rejection

Francesco Guzzi [1,2,*], Luigi Cirillo [1,2], Elisa Buti [2], Francesca Becherucci [2], Carmela Errichiello [2], Rosa Maria Roperto [2], James P. Hunter [3] and Paola Romagnani [1,2]

1 Department of Experimental and Clinical Biomedical Sciences "Mario Serio", University of Florence, 50134 Florence, Italy; luigi.cirillo@unifi.it (L.C.); paola.romagnani@unifi.it (P.R.)
2 Nephrology and Dialysis Unit, Meyer Children's University Hospital, 50139 Florence, Italy; elisa.buti@meyer.it (E.B.); francesca.becherucci@meyer.it (F.B.); carmela.errichiello@meyer.it (C.E.); rosa.roperto@meyer.it (R.M.R.)
3 Nuffield Department of Surgical Sciences, Oxford Transplant Centre, Churchill Hospital, University of Oxford, Oxford OX3 7LJ, UK; james.hunter@nds.ox.ac.uk
* Correspondence: francesco.guzzi@gmail.com

Abstract: Noninvasive tools for diagnosis or prediction of acute kidney allograft rejection have been extensively investigated in recent years. Biochemical and molecular analyses of blood and urine provide a liquid biopsy that could offer new possibilities for rejection prevention, monitoring, and therefore, treatment. Nevertheless, these tools are not yet available for routine use in clinical practice. In this systematic review, MEDLINE was searched for articles assessing urinary biomarkers for diagnosis or prediction of kidney allograft acute rejection published in the last five years (from 1 January 2015 to 31 May 2020). This review follows the Preferred Reporting Items for Systematic Reviews and Meta-analysis (PRISMA) guidelines. Articles providing targeted or unbiased urine sample analysis for the diagnosis or prediction of both acute cellular and antibody-mediated kidney allograft rejection were included, analyzed, and graded for methodological quality with a particular focus on study design and diagnostic test accuracy measures. Urinary C-X-C motif chemokine ligands were the most promising and frequently studied biomarkers. The combination of precise diagnostic reference in training sets with accurate validation in real-life cohorts provided the most relevant results and exciting groundwork for future studies.

Keywords: kidney transplantation; kidney graft; T-cell-mediated rejection; antibody-mediated rejection; diagnostic test accuracy

---

1. Introduction

The growing call for precision medicine justifies a trend shift towards the implementation of new prognostic and diagnostic biomarkers in many fields of medicine. Progress in molecular and biomarker technology now permits the possibility to tailor and customize clinical and therapeutic approaches to the specific needs of a single patient, for a variety of medical conditions. Kidney diseases are no exception, with biomarkers constantly gaining more ground in the management of acute kidney injury (AKI), glomerulopathies, and chronic kidney disease (CKD) [1–3]. Also, in the setting of kidney transplantation, precision medicine is rapidly moving forward, with biomarkers a significant part of this trend. In kidney transplantation, biomarkers have been studied for early recognition and diagnosis of disease recurrence, delayed graft function (DGF), infections, and acute and chronic allograft rejection [4]. Since the 1970s, biomarkers have been studied for organ quality assessment prior to transplantation [5,6] and post-transplant evaluation [7]. However, in clinical practice, few genuine biomarkers have emerged, and clinicians still largely rely on serum creatinine and proteinuria monitoring. Novel biomarkers could be of great help not only for early recognition of allograft disease, but also for monitoring disease activity, optimizing the need for invasive biopsies, predicting the effectiveness and safety of a certain treatment, and tailoring the management of each single patient to their specific needs [4,8].

Despite near-optimal immunosuppressive regimens and accurate therapy compliance, kidney transplants still suffer from potentially preventable acute rejection (AR) episodes. AR early identification is important for preserving nephron mass and aiding long-term allograft survival [9]. The gold standard for AR diagnosis is histological examination of a kidney biopsy. The biopsy can then be interpreted with the help of the Banff classification (created in the 1990s and periodically revised), which describes acute lesions according to two mechanistic pathways: T-cell-mediated rejection (TCMR) and antibody-mediated rejection (ABMR) [10]. However, a biopsy is an invasive procedure, may not be straightforward to perform and can be complicated by major bleeding. In addition, potential sampling errors, inter-observer variability, and elevated costs make allograft biopsy impractical for continuous monitoring of the graft over time. Urine samples, as a readily available and direct product of the allograft, with minimal influence from systemic inflammation, are a more desirable source for AR biomarkers. Very recently, narrative reviews explored the use of biomarkers in the diagnosis of AR [11,12]. However, to our knowledge, the most recent systematic review assessing urinary biomarkers' ability for allograft AR diagnosis in kidney transplant patients included papers published until 2015 [7]. The most relevant articles and findings in the field before 2015 have been also thoroughly summarized elsewhere [13–15]. Up to 2015, no urinary biomarker was validated in sufficiently robust trials to be translated into clinical practice independent of traditional surveillance and diagnostic methods.

The aim of this systematic review is to perform a methodical analysis and to summarize important results coming from the most recent literature (2015–present) evaluating urinary biomarkers and their performance as diagnostic and/or predictive tools for kidney allograft acute rejection.

2. Results

2.1. Included Studies

The original literature search yielded a total of 314 citations. Of these, 251 studies were discarded after evaluation of title and abstract in the eligibility process. The remaining 63 studies were reviewed full-text for inclusion in the study. Twenty-five studies were excluded, as detailed in Figure 1.

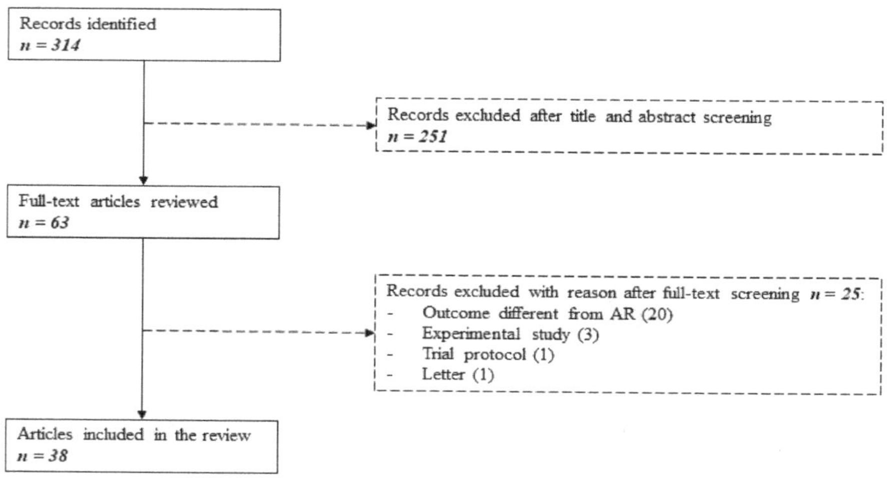

Figure 1. Search flowchart as per PRISMA guidelines. Three hundred fourteen studies were identified searching MEDLINE between January 2015 and May 2020. After evaluating for eligibility and inclusion, 38 articles were selected.

The main reason for exclusion was the evaluation of a different outcome instead of AR (e.g., chronic or late rejection, graft dysfunction, graft failure). Experimental studies, one trial protocol, and one letter were also excluded. A total of 38 remaining articles, published between 1 January 2015 and 31 May 2020, were finally included. No additional articles were included from the reference lists.

2.2. Study Characteristics

Table 1 summarizes the most relevant characteristics of each of the 38 included studies. Twenty-nine were single center studies, while nine were multicenter collaborations. Among the 32 studies assessing urinary biomarkers in the diagnosis of acute rejection, the majority of them, 18/32, were designed as case-control, while 14/32 as cross-sectional studies. Among the six studies assessing the ability of urinary biomarkers to predict acute rejection at variable time-points before the episode, five studies analyzed prospectively collected data and one study analyzed retrospectively collected data. Population characteristics, patient selection protocols, inclusion and exclusion criteria, as well as sample size, were heterogeneous between studies. Sample size varied from 15 to 396 kidney transplant patients, and occasionally more than one urine sample was obtained from the same patient. Although all of the included studies were published after January 2015, some of them enrolled patients transplanted from the early 2000's. Table 1 also highlights the year of study population enrolment to help the identification of possibly overlapping populations and to assess the appropriateness of the Banff classification used in each study. The majority of the included studies applied up to date Banff classification, with ten studies apparently using the 1997 version or not reporting the year. Using an outdated classification could be a source of bias mostly for studies assessing ABMR, as discussed later. For one study, the application of the Banff classification was not clearly stated. Studies were also heterogeneous in terms of the considered outcome. Among the 38 included studies, 15 specifically addressed TCMR only, whereas just two exclusively focused on ABMR. Sixteen studies assessed the combination of TCMR and ABMR, while five studies did not specify the characteristics of the observed acute rejection (Table 1).

Table 1. Description of the study characteristics. The table summarizes the main characteristics of the 38 included studies.

Ref	Study Design	Single/Multicenter	Patients (n)	Enrolment (years)	Urinary Biomarker(s)	Ref. Standard	Outcome
Tinel [16]	Cross-sectional	Single center	329	2011–2016	CXCL9, CXCL10	Banff '15	TCMR, ABMR
Yang [17]	Cross-sectional	Multicenter	364	2010–2018	*Q score*	Banff '17	TCMR, ABMR
Kalantari [18]	Case-control	Single center	22	2016–2018	Unbiased metabolomics [1]	Banff '97	TCMR
Verma [19]	Case-control	Single center	53	N/R	RNA-Seq signature	Banff '17	TCMR
Goerlich [20]	Case-control	Single center	39	2016–2017	T cells, TEC, PDX	Banff '13	TCMR, ABMR
Banas [21]	Cross-sectional	Single center	109	2011–2012	Unbiased metabolomics [2]	Banff '09	TCMR, ABMR
Tajima [22]	Cross-sectional	Single center	80	2014–2016	LC3, CCL2, LFABP, NGAL, HE4	Banff '09	TCMR, ABMR
Kolling [23]	Case-control	Single center	93	N/R	Circular RNAs	Banff '09	TCMR
Sigdel [24]	Cross-sectional	Multicenter	150	2000–2016	*uCRM score*	Banff '09	TCMR, ABMR
Kim [25]	Case-control	Multicenter	23	N/R	Unbiased metabolomics [3]	Banff '07	TCMR
Ciftci [26] *	Prospective	Single center	85	2014–2017	CXCL9, CXCL10	Banff '13	TCMR, ABMR
Banas [27]	Case-control	Single center	358	2008–2010; 2015–2016	Unbiased metabolomics [2]	Banff '97	TCMR
Lim [28]	Case-control	Multicenter	47	2013–2015	Exosome proteins	Banff '07	TCMR
Chen [29]	Case-control	Single center	49	2006–2009	CXCL13	Banff '97	TCMR, ABMR
Barabadi [30] §	Cross-sectional	Single center	91	2013–2015	FOXP3	Banff '13	AR
Mockler [31] *§	Prospective	Single center	38	N/R	CCL2	Banff '13	TCMR
Ciftci [32] *	Prospective	Single center	65	2013–2015	TNFα	Banff '97	AR
Park [33]	Case-control	Single center	44	N/R	Exosome proteins	Banff (N/R)	TCMR
Millan [34] *	Prospective	Multicenter	80	N/R	miR-155-5p, CXCL10	Banff '97	TCMR

Table 1. *Cont.*

Ref	Study Design	Single/Multicenter	Patients (*n*)	Enrolment (years)	Urinary Biomarker(s)	Ref. Standard	Outcome
Seo [35]	Case-control	Multicenter	88	2013–2015	*CTOT4 formula*	Banff (N/R)	TCMR, ABMR
Gandolfini [36] §	Case-control	Multicenter	56	N/R	CXCL9	Banff '13	TCMR
Chen [37]	Case-control	Single center	156	2006–2009	sTim3	Banff '97	TCMR, ABMR
Domenico [38] §	Case-control	Single center	49	N/R	miRNA-142-3p	Banff '07	AR
Lee [39] §	Case-control	Single center	34	N/R	Donor-derived cfDNA	unclear	AR
Seeman [40] §	Case-control	Single center	15	2013–2014	NGAL	Banff '09	TCMR, ABMR
Blydt-H. [41]	Cross-sectional	Multicenter	59	2002–N/R	*ABMR score*	Banff '13	ABMR
Belmar V. [42] *	Retrospective	Single center	86	2012–2015	Albumin	Banff (N/R)	ABMR
Raza [43]	Cross-sectional	Single center	300	2009–2014	CCL2	Banff '97	TCMR
Galichon [44]	Cross-sectional	Multicenter	108	N/R	*CTOT4 formula*	Banff '09	TCMR, ABMR
Sigdel [45]	Cross-sectional	Single center	396	2000–2011	Unbiased proteomics	Banff '07	TCMR, ABMR
Garcìa-C. [46] §	Cross-sectional	Single center	50	N/R	IL10, IFNγ	Banff '09	TCMR, ABMR
Ho [47] §	Cross-sectional	Single center	133	N/R	MMP7, CXCL10	Banff '07	TCMR
A. Elaziz [48]	Cross-sectional	Single center	54	2011–2014	PD1, FOXP3	Banff '07	TCMR
Lorenzen [49]	Cross-sectional	Single center	93	N/R	LncRNAs	Banff '09	TCMR
Rabant [50] *	Prospective	Single center	300	2010–2012	CXCL9, CXCL10	Banff '07	TCMR, ABMR
Rabant [51]	Cross-sectional	Single center	244	2011–2013	CXCL9, CXCL10	Banff '07	TCMR, ABMR
Blydt-H. [52]	Cross-sectional	Single center	51	2002–N/R	CXCL10	Banff '07	TCMR
Sigdel [53] §	Case-control	Single center	30	2000–2009	Exosome proteins	Banff '07	AR

Unbiased metabolomics: [1] (NAD, NADP, nicotinic acid, MNA, GABA, cholesterol sulfate, homocysteine); [2] (alanine, citrate, lactate, urea); [3] (guanidoacetic acid, methylimidazoleacetic acid, dopamine, 4-guanidinobutyric acid, and L-tryptophan). * Prediction study; § Diagnostic Test Accuracy analysis not present. N/R, not reported.

2.3. Biomarkers

The included studies were split into diagnostic and prediction studies. To be considered a diagnostic study, the collection of a urine sample should be performed on the day that AR was suspected or when per-protocol biopsies were planned. There were a few exceptions to this rule where sample collection occasionally occurred up to seven days before biopsy. For prediction studies, urine samples were collected at any time point post-transplant and, in this analysis, these ranged from day one up to six months post-transplantation. Among the various techniques for targeted analysis of known urinary biomarkers, ELISA and RT-PCR were the most frequently utilized. Mass spectrometry, nuclear magnetic resonance spectroscopy, liquid chromatography, RNA expression, and transcriptome analysis by RNA-Seq were employed for unbiased metabolomics, proteomics, and genomic profiling and for detection and identification of urinary exosome proteins. All biomarkers are detailed per category in Table 2.

In accordance with previous studies, the most extensively assessed urinary biomarkers were C-X-C motif chemokine ligand 9 (CXCL9) and 10 (CXCL10), usually adjusted for urinary creatinine concentration. In detail, 12/38 (32%) studies either addressed CXCL9 and CXCL10 alone, in combination, or in the context of particular scores or formulas [16,17,24,26,34–36,44,47,50–52]. Other directly targeted cytokines and interleukins were chemokine ligand 2 (CCL2), also known as monocyte chemoattractant protein 1 [22,31,43], CXCL13 [29], interleukin 10 (IL10) with interferon gamma (IFNγ) [46] and tumor necrosis factor alpha (TNFα) [32].

Table 2. Urinary biomarkers. Table illustrating all urinary biomarkers divided per category and in alphabetic order. Specific formulas and scores are also detailed.

Category	Biomarkers
Cytokines	
Chemokines	CCL2, CXCL9, CXCL10, CXCL13
Other	IFNγ, IL10, TNFα
Metabolites	
Nucleotides	NAD, NADP
Amino acids and Organic acids	Alanine, Citrate, GABA, 4-Guanidinobutyric Acid, Guanidoacetic Acid, Homocysteine, Lactate, Methylimidazoleacetic Acid, Nicotinic Acid, L-Tryptophan
Other small molecules	Cholesterol Sulfate, Dopamine, MNA, Urea
Proteins	Albumin, LFAPB, HE4, LC3, MMP7, NGAL, sTIM3, Urinary extracellular vesicle (exosome) proteins (HPX, TSPAN1)
RNAs	Circular RNAs, FOXP3 mRNA, LncRNAs, PD1 mRNA, RNA-seq
micro RNAs	miR-142-3p, miR-155-5p
Urinary Cells	CD4+/CD8+ T cells, CD10+/EPCAM+ cells, PDX+ cells, TEC
Scores and Formulas	
ABMR score [41]	Signature of 133 unique metabolites
CTOT-4 formula [54]	CD3ε mRNA + CXCL10 mRNA + 18S rRNA
Q score [17]	Cell-free DNA + Clusterin + Creatinine + CXCL10 + Methylated Cell-free DNA + Total Urinary Protein
uCRM score [24]	11 genes expression score on urinary cell pellet (including CXCL9 and CXCL10)

Unbiased metabolomic analysis and untargeted profiling revealed multiple urinary metabolites as potential biomarkers of AR: nicotinamide adenine dinucleotide (NAD), nicotinamide adenine dinucleotide phosphate (NADP), nicotinic acid, 1-methylnicotinamide (MNA), gamma-aminobutyric acid (GABA), cholesterol sulfate, homocysteine [18], the combination of alanine, citrate, lactate, and urea [21,27], and the combination of guanidoacetic acid, methylimidazoleacetic acid, dopamine, 4-guanidinobutyric acid, and L-tryptophan [25].

Urinary proteins of interest were neutrophil gelatinase-associated lipocalin (NGAL) [22,40], liver-type fatty acid-binding protein (LFABP) [22], human epididymis protein 4 (HE4) [22], matrix metalloproteinase 7 (MMP7) [47], soluble T cell immunoglobulin mucin domain 3 (sTIM3) [37]. The presence and diagnostic performance of urinary extracellular vesicle (exosome) proteins, derived from inflammatory cells and collected with the help of nano-membrane or immune-magnetic capture, was investigated by three studies [28,32,52].

Direct RT-PCR was used to identify targeted RNAs like programmed cell death protein1 (PD1) mRNA, forkhead box P3 (FOXP3) mRNA, and micro (mi) RNAs (miR-142-3p, miR-155-5p) [30,34,38,48], while genome-wide or transcriptome analysis were applied for the unbiased identification of circular and long noncoding RNAs [23,49].

The amount of urinary CD4+ and CD8+ T cells, tubular epithelial cells (TEC), podocalyxin (PDX)-positive, CD10+ or epithelial cell adhesion molecule (EPCAM)-positive cells was determined by flow cytometry and compared with biopsy results [20].

Two studies [35,44] investigated the diagnostic accuracy of the *CTOT4 formula* (CXCL10 mRNA, CD3ε mRNA, 18S rRNA), previously validated by the CTOT-4 (clinical trials in organ transplantation-4) multicenter study group [54]. CXCL10 was also included in newly derived scores such as the *Q score*, composed of six DNA, protein, and metabolite urinary biomarkers (cell-free DNA, methylated cell-free DNA, clusterin, total protein, creatinine, and CXCL10) [17], while CXCL9 and CXCL10 genes were included in the *uCRM score* [24]. Finally, the *ABMR score* comprised more than 130 unique metabolites [41].

2.4. Quality Assessment

Studies reporting diagnostic test accuracy (DTA) analysis (29/38) were graded for risk of bias and applicability concerns according to the QUADAS-2 tool (Table 3). Risk of bias was frequently high for patient selection (14/29, 48%) and index test (23/29, 79%).

Table 3. QUADAS-2 tool assessment for DTA studies. Table illustrating risk of bias and applicability concerns evaluation as per QUADAS-2 tool for 29 studies providing diagnostic test accuracy data.

Ref	Risk of Bias				Applicability Concerns		
	Patient Selection	Index Test	Reference Standard	Flow and Timing	Patient Selection	Index Test	Reference Standard
Tinel [16]	☺	☺	☺	☺	☺	☺	☺
Yang [17]	☺	☺	☺	☺	☺	☺	☺
Kalantari [18]	☹	☹	☺	?	☹	☹	☺
Verma [19]	☹	☹	☺	☺	☹	☺	☺
Goerlich [20]	☹	☹	☺	☺	☹	☺	☺
Banas [21]	☺	☺	☺	?	☺	☺	☺
Tajima [22]	☺	☹	☺	☺	☹	☺	☺
Kolling [23]	☹	☹	☺	☺	☹	☺	☺
Sigdel [24]	☺	☹	☺	☺	☺	☺	☺
Kim [25]	☹	☹	☺	☺	☹	☺	☺
Ciftci [26] *	☹	☹	☺	?	☹	☺	☺
Banas [27]	☹	☹	☺	☺	☹	☺	☺
Lim [28]	☹	☹	☺	☺	☹	☺	☺
Chen [29]	☹	☹	?	☺	☹	☺	☺
Ciftci [31] *	☹	☹	?	?	☹	☺	☺
Park [33]	☹	☺	☺	☺	☹	☺	☺
Millan [34] *	?	☹	☺	?	☺	☺	☺
Seo [35]	☹	☹	☺	☹	☹	☺	☺
Chen [37]	☹	☹	?	☺	☹	☺	☺
Blydt-H. [41]	☺	☺	☺	☺	☺	☺	☺
Belm.V. [42] *	☹	☹	?	☺	☹	☺	☺
Raza [43]	☺	☹	☺	☹	☹	☺	☺
Galichon [44]	☺	☹	?	☺	☺	☺	☺
Sigdel [45]	☺	☺	☺	☺	☺	☺	☺
A. Elaziz [48]	?	☹	☺	☺	☺	☺	☺
Lorenzen [49]	☺	☹	☺	☺	☺	☺	☺
Rabant [50] *	☺	☹	☺	☺	☺	☺	☺
Rabant [51]	☺	☹	☺	☺	☺	☺	☺
Blydt-H. [52]	☺	☹	☺	☹	☺	☺	☺

*, Prediction study; ☺, Low Risk; ☹, High Risk; ?, Unclear Risk.

The most frequent reasons for high risk of bias were the selection of the study population by case-control design, which was the case for the majority of the studies, the exclusion of the typical confounding of a real-life setting, the absence of threshold definition and independent validation. For example, when control patients were selected among stable patients without performing allograft biopsy, or only among normal histology patients, and the obtained thresholds were not tested in a randomly selected validation group, the study was highlighted for high risk of bias in patient selection and index test (Table 3). This then raised the possibility of an increased risk of over-fitting association and unrealistic DTA performance and, therefore, concerns for applicability. The ideal control patients were randomly (or in a cross-sectional fashion) selected, all having had an allograft biopsy (per indication or per protocol) with various histological diagnosis (e.g., normal histology; acute tubular necrosis, ATN; interstitial fibrosis and tubular atrophy, IFTA; chronic allograft nephropathy, CAN; BK virus nephropathy, BKVN; recurrence of the primary disease on the allograft). Only 5/29 studies were found to have a low risk of bias in both patient selection and index test. Allograft histology, according to Banff classification, was the reference standard for AR diagnosis, with histology grading usually assigned in a blinded fashion with respect to the index test results. Since urinary samples were frequently obtained for all included patients, prior to a diagnostic allograft biopsy, and all included patients were evaluated in the DTA analysis, a low risk of bias was frequently identified in the flow and timing domain. The QUADAS-2 tool does not include publication bias (PB) as one of the variables and, in the context of this review, it is difficult to formally assess PB. Given the broad variety of different biomarkers that were assessed and the absence of a meta-analysis, performing formal PB assessment such as Egger's test, Deek's test or the construction of a funnel plot was not possible. It is also recognized that the assessment of PB in data synthesis of DTA data is challenging with limited reliability [55].

2.5. *Summary of the Results*

Tables 4–6 provide a detailed summary of each study results. When DTA analysis was available (29 studies), the results are summarized in Table 4 for diagnostic studies (24/38) and Table 5 for prediction studies (5/38). Descriptive results from the remaining nine studies are briefly reported in Table 6. For each DTA study, the particular outcome of interest and characteristics of the control population are reported with sample size for each group included in the final DTA analysis. The urinary biomarker of interest, thresholds (when available) and test design (training, validation, or particular comparisons between groups) are also detailed. For prediction studies, time from transplantation to urinary biomarker analysis is also reported (between 1 day to 6 months post-transplantation). Sensitivity, specificity, positive and negative predictive values (PPV, NPV), and area under the receiver operating characteristic curve (AUC) are reported as measures of diagnostic test accuracy when available (Tables 4 and 5) and results are in bold text when arising from validation cohorts. Results confirmation in at least one validation cohort was available in less than one third of studies (7/29, 24%). Of these, two were case-control studies [25,33], while the others were the previously mentioned five cross-sectional studies with the lowest risk of bias score [16,17,21,41,45]. Sensitivity and specificity values were highly variable between studies, ranging from 9% to 100% and from 34% and 100%, respectively. PPV and NPV were also variable, ranging from 15% to 98% and from 32% to 100%, respectively.

Table 4. Summary of the study results—Diagnostic studies with DTA. This table shows the outcome of diagnostic studies. Outcome and control group for the DTA analysis are reported (sample size when available), followed by test design, studied urinary biomarker(s), and thresholds when provided.

Ref.	Outcome (*n*)	Control Group (*n*)	Test Design, Biomarkers, Thresholds	Diagnostic Test Accuracy (95%CI)				
				Sens.	Spec.	PPV	NPV	AUC–Accuracy(%)
Tinel [16]	TCMR (17), ABMR (64), mixed (14)	ALL-B (normal, 21; IFTA, 154; BKVN, 23; ATN, 11; recurrent disease, 9; other, 78)	CXCL9 + CXCL10 for AR	62%	72%	41%	86%	**0.70 (0.64–0.76)**
			CXCL9 + CXCL10 for TCMR	79%	74%	21%	98%	**0.81 (0.73–0.89)**
			CXCL9 + CXCL10 for ABMR	72%	54%	28%	88%	**0.67 (0.61–0.74)**
Yang [17]	TCMR + ABMR (103)	ALL-B (normal, 170; bAR, 50; BKVN, 9)	Training: AR vs normal (Q score ≥ 32)	95%	100%	-	-	0.99 (0.99–1.00)
			Validation 1: AR vs normal	91%	92%	-	-	**0.98 (0.96–1.00)**
			Validation 2: AR vs normal	100%	96%	-	-	**1.00 (1.00–1.00)**
			All AR vs All normal	95%	96%	87%	98%	**0.99(0.98–0.99)**
			All AR vs ALL-B	-	-	-	-	**0.96 (0.94–0.98)**
Kalantari [18]	TCMR (7)	DYS-B (normal, 15)	Unbiased metab.[1]	67–71%	40–100%	-	-	0.51–0.71
Verma [19]	TCMR (22)	ALL-B (normal, 28)	13-gene urinary cell signature	-	-	-	-	0.92 (0.85–0.99)
Goerlich [20]	TCMR (14) + ABMR (7)	DYS-B (normal, 18)	T cells + total TEC	-	-	-	-	0.90
			T cells + CD10+ TEC	-	-	-	-	0.89
			T cells + ECPAM+ TEC	-	-	-	-	0.91
			T cells + PDX+ cells	-	-	-	-	0.89
Banas [21]	TCMR + ABMR + mixed	ALL-B (normal) + STA	Unbiased metab.[2]	-	-	-	-	0.75 (0.68–0.83)
			Score = 3.0	91% (79–98)	34% (30–38)	-	-	-
			Score = 13.0	48% (33–63)	89% (86–91)	-	-	-
	+ bAR	+ (IFTA + other)		-	-	-	-	**0.71 (0.64–0.79)**
Tajima [22]	TCMR + ABMR (subclinical, 11)	STA-B (normal or borderline AR, 69)	LC3 (517.9 pg/mg)	64% (31–89)	78% (67–87)	32%	93%	0.73 (0.55–0.90)
			CCL2 (226.0 pg/mg)	82% (48–98)	57% (44–68)	23%	95%	0.69 (0.54–0.84)
			L-FABP (7.6 ng/mg)	9% (0–41)	88% (78–94)	15%	100%	0.61 (0.45–0.77)
			NGAL (12.8 ng/mg)	100% (72–100)	48% (36–60)	23%	100%	0.72 (0.59–0.84)
			HE4 (789.1 ng/mg)	100% (72–100)	54% (41–66)	26%	100%	0.81 (0.70–0.92)
Kolling [23]	TCMR (11; subclinical, 51)	STA-B (normal, 31)	hsa_circ_0001334 (2.41)	70% (59–80)	92% (64–100)	98%	32%	0.85 ($p < 0.0001$)
Sigdel [24]	TCMR + ABMR (45)	ALL-B (normal, 43; bAR, 19; BKVN, 43)	AR vs normal (uCRM score = 3.63)	95%	98%	-	-	0.99, $p < 0.0001$

Table 4. *Cont.*

Ref.	Outcome (*n*)	Control Group (*n*)	Test Design, Biomarkers, Thresholds	Diagnostic Test Accuracy (95%CI)				
				Sens.	Spec.	PPV	NPV	AUC–Accuracy(%)
			AR vs normal + bAR	87%	98%	-	-	-
			AR vs normal + bAR + BKVN	77%	98%	-	-	96.6%
			Unbiased metab.[3]	-	-	-	-	-
Kim [25]	TCMR (14)	STA-B (normal, 17)	Training: TCMR (10) vs STA-B (13)	90%	85%	-	-	0.93 (0.72–1.00) - 87%
			Validation: TCMR (4) vs STA-B (4)	-	-	-	-	**62.5%**
Banas [27]	TCMR	ALL-B (normal) + STA (extended)	Unbiased metab.[2], train (180)	-	-	-	-	0.76 (0.69–0.82)
			Test (178) strict/extended cohort	-	-	-	-	0.72 (0.58–0.86)/ 0.74 (0.62–0.86)
Lim [28]	TCMR (25)	STA-B (normal, 22)	TSPAN1 + HPX	64%	73%	-	-	0.74
Chen [29]	TCMR (37) + ABMR (12)	ALL-B (normal, 58; CAN, 29; ATN, 10)	CXCL13 for AR vs. normal	84%	79%	-	-	0.82 (0.73–0.90)
			CXCL13 for AR vs. CAN + ATN	-	-	-	-	0.63 (0.52–0.75)
			iKEA					
Park [33]	TCMR (22)	DYS-B (normal, 22)	Training: TCMR (15) vs normal (15)	93%	88%	-	-	0.91 ± 0.02 - 90%
			Validation: TCMR (7) vs normal (7)	64%	100%	-	-	**0.84 ± 0.11 - 71%**
Seo [35]	TCMR (27) + ABMR (13)	STA-B (normal, 17); STA (22)	CTOT4 formula	-	-	-	-	0.72 (0.60–0.83)
			CXCL10 mRNA	-	-	-	-	0.72 (0.60–0.83)
			CD3ε mRNA	-	-	-	-	0.71 (0.60–0.83)
			18S rRNA	-	-	-	-	0.47 (0.33–0.60)
Chen [37]	TCMR (37) + ABMR (12)	STA-B (normal, 58)	sTim-3 (1.836 ng/mmol)	90%	83%	-	-	0.88 (0.81–0.95)
Blydt-H. [41]	ABMR (10)	ALL-B (normal, TCMR, transplant glomerulopathy, IFTA, other, 49)	ABMR score = 0.23	78%	83%	40%	96%	0.84 (0.77–0.91)
			ABMR score with top 10 metabolites	-	-	-	-	0.80 (0.73–0.88)
			Validation	-	-	-	-	**0.76 (0.67–0.84)**
Raza [43]	TCMR (acute, 101; borderline, 47; vascular, 17)	DYS-B (normal, 47; IFTA, 46) + STA (42)	CCL2 (198 pg/mL)	87%	62%	-	-	0.81 (0.76–0.86)
Galichon [44]	TCMR (11) + bAR (3) + ABMR (28) + mixed (9)	ALL-B (56)	CTOT4 formula	-	-	-	-	0.72 (0.61–0.82)
			CXCL10 mRNA	-	-	-	-	0.76 (0.66–0.86)
			CD3ε mRNA	-	-	-	-	0.67 (0.56–0.78)
			18S rRNA	-	-	-	-	0.63 (0.53–0.74)

Table 4. *Cont.*

Ref.	Outcome (*n*)	Control Group (*n*)	Test Design, Biomarkers, Thresholds	Diagnostic Test Accuracy (95%CI)				
				Sens.	Spec.	PPV	NPV	AUC–Accuracy(%)
Sigdel [45]	TCMR + ABMR (42)	ALL-B (normal, 47; CAN, 46; BKVN, 16)	Unbiased proteomics (11 peptides) Validation: AR (20) vs normal (27), CAN (15), BKVN (16)	-	-	-	-	**0.94 (0.93–0.95)**
A. Elaziz [48]	TCMR (31)	STA-B (normal, 23)	PD1 mRNA (2.6)	80%	84%	-	-	0.81
			FOXP3 mRNA (1.5)	83%	90%	-	-	0.91
			PD1 + FOXP3 mRNA	94%	97%	-	-	0.98
Lorenzen [49]	TCMR (11; subclinical 51)	STA-B (normal, 31)	RNA L328 (9.556)	49%	96%	49%	93%	0.76 ($p < 0.001$)
Rabant [51]	TCMR (10) + ABMR (37) + mixed (31)	DYS-B (203)	CXCL9	58%	85%	59%	84%	0.71 (0.64–0.78)
			CXCL10	59%	83%	58%	84%	0.74 (0.68–0.80)
Blydt-H. [52]	TCMR (subclinical, 17; clinical, 9)	ALL-B (normal, 21; IFTA, 31)	CXCL10, subclinical (4.82 ng/mL)	59%	67%	-	-	0.81 (0.70–0.92)
			Clinical (4.72 ng/mL)	77%	60%	-	-	0.88 (0.73–1.0)

Results from a validation group are shown in **bold**. Unbiased metabolomics: [1] (NAD, NADP, nicotinic acid, MNA, GABA, cholesterol sulfate, homocysteine); [2] (alanine, citrate, lactate, urea); [3] (guanidoacetic acid, methylimidazoleacetic acid, dopamine, 4-guanidinobutyric acid, and L-tryptophan). ALL, all patients irrespectively of allograft function (-B, biopsied); DYS, dysfunctional graft patients (-B, biopsied); STA, stable graft patients (-B, biopsied).

Table 5. Summary of the study results—Predictive studies with DTA. This table shows the outcome of prediction studies. Outcome and control group for the DTA analysis are reported (sample size when available), followed by the studied urinary biomarker(s), thresholds and time from transplant to test.

Ref.	Outcome (n)	Control Group (*n*)	Biomarkers, Thresholds and Time Post-Transplant	Diagnostic Test Accuracy (95%CI)				
				Sens.	Spec.	PPV	NPV	AUC
Ciftci [26]	TCMR (9) + ABMR (6)	STA (70)	CXCL9, 1 day - 3 months	70–85%	37–88%	60–71%	71–90%	0.71–0.95
			CXCL10, 1 day - 3 months	78–82%	58–85%	59–73%	74–87%	0.75–0.97
			TNF-α (12.08 pg/mL), 1 day	71%	57%	-	-	0.74 (0.51–0.97)
Ciftci [32]	AR (9)	STA (56)	TNF-α (11.03), 7 days	100%	84%	-	-	0.95 (0.88–1.00)
			TNF-α (9.85), 1 month	100%	83%	-	-	0.91 (0.81–1.00)
			TNF-α (9.13), 3 months	100%	71%	-	-	0.83 (0.75–0.98)
			TNF-α (7.42), 6 months	100%	62%	-	-	0.82 (0.69–0.95)
Millan [34]	TCMR (8)	STA (72)	miR-155-5p (0.51), 1wk-6m	85%	86%	88%	100%	0.88 (0.78–0.97)
			CXCL10 (84.73 pg/mL),1wk-6m	84%	80%	90%	85%	0.87 (0.81–0.92)
			CXCL10:Cr (0.43), 1wk-6m	72%	73%	90%	96%	0.75 (0.67–0.83)
Belm.V. [42]	ABMR (subclinical)	ALL-B	Albuminuria (> 30 mg/g), 6m	-	-	-	-	0.75 (0.55–0.95)
Rabant [50]	AR (TCMR + ABMR + mixed, 76)	ALL-B	CXCL9:Cr (1.78 ng/mmoL),10d	61%	50%	24%	84%	0.58 (0.47–0.68)
			CXCL9:Cr (0.96), 1 month	81%	35%	23%	89%	0.50 (0.37–0.62)
			CXCL9:Cr (1.67), 3 months	57%	62%	18%	91%	0.57 (0.39–0.75)
			CXCL10:Cr (4.80), 10 days	57%	52%	23%	83%	0.54 (0.43–0.65)
			CXCL10:Cr (2.79), 1 month	83%	51%	29%	93%	0.72 (0.61–0.80)
			CXCL10:Cr (5.32), 3 months	54%	77%	25%	92%	0.68 (0.55–0.80)

ALL, all patients irrespectively of allograft function (-B, biopsied); STA, stable graft patients (-B, biopsied).

2.5.1. Acute Rejection Diagnosis

Among studies with the lowest risk of bias, only three studies [16,17,45] yielded a very good (0.8–0.9) or excellent (> 0.9) performance as diagnostic AUC (Table 4). All of these studies provided diagnostic accuracy measure for the diagnosis of AR, considering both TCMR and ABMR as outcome of interest. Tinel et al. found that the combination of urinary CXCL9 and CXCL10 could distinguish AR patients among almost three-hundred heterogeneous patients with an AUC of 0.70 [16]. These results strengthened the good performance previously described, among dysfunctional allografts, separately for CXCL9 (AUC 0.71) and CXCL10 (AUC 0.74) by Rabant and colleagues [51]. Yang et al. separately validated the so-called *Q score* in two validation cohorts for the diagnosis of AR. A *Q score* ≥ 32 maintained an excellent diagnostic performance (AUC 0.96) also when validated in the entire study population (n = 364), with high PPV and NPV (87–98%) [17]. Banas et al., after identifying a urinary metabolite signature with good diagnostic performance for TCMR [27], validated it in a cohort of 109 patients for the diagnosis of AR with and AUC of 0.71 [21]. Through unbiased metabolomics, Sigdel et al. identified a signature of eleven urinary peptides able to segregate AR patients from normal histology, chronic allograft nephropathy and BK virus nephropathy patients with an excellent AUC of 0.94 in validation cohort [45]. The same authors proved a urine cell sediment gene expression-based score (*uCRM score*) able to diagnose AR with 96.6% accuracy and potentially quantify the degree of injury [24].

Table 6. Summary of the study results—Studies with no DTA. This table describes the main results from studies with no DTA. Sample size is reported for the outcome and control group when available.

Ref.	Outcome (n)	Control Group (*n*)	Biomarkers, Thresholds and Main Results
Barabadi [30]	AR (27)	ALL-B (normal, 45; CAN, 19)	FOXP3 mRNA expression was significantly higher in AR (***p* < 0.001**)
Mockler [31] *	TCMR (5; borderline, 3)	STA-B	There was no significant association between 6 months post-transplant CCL2 and TCMR changes ($p = 0.46$)
Gandolfini [36]	TCMR (22)	ALL-B (normal, 19)	CXCL9 > 200 pg/mL in TCMR, 100-200 in dysfunction graft, and < 100 pg/mL in stable graft (***p* < 0.01**)
Domenico [38]	AR (23)	ALL-B (ATN, 18; normal, 8)	mirRNA 142-3p was significantly higher in AR compared to stable graft (***p* < 0.001**); not compared to ATN (***p* = 0.079**)
Lee [39]	AR (8)	STA (8); DYS-B (ATN, 8; other, 4)	Donor-derived cfDNA was not significantly different between groups ($p = 0.95$)
Seeman [40]	TCMR (2) + ABMR (2)	DYS-B (11)	NGAL was not significantly different between groups ($p = 0.48$)
Garcìa-C. [46]	AR (9)	ALL-B (fibrosis, 31; other, 10)	IL10 and IFNγ were not significantly different between groups ($p = 0.95$, $p = 0.1$)
Ho [47]	TCMR (17; subclinical, 17)	ALL-B (normal, 22)	MMP7 and CXCL10 were significantly elevated in subclinical (***p* = 0.01, *p* < 0.0001**) and clinical (***p* < 0.001**) TCMR
Sigdel [53]	AR (10)	DYS-B (IFTA, BKVN, 20)	Ten urinary exosomal proteins were significantly increased in AR (***p* < 0.05**)

Statistically significant ($p < 0.05$) results are shown in **bold**. * Prediction study. ALL, all patients irrespectively of allograft function (-B, biopsied); DYS, dysfunctional graft patients (-B, biopsied); STA, stable graft patients (-B, biopsied).

2.5.2. T-Cell-Mediated Rejection Diagnosis

The previously mentioned study by Tinel et al. also provided separate outcome analysis for CXCL9 and CXCL10, with the best performance for TCMR diagnosis with a NPV of 98% and a very good AUC of 0.81 [16]. Also of note, CCL2, at a threshold level of 198 pg/mL, yielded very good performance (AUC 0.81) for TCMR identification among a population of 300 normal and dysfunctional grafts in the study by Raza et al. [43]. Urinary exosome proteins were investigated in two case-control studies for the diagnosis of TCMR. Lim et al. found significantly higher urinary tetraspanin-1 (TSPAN1) and hemopexin (HPX) expression levels in TCMR patients with good diagnostic performance (AUC 0.74) [28], while Park et al. reported the initial results of an optimized integrated kidney exosome analysis (iKEA) able to distinguish TCMR from normal histology patients, with a very good performance (AUC 0.84) in a small validation cohort [33].

2.5.3. Antibody-Mediated Rejection Diagnosis

The study from Blydt-Hansen et al. was the only one to specifically evaluate the diagnostic performance for ABMR diagnosis [41]. The authors tested and validated the use of the *ABMR score*, with a good sensitivity (78%) and specificity (83%), NPV of 96%, a good performance (AUC 0.76 in validation), and the ability to provide a stratification from negative—indeterminate—to positive ABMR patients [41].

2.5.4. Acute Rejection, TCMR, and ABMR Prediction

Among prediction studies (Table 5), high risk of bias was often identified for patient selection and index test. However, good performances for AR prediction were obtained by three months post-transplant for CXCL9 and CXCL10 levels [26], and seven days and one month post-transplant for TNF-alpha levels [32]. The well-conducted study by Rabant et al. found both urinary CXCL9 and CXCL10, adjusted for urinary creatinine concentration, to have high NPV (89 to 93%) for AR at one and three months post-transplantation. CXCL10 yielded the best predictive performance (AUC 0.72) at one month post-transplantation, at the threshold of 2.79 ng/mmoL [50]. For TCMR prediction, post-transplant CXCL10 and miR-155-5p levels yielded positive results [34], while for ABMR prediction six months albuminuria was investigated [42].

3. Discussion

With this systematic review, we critically summarize the results of the last five years research, the latest advances, and highlight the most frequent limitations of studies assessing urinary biomarkers for the diagnosis or prediction of acute allograft rejection. We focused on study design, distinction between TCMR and ABMR setting, evaluation of confounding (e.g., DGF, infections, calcineurin inhibitors nephrotoxicity), comparison with the gold standard of diagnosis (both for cases and controls), and presence of estimates of the biomarker(s) performance in validation.

The main finding was the strengthening in evidence for the clinical utility of urinary C-X-C motif chemokine ligands (in particular for the diagnosis of TCMR) alone or in combination with other biomarkers as in the *Q score* (cell-free DNA, methylated cell-free DNA, clusterin, total protein, creatinine, and CXCL10) or in the CTOT-4 formula. CXCL9 and CXCL10 had AUC ranging from 0.67–0.88 with a NPV ranging from 84–98% for AR diagnosis and AUC ranging from 0.50–0.97 with a NPV ranging from 71–96% for AR prediction. Signatures of urinary peptides and metabolites identified through unbiased proteomic and metabolomics, and a cluster of urinary cell pellet genes (*uCRM score*) were also established for the diagnosis of AR, net of some limitations for their introduction in clinical practice. Confounding outcomes need always to be considered due to potential overlap in diagnosis. For example, urinary chemokines are also elevated in allograft BK virus nephropathy (as discussed below), urinary NGAL was proposed as early predictor of DGF [56], and as a biomarker of CNI toxicity [57], while urinary miRNAs dysregulation has been linked to interstitial inflammation and tubular atrophy [58]. For the first time Tinel and colleagues demonstrated that considering (instead of excluding) potential confounding factors (i.e., urinary tract infection and BK virus reactivation) in a diagnostic multi-parametric model could optimize its performance [16]. A model combining eight parameters (recipient age, sex, eGFR, DSA presence, signs of urinary tract infection, BKV blood viral load, CXCL9, and CXCL10) could reach AR diagnosis with high accuracy (AUC: 0.85, 0.80–0.89), paving the way for new studies combining urinary biomarkers with clinical characteristics to reach the highest clinical relevance and provide targeted therapy for our patients.

Up to 2015, almost ninety non-redundant molecules were identified as urinary biomarkers of AR, participating in different pathways such as complement activation, antigen presentation, and inflammation signaling [15]. Urine was the most frequent matrix of choice for these analyses, and studies were often limited by small sample size and case-control design, no histology in the control cohorts, lack of confounding adjustment, lack of a validation set, and technical difficulties with procedure standardization and costs [15]. Although serum creatinine levels and proteinuria monitoring are well established biomarkers used by transplant physicians to suspect AR, they lack both sensitivity and specificity, and they are of little help in the prediction phase, in detecting subclinical rejection, and in differential diagnosis between AR, infections, drug toxicity, and acute tubular necrosis [14,59]. In a study of 281 consecutive biopsies, indicated by an increase in serum creatinine levels, only 27.8% revealed any sign of AR [51]. Conversely, subclinical rejection (i.e., rejection without clinical dysfunction) was found in over 40% of patients with normal renal function in the presence of anti-HLA de novo donor-specific antibodies (DSA) [60]. Proteinuria is common after kidney transplant and, although widely used as a biomarker of renal disease and despite its value as an independent predictor of long-term graft survival, it could also be sign of post-transplant primary disease recurrence (e.g., focal-segmental glomerulosclerosis), infections (e.g., CMV), immunosuppressive medication toxicity, or systemic (e.g., new-onset diabetes) and urologic complications (e.g., ureteral stenosis) [59,61]. DSA monitoring is currently considered the primary biomarker for ABMR but, despite the increasing ability to detect low level of DSAs, their positive predictive value is low, so that up to 60% of patients showing de novo DSA do not show any sign of AR at biopsy [60].

Continuous advances in molecular techniques and the "-omics" sciences have helped to identify many potential new blood and urine biomarkers for the diagnosis and prediction of kidney allograft AR in the last two decades. Of note, elevated pretransplant serum CXCL9 and CXCL10 levels were found to be associated to increased risk of early and severe AR and graft failure [62–64]. Subsequently, among urine-derived proteins, a 2012 study found CXCL9 and CXCL10 to be considerably elevated in patients experiencing either AR (clinical or subclinical) or BK virus infection (86% sensitivity and 80% specificity for CXCL9; 80% sensitivity and 76% specificity for CXCL10), but they were not able to distinguish between the two conditions [65]. These results were reinforced by the 2013 CTOT-1 study, which found that low urine CXCL9 measured at 6 months post-transplant identified a subset of patients at low-risk for AR development (92% NPV for Banff ≥1A TCMR) and predicted allograft stability up to 24 months post-transplant (93-99% NPV) [66]. With the help of mass spectroscopy, elevated beta2-microglobulin levels were identified as strongly correlated with AR (83% sensitivity, 80% specificity, 89% PPV, 71% NPV) and then validated by ELISA in the urine of AR patients [67]. Cytotoxic proteins perforine and granzyme B urine mRNAs were proposed to noninvasively diagnose AR (respectively with 83% sensitivity, 83% specificity, and 79% sensitivity, 77% specificity) [68] and Treg marker FOXP3 was shown to predict reversal of AR (90% sensitivity, 73% specificity) [69]. T-cell immunoglobulin-3 domain, mucin domain mRNA expression (Tim-3, also known as hepatitis A virus cellular receptor 2) in urinary cells was found to be able to discriminate AR from other causes of acute graft dysfunction (calcineurin inhibitor nephrotoxicity or interstitial fibrosis and tubular atrophy) with an AUC of 0.96, 89% PPV and 94% NPV [70]. A 2013 multicenter study from the CTOT-4 study group later identified a 3-gene urinary mRNA signature (CD3ε mRNA, CXCL10 mRNA, 18S rRNA) able to discriminate acute TCMR from no rejection in indication biopsies, with an AUC of 0.74, 79% sensitivity and 78% specificity in a validation set [54]. Also, noncoding miRNAs (e.g., miRNA-10a, miRNA-10b, miRNA-210), although limited by the easy degradation, proved to be detectable in the urine, and in particular low miRNA-210 levels discriminated patients affected by AR from stable control transplant patients (74% sensitivity, 52% specificity) [71].

Our systematic analysis of the more recent literature details the accuracy of a variety of urinary biomarkers for allograft AR with the objective of allowing transplant physicians early diagnosis and prediction of rejection episodes, and differential diagnosis with other causes of allograft dysfunction. A correct histologic diagnosis of AR is essential during the process of new biomarkers validation and the Banff criteria are considered the gold standard for biopsy evaluation. The diagnostic criteria for TCMR have essentially undergone no major change in the last decade with lymphocytic infiltrate of tubules (tubulitis) and larger vessels (vasculitis) being the main descriptive features. The severity of these lesions is graded according to the degree of lymphocytic infiltrate per high-powered field. On the other hand, ABMR criteria has continuously evolved in recent years–thus highlighting the great importance of applying an up to date classification in this setting–with the recognition of its variable histologic presentation [72,73]. Original criteria established in 2000s included active tissue injury, immunohistologic evidence of peritubular capillary complement split-product C4d deposition and circulating DSA. Subsequent studies demonstrating the presence of ABMR also in lacking detectable C4d staining biopsies [74], pushed the Banff Working Group in 2013 to the major change in the ABMR criteria, removing the requirement for C4d detection [75]. The most recent changes in 2017 included removing the requirement for documented circulating DSA in the setting of positive C4d staining and microvascular inflammation and included the use of AMR-associated gene transcripts panels [10].

The ideal biomarker should be readily available, accurate, inexpensive, standardized, repeatable, and noninvasive and would be useful to reduce the need for protocol biopsy and enable early targeted intervention. The chance of finding an ideal biomarker with high sensitivity, specificity, PPV and NPV is small. However, not all biomarkers need to be highly sensitive and highly specific at the same time, depending on the clinical question they are going to answer. Therefore, targeting specific populations and accepting lower predictive values in certain variables may be a better strategy. For example, to confirm the need for allograft biopsy in a population at high risk for AR (thus providing biopsy to the correct patients), a test with high sensitivity, and low false negative rate, would be the most useful. On the contrary, to propose diagnostic biopsies in a population at low risk for AR (thus avoiding unnecessary per-protocol biopsies), a test with high specificity, and low false positive rate, would be the test of choice. Also, TCMR and ABMR are different clinical entities and it is unrealistic, on current evidence, to hope for a biomarker that will accurately predict AR in both forms in a typical population of transplant patients with possible confounding.

Our systematic review has some limitations. The heterogeneity of the included studies did not permit to detail the many facets of individual study results, especially the more complex ones, to stick with the systematic review question. For space restraints, tables only report the major findings of each study, limited to urinary biomarkers. A narrative synthesis of the most promising results was applied to improve readability and a meta-analysis could not be performed. From our work, overall good quality studies emerged, many with DTA analysis and some comprising a thorough validation process yielding a very good to excellent diagnostic performance. Although specific forms of bias were assessed using QUADAS-2 publication bias could not be formally assessed and the authors acknowledge this can overestimate the weight of positive results. Weaknesses of the included studies were often the use of small cohorts obtained by case-control selection yielding inflated predictive values, the exclusion of confounding, unclear or out of date Banff classification application, the absence of validation cohorts, and lack of hypothesis-driven approach. In fact, the biomarker discovery process should not only consist of a training phase (i.e., a case-control study), but also comprise independent validation in a prospective study and confrontation with real-life clinical setting.

4. Materials and Methods

4.1. Literature Search

This review follows the Preferred Reporting Items for Systematic Reviews and Meta-Analysis (PRISMA) guidelines [76]. The objective of the study, search strategy, inclusion and exclusion criteria, and study evaluation method were planned in advance, refined, and approved by all authors. MEDLINE was searched from 1 January 2015 to 31 May 2020. Key terms like "kidney", "renal", "transplant/transplantation", "urine/urinary", "marker/biomarker", and "rejection" were combined in the search strategy. Additional relevant articles were searched from scanning reference lists of included studies and added if not detected by the original literature search.

4.2. Selection Process

The first screening by title and abstract was separately performed by two authors (F.G., L.C.) in the eligibility process. Original articles were selected if they assessed one, more, or a combination of urinary biomarker(s) and their performance in diagnosis or prediction of kidney allograft AR. Abstracts, reviews, studies assessing biomarkers from other matrix (e.g., blood samples or histology staining), and studies specifically evaluating different outcomes (e.g., chronic rejection, infection, or allograft survival) were excluded. In the inclusion process, selected articles were then independently full-text reviewed by two authors (F.G., L.C.). Any disagreement between the two investigators was discussed and solved with the help of all authors.

4.3. Data Collection and Analysis

Data from each of the included studies were collected with the help of a pre-specified spreadsheet and extraction table refined by all authors. Study design, single or multicenter patient collection, sample size, years of enrollment, urinary biomarker(s) of interest (i.e., index test), the Banff classification used for histological AR diagnosis (i.e., reference standard) and the addressed outcome(s) were collected in a descriptive table. Studies were distinguished between diagnostic and predictive. Diagnostic studies were usually collecting urine samples on the day of the diagnostic biopsy while predictive studies were analyzing urine samples collected before AR development. Studies that reported DTA data, such as sensitivity, specificity, PPV, NPV, and AUC were evaluated for risk of bias and applicability concern using the Quality Assessment Tool for Diagnostic Accuracy Studies-2 (QUADAS-2), a tool for quality evaluation of diagnostic accuracy studies [77]. The most important items for a positive evaluation included; a cross-sectional study design; avoiding patient selection bias and inappropriate exclusion; the definition of the index test (biomarker) threshold in a training set and its validation in a separate set of patients; and compliance with the correct histological definition of AR as a standard reference for all patients included in the analysis. Due to the great heterogeneity of the included studies, a meta-analysis was not performed, and a narrative synthesis of the results was preferred.

5. Conclusions

In recent years, numerous studies joined the challenging quest for urinary biomarkers in diagnosis and prediction of acute kidney allograft rejection. Authors must face the difficult task to allow for mediating between the need for a precise setting and reference standard diagnosis (to develop the most precise biomarkers), and the need for their validation in the most heterogeneous population of kidney allograft patients (to increase clinical utility). Urinary chemokines CXCL9 and CXCL10, alone or in combination with others, are the most frequently used and the most promising biomarkers, but multi-parametric clinical and laboratory models could represent the best strategy for future studies. Remarkable advances have been made on the path of allowing a more precise allocation of resources, helping clinicians to move from the standard protocol/indication biopsy dichotomy, to reduce unnecessary immunosuppression, and to improve kidney allograft outcomes in the long-term.

Author Contributions: Conceptualization, investigation, resources, F.G. and L.C.; methodology, data curation, formal analysis, visualization F.G.; writing—original draft preparation, F.G. and L.C.; writing—review and editing, E.B., F.B., C.E., R.M.R., J.P.H.; supervision J.P.H., P.R.; funding acquisition, P.R. All authors made a significant contribution to the content of this manuscript as per ICJME recommendations. All authors have read and agreed to the published version of the manuscript.

Acknowledgments: We thank the Meyer Children's Hospital and the Meyer Children's Hospital Foundation.

Abbreviations

ABMR	Antibody-mediated rejection
AKI	Acute kidney injury
AR	Acute rejection
ATN	Acute tubular necrosis
AUC	Area under the ROC curve
BKVN	BK virus nephropathy
CAN	Chronic allograft nephropathy
CCL2	Chemokine ligand 2
cfDNA	Cell free DNA
CKD	Chronic kidney disease
CTOT	Clinical trials in organ transplantation
CXCL	C-X-C motif chemokine ligands
DGF	Delayed graft function
DSA	Donor-specific antibodies
DTA	Diagnostic test accuracy
EPCAM	Epithelial cell adhesion molecule
FOXP3	Forkhead box P3
GABA	Gamma-aminobutyric acid
HE4	Human epididymis protein 4
HPX	Hemopexin

IFNγ	Interferon gamma
IFTA	Interstitial fibrosis and tubular atrophy
iKEA	Integrated kidney exosome analysis
IL	Interleukin
LC3	Microtubule-associated protein 1A/1B-light chain 3
LFABP	Liver-type fatty acid-binding protein
MMP7	Matrix metalloproteinase 7
MNA	1-methylnicotinamide
NAD	Nicotinamide adenine dinucleotide
NADP	Nicotinamide adenine dinucleotide phosphate
NGAL	Neutrophil gelatinase-associated lipocalin
NPV	Negative predictive value
PB	Publication bias
PD1	Programmed cell death protein 1
PDX	Podocalyxin
PPV	Positive predictive value
PRISMA	Preferred reporting items for systematic reviews and meta-analysis
QUADAS	Quality assessment tool for diagnostic accuracy studies
Sens	Sensitivity
Spec	Specificity
sTIM3	Soluble T cell immunoglobulin mucin domain 3
TCMR	T-cell mediated rejection
TEC	Tubular epithelial cells
TNFα	Tumor necrosis factor alpha
TSPAN1	Tetraspanin 1
uCRM	Urinary common rejection module

References

1. Ronco, C.; Bellomo, R.; Kellum, J.A. Acute kidney injury. *Lancet* **2019**, *394*, 1949–1964. [CrossRef]
2. Yang, J.Y.C.; Sarwal, R.D.; Fervenza, F.C.; Sarwal, M.M.; Lafayette, R.A. Noninvasive Urinary Monitoring of Progression in IgA Nephropathy. *Int. J. Mol. Sci.* **2019**, *20*, 4463. [CrossRef] [PubMed]
3. Kwan, B.; Fuhrer, T.; Zhang, J.; Darshi, M.; Van Espen, B.; Montemayor, D.; de Boer, I.H.; Dobre, M.; Hsu, C.-Y.; Kelly, T.N.; et al. Metabolomic Markers of Kidney Function Decline in Patients With Diabetes: Evidence From the Chronic Renal Insufficiency Cohort (CRIC) Study. *Am. J. Kidney Dis.* **2020**. S0272-6386(20)30572-2. [CrossRef] [PubMed]
4. Naesens, M.; Anglicheau, D. Precision Transplant Medicine: Biomarkers to the Rescue. *J. Am. Soc. Nephrol.* **2018**, *29*, 24–34. [CrossRef]
5. Guzzi, F.; Knight, S.R.; Ploeg, R.J.; Hunter, J.P. A systematic review to identify whether perfusate biomarkers produced during hypothermic machine perfusion can predict graft outcomes in kidney transplantation. *Transpl. Int.* **2020**, *33*, 590–602. [CrossRef]
6. Jochmans, I.; Pirenne, J. Graft quality assessment in kidney transplantation: Not an exact science yet! *Curr. Opin. Organ Transplant.* **2011**, *16*, 174–179. [CrossRef]
7. Jamshaid, F.; Froghi, S.; Cocco, P.D.; Dor, F.J. Novel non-invasive biomarkers diagnostic of acute rejection in renal transplant recipients: A systematic review. *Int. J. Clin. Pract.* **2018**, *72*, e13220. [CrossRef]
8. Wiebe, C.; Ho, J.; Gibson, I.W.; Rush, D.N.; Nickerson, P.W. Carpe diem-Time to transition from empiric to precision medicine in kidney transplantation. *Am. J. Transplant.* **2018**, *18*, 1615–1625. [CrossRef]
9. Thierry, A.; Thervet, E.; Vuiblet, V.; Goujon, J.-M.; Machet, M.-C.; Noel, L.-H.; Rioux-Leclercq, N.; Comoz, F.; Cordonnier, C.; François, A.; et al. Long-term impact of subclinical inflammation diagnosed by protocol biopsy one year after renal transplantation. *Am. J. Transplant.* **2011**, *11*, 2153–2161. [CrossRef]
10. Haas, M.; Loupy, A.; Lefaucheur, C.; Roufosse, C.; Glotz, D.; Seron, D.; Nankivell, B.J.; Halloran, P.F.; Colvin, R.B.; Akalin, E.; et al. The Banff 2017 Kidney Meeting Report: Revised diagnostic criteria for chronic active T cell-mediated rejection, antibody-mediated rejection, and prospects for integrative endpoints for next-generation clinical trials. *Am. J. Transplant.* **2018**, *18*, 293–307. [CrossRef]

11. Singh, N.; Samant, H.; Hawxby, A.; Samaniego, M.D. Biomarkers of rejection in kidney transplantation. *Curr Opin Organ Transplant* **2019**, *24*, 103–110. [CrossRef] [PubMed]
12. Quaglia, M.; Merlotti, G.; Guglielmetti, G.; Castellano, G.; Cantaluppi, V. Recent Advances on Biomarkers of Early and Late Kidney Graft Dysfunction. *Int. J. Mol. Sci.* **2020**, *21*, 5404. [CrossRef] [PubMed]
13. Anglicheau, D.; Naesens, M.; Essig, M.; Gwinner, W.; Marquet, P. Establishing Biomarkers in Transplant Medicine: A Critical Review of Current Approaches. *Transplantation* **2016**, *100*, 2024–2038. [CrossRef]
14. Lo, D.J.; Kaplan, B.; Kirk, A.D. Biomarkers for kidney transplant rejection. *Nat. Rev. Nephrol.* **2014**, *10*, 215–225. [CrossRef] [PubMed]
15. Gwinner, W.; Metzger, J.; Husi, H.; Marx, D. Proteomics for rejection diagnosis in renal transplant patients: Where are we now? *World J. Transplant* **2016**, *6*, 28–41. [CrossRef] [PubMed]
16. Tinel, C.; Devresse, A.; Vermorel, A.; Sauvaget, V.; Marx, D.; Avettand-Fenoel, V.; Amrouche, L.; Timsit, M.-O.; Snanoudj, R.; Caillard, S.; et al. Development and validation of an optimized integrative model using urinary chemokines for noninvasive diagnosis of acute allograft rejection. *Am. J. Transplant.* **2020**. [CrossRef]
17. Yang, J.Y.C.; Sarwal, R.D.; Sigdel, T.K.; Damm, I.; Rosenbaum, B.; Liberto, J.M.; Chan-On, C.; Arreola-Guerra, J.M.; Alberu, J.; Vincenti, F.; et al. A urine score for noninvasive accurate diagnosis and prediction of kidney transplant rejection. *Sci. Transl. Med.* **2020**, *12*, eaba2501. [CrossRef]
18. Kalantari, S.; Chashmniam, S.; Nafar, M.; Samavat, S.; Rezaie, D.; Dalili, N. A Noninvasive Urine Metabolome Panel as Potential Biomarkers for Diagnosis of T Cell-Mediated Renal Transplant Rejection. *OMICS A J. Integr. Biol.* **2020**, *24*, 140–147. [CrossRef]
19. Verma, A.; Muthukumar, T.; Yang, H.; Lubetzky, M.; Cassidy, M.F.; Lee, J.R.; Dadhania, D.M.; Snopkowski, C.; Shankaranarayanan, D.; Salvatore, S.P.; et al. Urinary cell transcriptomics and acute rejection in human kidney allografts. *JCI Insight* **2020**, *5*, e131552. [CrossRef]
20. Goerlich, N.; Brand, H.A.; Langhans, V.; Tesch, S.; Schachtner, T.; Koch, B.; Paliege, A.; Schneider, W.; Grützkau, A.; Reinke, P.; et al. Kidney transplant monitoring by urinary flow cytometry: Biomarker combination of T cells, renal tubular epithelial cells, and podocalyxin-positive cells detects rejection. *Sci. Rep.* **2020**, *10*, 796. [CrossRef]
21. Banas, M.C.; Neumann, S.; Pagel, P.; Putz, F.J.; Krämer, B.K.; Böhmig, G.A.; Eiglsperger, J.; Schiffer, E.; Ruemmele, P.; Banas, B. A urinary metabolite constellation to detect acute rejection in kidney allografts. *EBioMedicine* **2019**, *48*, 505–512. [CrossRef] [PubMed]
22. Tajima, S.; Fu, R.; Shigematsu, T.; Noguchi, H.; Kaku, K.; Tsuchimoto, A.; Okabe, Y.; Masuda, S. Urinary Human Epididymis Secretory Protein 4 as a Useful Biomarker for Subclinical Acute Rejection Three Months after Kidney Transplantation. *Int. J. Mol. Sci.* **2019**, *20*, 4699. [CrossRef]
23. Kölling, M.; Haddad, G.; Wegmann, U.; Kistler, A.; Bosakova, A.; Seeger, H.; Hübel, K.; Haller, H.; Mueller, T.; Wüthrich, R.P.; et al. Circular RNAs in Urine of Kidney Transplant Patients with Acute T Cell-Mediated Allograft Rejection. *Clin. Chem.* **2019**, *65*, 1287–1294. [CrossRef] [PubMed]
24. Sigdel, T.K.; Yang, J.Y.C.; Bestard, O.; Schroeder, A.; Hsieh, S.-C.; Liberto, J.M.; Damm, I.; Geraedts, A.C.M.; Sarwal, M.M. A urinary Common Rejection Module (uCRM) score for non-invasive kidney transplant monitoring. *PLoS ONE* **2019**, *14*, e0220052. [CrossRef] [PubMed]
25. Kim, S.-Y.; Kim, B.K.; Gwon, M.-R.; Seong, S.J.; Ohk, B.; Kang, W.Y.; Lee, H.W.; Jung, H.-Y.; Cho, J.-H.; Chung, B.H.; et al. Urinary metabolomic profiling for noninvasive diagnosis of acute T cell-mediated rejection after kidney transplantation. *J. Chromatogr. B Analyt. Technol. Biomed. Life Sci.* **2019**, *1118–1119*, 157–163. [CrossRef] [PubMed]
26. Ciftci, H.S.; Tefik, T.; Savran, M.K.; Demir, E.; Caliskan, Y.; Ogret, Y.D.; Oktar, T.; Sanlı, O.; Kocak, T.; Ozluk, Y.; et al. Urinary CXCL9 and CXCL10 Levels and Acute Renal Graft Rejection. *Int. J. Organ Transplant. Med.* **2019**, *10*, 53–63.
27. Banas, M.; Neumann, S.; Eiglsperger, J.; Schiffer, E.; Putz, F.J.; Reichelt-Wurm, S.; Krämer, B.K.; Pagel, P.; Banas, B. Identification of a urine metabolite constellation characteristic for kidney allograft rejection. *Metabolomics* **2018**, *14*, 116. [CrossRef] [PubMed]
28. Lim, J.-H.; Lee, C.-H.; Kim, K.Y.; Jung, H.-Y.; Choi, J.-Y.; Cho, J.-H.; Park, S.-H.; Kim, Y.-L.; Baek, M.-C.; Park, J.B.; et al. Novel urinary exosomal biomarkers of acute T cell-mediated rejection in kidney transplant recipients: A cross-sectional study. *PLoS ONE* **2018**, *13*, e0204204. [CrossRef]
29. Chen, D.; Zhang, J.; Peng, W.; Weng, C.; Chen, J. Urinary C-X-C motif chemokine 13 is a noninvasive biomarker of antibody-mediated renal allograft rejection. *Mol. Med. Rep.* **2018**, *18*, 2399–2406. [CrossRef]

30. Barabadi, M.; Shahbaz, S.K.; Foroughi, F.; Hosseinzadeh, M.; Nafar, M.; Yekaninejad, M.S.; Amirzargar, A. High Expression of FOXP3 mRNA in Blood and Urine as a Predictive Marker in Kidney Transplantation. *Prog. Transplant.* **2018**, *28*, 134–141. [CrossRef]
31. Mockler, C.; Sharma, A.; Gibson, I.W.; Gao, A.; Wong, A.; Ho, J.; Blydt-Hansen, T.D. The prognostic value of urinary chemokines at 6 months after pediatric kidney transplantation. *Pediatr. Transplant.* **2018**, *22*, e13205. [CrossRef] [PubMed]
32. Senturk Ciftci, H.; Demir, E.; Savran Karadeniz, M.; Tefik, T.; Yazici, H.; Nane, I.; Savran Oguz, F.; Aydin, F.; Turkmen, A. Serum and Urinary Levels of Tumor Necrosis Factor-Alpha in Renal Transplant Patients. *Exp. Clin. Transplant.* **2018**, *16*, 671–675. [CrossRef] [PubMed]
33. Park, J.; Lin, H.-Y.; Assaker, J.P.; Jeong, S.; Huang, C.-H.; Kurdi, A.; Lee, K.; Fraser, K.; Min, C.; Eskandari, S.; et al. Integrated Kidney Exosome Analysis for the Detection of Kidney Transplant Rejection. *ACS Nano* **2017**, *11*, 11041–11046. [CrossRef] [PubMed]
34. Millán, O.; Budde, K.; Sommerer, C.; Aliart, I.; Rissling, O.; Bardaji, B.; Matz, M.; Zeier, M.; Silva, I.; Guirado, L.; et al. Urinary miR-155-5p and CXCL10 as prognostic and predictive biomarkers of rejection, graft outcome and treatment response in kidney transplantation. *Br. J. Clin. Pharmacol.* **2017**, *83*, 2636–2650. [CrossRef]
35. Seo, J.-W.; Moon, H.; Kim, S.-Y.; Moon, J.-Y.; Jeong, K.H.; Lee, Y.-H.; Kim, Y.-G.; Lee, T.-W.; Ihm, C.-G.; Kim, C.-D.; et al. Both absolute and relative quantification of urinary mRNA are useful for non-invasive diagnosis of acute kidney allograft rejection. *PLoS ONE* **2017**, *12*, e0180045. [CrossRef]
36. Gandolfini, I.; Harris, C.; Abecassis, M.; Anderson, L.; Bestard, O.; Comai, G.; Cravedi, P.; Cremaschi, E.; Duty, J.A.; Florman, S.; et al. Rapid Biolayer Interferometry Measurements of Urinary CXCL9 to Detect Cellular Infiltrates Noninvasively After Kidney Transplantation. *Kidney Int. Rep.* **2017**, *2*, 1186–1193. [CrossRef]
37. Chen, D.; Peng, W.; Jiang, H.; Yang, H.; Wu, J.; Wang, H.; Chen, J. Noninvasive detection of acute renal allograft rejection by measurement of soluble Tim-3 in urine. *Mol. Med. Rep.* **2017**, *16*, 915–921. [CrossRef]
38. Domenico, T.D.; Joelsons, G.; Montenegro, R.M.; Manfro, R.C. Upregulation of microRNA 142-3p in the peripheral blood and urinary cells of kidney transplant recipients with post-transplant graft dysfunction. *Braz. J. Med. Biol. Res.* **2017**, *50*, e5533. [CrossRef]
39. Lee, H.; Park, Y.-M.; We, Y.-M.; Han, D.J.; Seo, J.-W.; Moon, H.; Lee, Y.-H.; Kim, Y.-G.; Moon, J.-Y.; Lee, S.-H.; et al. Evaluation of Digital PCR as a Technique for Monitoring Acute Rejection in Kidney Transplantation. *Genomics Inform.* **2017**, *15*, 2–10. [CrossRef]
40. Seeman, T.; Vondrak, K.; Dusek, J.; Simankova, N.; Zieg, J.; Hacek, J.; Chadimova, M.; Sopko, B.; Fortova, M. Urinary Neutrophil Gelatinase-Associated Lipocalin Does Not Distinguish Acute Rejection from Other Causes of Acute Kidney Injury in Pediatric Renal Transplant Recipients. *Clin. Lab.* **2017**, *63*, 111–114. [CrossRef]
41. Blydt-Hansen, T.D.; Sharma, A.; Gibson, I.W.; Wishart, D.S.; Mandal, R.; Ho, J.; Nickerson, P.; Rush, D. Urinary Metabolomics for Noninvasive Detection of Antibody-Mediated Rejection in Children After Kidney Transplantation. *Transplantation* **2017**, *101*, 2553–2561. [CrossRef] [PubMed]
42. Belmar Vega, L.; Rodrigo Calabia, E.; Gómez Román, J.J.; Ruiz San Millán, J.C.; Martín Penagos, L.; Arias Rodríguez, M. Relationship Between Albuminuria During the First Year and Antibody-Mediated Rejection in Protocol Biopsies in Kidney Transplant Recipients. *Transplant. Proc.* **2016**, *48*, 2950–2952. [CrossRef] [PubMed]
43. Raza, A.; Firasat, S.; Khaliq, S.; Khan, A.R.; Mahmood, S.; Aziz, T.; Mubarak, M.; Naqvi, S.A.A.; Rizvi, S.A.H.; Abid, A. Monocyte Chemoattractant Protein-1 (MCP-1/CCL2) Levels and Its Association with Renal Allograft Rejection. *Immunol. Investig.* **2017**, *46*, 251–262. [CrossRef]
44. Galichon, P.; Amrouche, L.; Hertig, A.; Brocheriou, I.; Rabant, M.; Xu-Dubois, Y.-C.; Ouali, N.; Dahan, K.; Morin, L.; Terzi, F.; et al. Urinary mRNA for the Diagnosis of Renal Allograft Rejection: The Issue of Normalization. *Am. J. Transplant.* **2016**, *16*, 3033–3040. [CrossRef]
45. Sigdel, T.K.; Gao, Y.; He, J.; Wang, A.; Nicora, C.D.; Fillmore, T.L.; Shi, T.; Webb-Robertson, B.-J.; Smith, R.D.; Qian, W.-J.; et al. Mining the human urine proteome for monitoring renal transplant injury. *Kidney Int.* **2016**, *89*, 1244–1252. [CrossRef] [PubMed]

46. García-Covarrubias, L.; Ventura, E.; Soto, V.; González, E.; García, A.; Aguilar, J.C.; Torres, J.M.; Hinojosa, H.; Fragoso, P.; De Los Santos, J.; et al. Lack of Association Between Elevated Urinary Levels of Interleukin-10 and Interferon Gamma With the Presence of Inflammation in Kidney Transplant Recipients. *Transplant. Proc.* **2016**, *48*, 583–587. [CrossRef]
47. Ho, J.; Rush, D.N.; Krokhin, O.; Antonovici, M.; Gao, A.; Bestland, J.; Wiebe, C.; Hiebert, B.; Rigatto, C.; Gibson, I.W.; et al. Elevated Urinary Matrix Metalloproteinase-7 Detects Underlying Renal Allograft Inflammation and Injury. *Transplantation* **2016**, *100*, 648–654. [CrossRef]
48. Abd Elaziz, M.M.; Bakry, S.; M Abd ElAal, A.E.; Rashed, L.; Hesham, D. Validation of Urinary PD-1 and FOXP3 mRNA in a Cohort of Egyptian Renal Allograft Recipients. *Ann. Transplant.* **2016**, *21*, 17–24. [CrossRef]
49. Lorenzen, J.M.; Schauerte, C.; Kölling, M.; Hübner, A.; Knapp, M.; Haller, H.; Thum, T. Long Noncoding RNAs in Urine Are Detectable and May Enable Early Detection of Acute T Cell-Mediated Rejection of Renal Allografts. *Clin. Chem.* **2015**, *61*, 1505–1514. [CrossRef]
50. Rabant, M.; Amrouche, L.; Morin, L.; Bonifay, R.; Lebreton, X.; Aouni, L.; Benon, A.; Sauvaget, V.; Le Vaillant, L.; Aulagnon, F.; et al. Early Low Urinary CXCL9 and CXCL10 Might Predict Immunological Quiescence in Clinically and Histologically Stable Kidney Recipients. *Am. J. Transplant.* **2016**, *16*, 1868–1881. [CrossRef]
51. Rabant, M.; Amrouche, L.; Lebreton, X.; Aulagnon, F.; Benon, A.; Sauvaget, V.; Bonifay, R.; Morin, L.; Scemla, A.; Delville, M.; et al. Urinary C-X-C Motif Chemokine 10 Independently Improves the Noninvasive Diagnosis of Antibody-Mediated Kidney Allograft Rejection. *J. Am. Soc. Nephrol.* **2015**, *26*, 2840–2851. [CrossRef] [PubMed]
52. Blydt-Hansen, T.D.; Gibson, I.W.; Gao, A.; Dufault, B.; Ho, J. Elevated urinary CXCL10-to-creatinine ratio is associated with subclinical and clinical rejection in pediatric renal transplantation. *Transplantation* **2015**, *99*, 797–804. [CrossRef] [PubMed]
53. Sigdel, T.K.; Ng, Y.W.; Lee, S.; Nicora, C.D.; Qian, W.-J.; Smith, R.D.; Camp, D.G., II; Sarwal, M.M. Perturbations in the urinary exosome in transplant rejection. *Front. Med. (Lausanne)* **2014**, *1*, 57. [CrossRef] [PubMed]
54. Suthanthiran, M.; Schwartz, J.E.; Ding, R.; Abecassis, M.; Dadhania, D.; Samstein, B.; Knechtle, S.J.; Friedewald, J.; Becker, Y.T.; Sharma, V.K.; et al. Urinary-cell mRNA profile and acute cellular rejection in kidney allografts. *N. Engl. J. Med.* **2013**, *369*, 20–31. [CrossRef] [PubMed]
55. van Enst, W.A.; Ochodo, E.; Scholten, R.J.P.M.; Hooft, L.; Leeflang, M.M. Investigation of publication bias in meta-analyses of diagnostic test accuracy: A meta-epidemiological study. *BMC Med. Res. Methodol.* **2014**, *14*, 70. [CrossRef]
56. Li, Y.M.; Li, Y.; Yan, L.; Wang, H.; Wu, X.J.; Tang, J.T.; Wang, L.L.; Shi, Y.Y. Comparison of urine and blood NGAL for early prediction of delayed graft function in adult kidney transplant recipients: A meta-analysis of observational studies. *BMC Nephrol.* **2019**, *20*, 291. [CrossRef]
57. Tsuchimoto, A.; Shinke, H.; Uesugi, M.; Kikuchi, M.; Hashimoto, E.; Sato, T.; Ogura, Y.; Hata, K.; Fujimoto, Y.; Kaido, T.; et al. Urinary Neutrophil Gelatinase-Associated Lipocalin: A Useful Biomarker for Tacrolimus-Induced Acute Kidney Injury in Liver Transplant Patients. *PLoS ONE* **2014**, *9*, e110527. [CrossRef]
58. Zununi Vahed, S.; Omidi, Y.; Ardalan, M.; Samadi, N. Dysregulation of urinary miR-21 and miR-200b associated with interstitial fibrosis and tubular atrophy (IFTA) in renal transplant recipients. *Clin. Biochem.* **2017**, *50*, 32–39. [CrossRef]
59. Naesens, M.; Lerut, E.; Emonds, M.-P.; Herelixka, A.; Evenepoel, P.; Claes, K.; Bammens, B.; Sprangers, B.; Meijers, B.; Jochmans, I.; et al. Proteinuria as a Noninvasive Marker for Renal Allograft Histology and Failure: An Observational Cohort Study. *J. Am. Soc. Nephrol.* **2016**, *27*, 281–292. [CrossRef]
60. Bertrand, D.; Gatault, P.; Jauréguy, M.; Garrouste, C.; Sayegh, J.; Bouvier, N.; Caillard, S.; Lanfranco, L.; Galinier, A.; Laurent, C.; et al. Protocol Biopsies in Patients with Subclinical De Novo DSA After Kidney Transplantation: A multicentric study. *Transplantation* **2020**, *104*, 1726–1737. [CrossRef]
61. Diena, D.; Messina, M.; De Biase, C.; Fop, F.; Scardino, E.; Rossetti, M.M.; Barreca, A.; Verri, A.; Biancone, L. Relationship between early proteinuria and long term outcome of kidney transplanted patients from different decades of donor age. *BMC Nephrol.* **2019**, *20*, 443. [CrossRef] [PubMed]
62. Rotondi, M.; Rosati, A.; Buonamano, A.; Lasagni, L.; Lazzeri, E.; Pradella, F.; Fossombroni, V.; Cirami, C.; Liotta, F.; La Villa, G.; et al. High pretransplant serum levels of CXCL10/IP-10 are related to increased risk of renal allograft failure. *Am. J. Transplant.* **2004**, *4*, 1466–1474. [CrossRef] [PubMed]

63. Lazzeri, E.; Rotondi, M.; Mazzinghi, B.; Lasagni, L.; Buonamano, A.; Rosati, A.; Pradella, F.; Fossombroni, V.; La Villa, G.; Gacci, M.; et al. High CXCL10 expression in rejected kidneys and predictive role of pretransplant serum CXCL10 for acute rejection and chronic allograft nephropathy. *Transplantation* **2005**, *79*, 1215–1220. [CrossRef] [PubMed]
64. Rotondi, M.; Netti, G.S.; Lazzeri, E.; Stallone, G.; Bertoni, E.; Chiovato, L.; Grandaliano, G.; Gesualdo, L.; Salvadori, M.; Schena, F.P.; et al. High pretransplant serum levels of CXCL9 are associated with increased risk of acute rejection and graft failure in kidney graft recipients. *Transpl. Int.* **2010**, *23*, 465–475. [CrossRef] [PubMed]
65. Jackson, J.A.; Kim, E.J.; Begley, B.; Cheeseman, J.; Harden, T.; Perez, S.D.; Thomas, S.; Warshaw, B.; Kirk, A.D. Urinary chemokines CXCL9 and CXCL10 are noninvasive markers of renal allograft rejection and BK viral infection. *Am. J. Transplant.* **2011**, *11*, 2228–2234. [CrossRef] [PubMed]
66. Hricik, D.E.; Nickerson, P.; Formica, R.N.; Poggio, E.D.; Rush, D.; Newell, K.A.; Goebel, J.; Gibson, I.W.; Fairchild, R.L.; Riggs, M.; et al. Multicenter validation of urinary CXCL9 as a risk-stratifying biomarker for kidney transplant injury. *Am. J. Transplant.* **2013**, *13*, 2634–2644. [CrossRef] [PubMed]
67. Oetting, W.S.; Rogers, T.B.; Krick, T.P.; Matas, A.J.; Ibrahim, H.N. Urinary beta2-microglobulin is associated with acute renal allograft rejection. *Am. J. Kidney Dis.* **2006**, *47*, 898–904. [CrossRef]
68. Li, B.; Hartono, C.; Ding, R.; Sharma, V.K.; Ramaswamy, R.; Qian, B.; Serur, D.; Mouradian, J.; Schwartz, J.E.; Suthanthiran, M. Noninvasive diagnosis of renal-allograft rejection by measurement of messenger RNA for perforin and granzyme B in urine. *N. Engl. J. Med.* **2001**, *344*, 947–954. [CrossRef]
69. Muthukumar, T.; Dadhania, D.; Ding, R.; Snopkowski, C.; Naqvi, R.; Lee, J.B.; Hartono, C.; Li, B.; Sharma, V.K.; Seshan, S.V.; et al. Messenger RNA for FOXP3 in the urine of renal-allograft recipients. *N. Engl. J. Med.* **2005**, *353*, 2342–2351. [CrossRef]
70. Manfro, R.C.; Aquino-Dias, E.C.; Joelsons, G.; Nogare, A.L.; Carpio, V.N.; Gonçalves, L.F.S. Noninvasive Tim-3 messenger RNA evaluation in renal transplant recipients with graft dysfunction. *Transplantation* **2008**, *86*, 1869–1874. [CrossRef]
71. Lorenzen, J.M.; Volkmann, I.; Fiedler, J.; Schmidt, M.; Scheffner, I.; Haller, H.; Gwinner, W.; Thum, T. Urinary miR-210 as a mediator of acute T-cell mediated rejection in renal allograft recipients. *Am. J. Transplant.* **2011**, *11*, 2221–2227. [CrossRef] [PubMed]
72. Cooper, J.E. Evaluation and Treatment of Acute Rejection in Kidney Allografts. *CJASN* **2020**, *15*, 430–438. [CrossRef] [PubMed]
73. Haas, M. Evolving criteria for the diagnosis of antibody-mediated rejection in renal allografts. *Curr. Opin. Nephrol. Hypertens.* **2018**, *27*, 137–143. [CrossRef]
74. Sis, B.; Jhangri, G.S.; Bunnag, S.; Allanach, K.; Kaplan, B.; Halloran, P.F. Endothelial gene expression in kidney transplants with alloantibody indicates antibody-mediated damage despite lack of C4d staining. *Am. J. Transplant.* **2009**, *9*, 2312–2323. [CrossRef]
75. Haas, M.; Sis, B.; Racusen, L.C.; Solez, K.; Glotz, D.; Colvin, R.B.; Castro, M.C.R.; David, D.S.R.; David-Neto, E.; Bagnasco, S.M.; et al. Banff 2013 meeting report: Inclusion of c4d-negative antibody-mediated rejection and antibody-associated arterial lesions. *Am. J. Transplant.* **2014**, *14*, 272–283. [CrossRef] [PubMed]
76. Moher, D.; Liberati, A.; Tetzlaff, J.; Altman, D.G. PRISMA Group Preferred reporting items for systematic reviews and meta-analyses: The PRISMA statement. *BMJ* **2009**, *339*, b2535. [CrossRef]
77. Whiting, P.F.; Rutjes, A.W.S.; Westwood, M.E.; Mallett, S.; Deeks, J.J.; Reitsma, J.B.; Leeflang, M.M.G.; Sterne, J.A.C.; Bossuyt, P.M.M. QUADAS-2 Group QUADAS-2: A revised tool for the quality assessment of diagnostic accuracy studies. *Ann. Intern. Med.* **2011**, *155*, 529–536. [CrossRef]

Permissions

All chapters in this book were first published by MDPI; hereby published with permission under the Creative Commons Attribution License or equivalent. Every chapter published in this book has been scrutinized by our experts. Their significance has been extensively debated. The topics covered herein carry significant findings which will fuel the growth of the discipline. They may even be implemented as practical applications or may be referred to as a beginning point for another development.

The contributors of this book come from diverse backgrounds, making this book a truly international effort. This book will bring forth new frontiers with its revolutionizing research information and detailed analysis of the nascent developments around the world.

We would like to thank all the contributing authors for lending their expertise to make the book truly unique. They have played a crucial role in the development of this book. Without their invaluable contributions this book wouldn't have been possible. They have made vital efforts to compile up to date information on the varied aspects of this subject to make this book a valuable addition to the collection of many professionals and students.

This book was conceptualized with the vision of imparting up-to-date information and advanced data in this field. To ensure the same, a matchless editorial board was set up. Every individual on the board went through rigorous rounds of assessment to prove their worth. After which they invested a large part of their time researching and compiling the most relevant data for our readers.

The editorial board has been involved in producing this book since its inception. They have spent rigorous hours researching and exploring the diverse topics which have resulted in the successful publishing of this book. They have passed on their knowledge of decades through this book. To expedite this challenging task, the publisher supported the team at every step. A small team of assistant editors was also appointed to further simplify the editing procedure and attain best results for the readers.

Apart from the editorial board, the designing team has also invested a significant amount of their time in understanding the subject and creating the most relevant covers. They scrutinized every image to scout for the most suitable representation of the subject and create an appropriate cover for the book.

The publishing team has been an ardent support to the editorial, designing and production team. Their endless efforts to recruit the best for this project, has resulted in the accomplishment of this book. They are a veteran in the field of academics and their pool of knowledge is as vast as their experience in printing. Their expertise and guidance has proved useful at every step. Their uncompromising quality standards have made this book an exceptional effort. Their encouragement from time to time has been an inspiration for everyone.

The publisher and the editorial board hope that this book will prove to be a valuable piece of knowledge for researchers, students, practitioners and scholars across the globe.

List of Contributors

Lilach O. Lerman
Division of Nephrology and Hypertension, Mayo Clinic, Rochester, MN 55905, USA

In O. Sun
Division of Nephrology and Hypertension, Mayo Clinic, Rochester, MN 55905, USA
Division of Nephrology, Department of Internal Medicine, Presbyterian Medical Center, Jeonju 54987, Korea

T.D.K.S.C. Gunasekara
Department of Zoology, Faculty of Science, University of Ruhuna, Matara 81000, Sri Lanka

P. Mangala C.S. De Silva
Department of Zoology, Faculty of Science, University of Ruhuna, Matara 81000, Sri Lanka
Renal Division, Brigham andWomen's Hospital, Harvard Medical School, Boston, MA 02115, USA

Chula Herath
Department of Nephrology, Sri Jayawardenapura General Hospital, Sri Jayawardenepura Kotte 10100, Sri Lanka

Sisira Siribaddana
Department of Medicine, Faculty of Medicine and Allied Sciences, Rajarata University of Sri Lanka, Mihintale 50300, Sri Lanka

Nipuna Siribaddana
Department of Parasitology, Faculty of Medicine and Allied Sciences, Rajarata University of Sri Lanka, Mihintale 50300, Sri Lanka

Channa Jayasumana
Department of Pharmacology, Faculty of Medicine and Allied Sciences, Rajarata University of Sri Lanka, Mihintale 50300, Sri Lanka

Sudheera Jayasinghe
Department of Pharmacology, Faculty of Medicine, University of Ruhuna, Matara 81000, Sri Lanka

Maria Cardenas-Gonzalez
Renal Division, Brigham andWomen's Hospital, Harvard Medical School, Boston, MA 02115, USA
Mexican Council of Science and Technology, Consejo Nacional de Ciencia y Tecnología, Mexico City 03940, Mexico

Nishad Jayasundara
The Nicholas School of the Environment, Duke University, Durham, NC 27708, USA
The School of Marine Sciences, University of Maine, Orono, ME 04469, USA

Sebastian Mertowski, Izabela Morawska, Ewelina Grywalska and Jacek Roliński
Department of Clinical Immunology and Immunotherapy, Medical University of Lublin, 20-093 Lublin, Poland

Paulina Lipa
Department of Genetics and Microbiology, Institute of Microbiology and Biotechnology, Faculty of Biology and Biotechnology, Maria Curie-Skłodowska University, Akademicka 19 St., 20-033 Lublin, Poland

Paulina Niedźwiedzka-Rystwej, Dominika Bębnowska and Rafał Hrynkiewicz
Institute of Biology, University of Szczecin, Felczaka 3c, 71-412 Szczecin, Poland

Wojciech Załuska
Department of Nephrology, Medical University of Lublin, 20-954 Lublin, Poland

Benjamin Miron, David Xu and Matthew Zibelman
Department of Hematology/Oncology, Fox Chase Cancer Center, Philadelphia, PA 19111, USA

Ming-Tsun Tsai
Division of Nephrology, Department of Medicine, Taipei Veterans General Hospital, Taipei 11217, Taiwan
Faculty of Medicine, School of Medicine, National Yang-Ming University, Taipei 11221, Taiwan
Institute of Clinical Medicine, School of Medicine, National Yang-Ming University, Taipei 11221, Taiwan

Wei-Cheng Tseng
Division of Nephrology, Department of Medicine, Taipei Veterans General Hospital, Taipei 11217, Taiwan
Faculty of Medicine, School of Medicine, National Yang-Ming University, Taipei 11221, Taiwan
Institute of Clinical Medicine, School of Medicine, National Yang-Ming University, Taipei 11221, Taiwan
Center for Intelligent Drug Systems and Smart Biodevices (IDS2B), National Chiao-Tung University, Hsinchu 30010, Taiwan

Nien-Jung Chen
Institute of Microbiology and Immunology, School of Life Sciences, National Yang-Ming University, Taipei 11221, Taiwan

Der-Cherng Tarng
Division of Nephrology, Department of Medicine, Taipei Veterans General Hospital, Taipei 11217, Taiwan
Faculty of Medicine, School of Medicine, National Yang-Ming University, Taipei 11221, Taiwan
Institute of Clinical Medicine, School of Medicine, National Yang-Ming University, Taipei 11221, Taiwan
Center for Intelligent Drug Systems and Smart Bio-devices (IDS2B), National Chiao-Tung University, Hsinchu 30010, Taiwan
Department and Institute of Physiology, School of Medicine, National Yang-Ming University, Taipei 11221, Taiwan
Department of Biological Science and Technology, College of Biological Science and Technology, National Chiao-Tung University, Hsinchu 30010, Taiwan

Félix Vargas and Isabel Rodríguez-Gómez
Depto. Fisiologia, Fac. Medicina, Universidad de Granada, 18071 Granada, Spain

Rosemary Wangesteen
Depto. Ciencias de la salud, Universidad de Jaén, 23071 Jaén, Spain

Joaquín García-Estañ
Depto. Fisiologia, Fac. Medicina, IMIB, Universidad de Murcia, 30120 Murcia, Spain

Tatiana N. Zamay
Laboratory for Biomolecular and Medical Technologies, Krasnoyarsk State Medical University Named after Prof. V.F. Voyno-Yasenetsky, 660022 Krasnoyarsk, Russia

Dmitry V. Veprintsev
Laboratory for Digital Controlled Drugs and Theranostics, Federal Research Center "Krasnoyarsk Science Center of the Siberian Branch of the Russian Academy of Science", 660036 Krasnoyarsk, Russia

Yury E. Glazyrin and Anna S. Kichkailo
Laboratory for Biomolecular and Medical Technologies, Krasnoyarsk State Medical University Named after Prof. V.F. Voyno-Yasenetsky, 660022 Krasnoyarsk, Russia
Laboratory for Digital Controlled Drugs and Theranostics, Federal Research Center "Krasnoyarsk Science Center of the Siberian Branch of the Russian Academy of Science", 660036 Krasnoyarsk, Russia

Irina A. Ler, Maria L. Rossovskaya and Svetlana A. Varygina
Department of Nephrology, Krasnoyarsk Interdistrict Clinical Hospital of Emergency Medical Care Named after N.S. Karpovich, 660062 Krasnoyarsk, Russia

Marina M. Petrova
Faculty of Medicine, Krasnoyarsk State Medical University Named after Prof. V.F. Voyno-Yasenetsky, 660022 Krasnoyarsk, Russia

Sofia L. Glizer
Department of Nephrology, Krasnoyarsk Interdistrict Clinical Hospital of Emergency Medical Care Named after N.S. Karpovich, 660062 Krasnoyarsk, Russia
Faculty of Medicine, Krasnoyarsk State Medical University Named after Prof. V.F. Voyno-Yasenetsky, 660022 Krasnoyarsk, Russia

Zoran Minic and Maxim V. Berezovski
Department of Chemistry and Biomolecular Sciences, University of Ottawa, Ottawa, ON K1N6N5, Canada

Takahiro Uchida and Takashi Oda
Kidney Disease Center, Department of Nephrology and Blood Purification, Tokyo Medical University Hachioji Medical Center, Hachioji, Tokyo 193-0998, Japan

Koen E. Groeneweg, Jacques M.G.J. Duijs, Barend W. Florijn, Cees van Kooten, Johan W. de Fijter, Anton Jan van Zonneveld, Marlies E.J. Reinders and Roel Bijkerk
Department of Internal Medicine (Nephrology) and the Einthoven Laboratory for Vascular and Regenerative Medicine, Leiden University Medical Center, Albinusdreef 2, 2333 ZA Leiden, Zuid Holland, The Netherlands

Wojciech Wołyniec and Marcin Renke
Department of Occupational, Metabolic and Internal Diseases, Institute of Maritime and Tropical Medicine, Medical University of Gdańsk, 9b Powstania Styczniowego Street, 81-519 Gdynia, Poland

Wojciech Ratkowski
Department of Athletics, Gda´nsk University of Physical Education and Sport, 1 Górskiego Street, 80-336 Gdańsk, Poland

Joanna Renke
Department of General and Medical Biochemistry, University of Gdansk, 59Wita Stwosza Street, 80- 308 Gdańsk, Poland

Michele Provenzano, Ida Gagliardi, Ashour Michael and Michele Andreucci
Renal Unit, Department of Health Sciences, "Magna Graecia" University of Catanzaro, I-88100 Catanzaro, Italy

Salvatore Rotundo and Daniela Foti
Department of Health Sciences, "Magna Graecia" University of Catanzaro, I-88100 Catanzaro, Italy

Paolo Chiodini
Medical Statistics Unit, University of Campania Luigi Vanvitelli, I-80138 Naples, Italy

Elvira Angotti
Clinical Biochemistry Unit, Azienda Ospedaliera Universitaria Mater Domini Hospital, I-88100 Catanzaro, Italy

Silvio Borrelli
Renal Unit, University of Campania "Luigi Vanvitelli", I-80138 Naples, Italy

Raffaele Serra
Interuniversity Center of Phlebolymphology (CIFL), "Magna Graecia" University of Catanzaro, I-88100 Catanzaro, Italy

Giovambattista De Sarro
Pharmacology Unit, Department of Health Sciences, School of Medicine, "Magna Graecia" University of Catanzaro, I-88100 Catanzaro, Italy

Špela Borštnar, Željka Večerić-Haler, Damjan Kovač and Jelka Lindič
Department of Nephrology, University Medical Centre Ljubljana, Zaloška 7, 1000 Ljubljana, Slovenia
Faculty of Medicine, University of Ljubljana, Vrazov trg 2, 1000 Ljubljana, Slovenia

Emanuela Boštjančič, Živa Pipan Tkalec and Nika Kojc
Institute of Pathology, Faculty of Medicine, University of Ljubljana, Korytkova 2, 1000 Ljubljana, Slovenia

Armando Coca, Carmen Aller, Jimmy Reinaldo Sánchez and Ana Lucía Valencia
Department of Nephrology, Hospital Clinico Universitario de Valladolid, 47003 Valladolid, Spain

Elena Bustamante-Munguira
Department of Intensive Care Medicine, Hospital Clinico Universitario de Valladolid, 47003 Valladolid, Spain

Juan Bustamante-Munguira
Department of Cardiac Surgery, Hospital Clinico Universitario de Valladolid, 47003 Valladolid, Spain

Hee-Sung Ahn and Jiyoung Yu
Asan Institute for Life Sciences, Asan Medical Center, Seoul 05505, Korea

Jong Ho Kim, Sang Heon Song, Sang Soo Kim and In Joo Kim
Department of Internal Medicine and Biomedical Research Institute, Pusan National University Hospital, Busan 49241, Korea

Hwangkyo Jeong
Department of Biomedical Sciences, University of Ulsan College of Medicine, Seoul 05505, Korea

Jeonghun Yeom
Convergence Medicine Research Center, Asan Institute for Life Sciences, Seoul 05505, Korea

Kyunggon Kim
Asan Institute for Life Sciences, Asan Medical Center, Seoul 05505, Korea
Department of Biomedical Sciences, University of Ulsan College of Medicine, Seoul 05505, Korea
Clinical Proteomics Core Laboratory, Convergence Medicine Research Center, Asan Medical Center, Seoul 05505, Korea
Bio-Medical Institute of Technology, Asan Medical Center, Seoul 05505, Korea

Francesco Guzzi, Luigi Cirillo and Paola Romagnani
Department of Experimental and Clinical Biomedical Sciences "Mario Serio", University of Florence, 50134 Florence, Italy
Nephrology and Dialysis Unit, Meyer Children's University Hospital, 50139 Florence, Italy

Elisa Buti, Francesca Becherucci, Carmela Errichiello and Rosa Maria Roperto
Nephrology and Dialysis Unit, Meyer Children's University Hospital, 50139 Florence, Italy

James P. Hunter
Nuffield Department of Surgical Sciences, Oxford Transplant Centre, Churchill Hospital, University of Oxford, Oxford OX3 7LJ, UK

Index

Printed in the USA
CPSIA information can be obtained
at www.ICGtesting.com
LVHW080037211023
761596LV00010BA/1804

9 781639 877911